Enhancing Resilience in Youth

Christoph Steinebach · Álvaro I. Langer
Editors

Enhancing Resilience in Youth

Mindfulness-Based Interventions in Positive Environments

Springer

Editors
Christoph Steinebach
School of Applied Psychology
ZHAW Zürich University
of Applied Sciences
Zürich, Switzerland

Álvaro I. Langer
Institute of Psychological Studies
Universidad Austral de Chile
Valdivia, Chile

ISBN 978-3-030-25512-1 ISBN 978-3-030-25513-8 (eBook)
https://doi.org/10.1007/978-3-030-25513-8

This Springer imprint is published by the registered company Springer Nature Switzerland AG
The registered company address is: Gewerbestrasse 11, 6330 Cham, Switzerland

Preface

Education, prevention, and therapeutic services aim to change individual behaviors and produce lasting changes in problematic emotions, cognitions, and social factors. It is becoming increasingly accepted that the consideration of individual needs, strengths, and resources must reorient the deficit-focused approach of interventions toward an approach that takes individual needs, strengths, and resources into account alongside any deficits. Improving mental health in children and adolescents is an urgent necessity which should be handled in an intersectoral and interdisciplinary way. Schools as institutions play a fundamental role in achieving this task. The educational system faces tremendous challenges linked to the need to develop not solely specific academic skills (e.g., language, maths), but also personal skills (i.e., socio-emotional and behavioral) which help adolescents to have a healthy relationship with themselves and others (including nature). This involves changes at several levels which should consequently be addressed via multilevel strategies. Otherwise, school-based interventions may fail to achieve their goal to deliver mental health promotion in a sustainable manner. Research on positive attitudes and emotions suggests that mindfulness-based interventions enhance positive qualities such as empathy and well-being. In addition, evaluations of interventions targeting prosocial behavior show sustainable effects on self-efficacy and resilience.

In this book, we combine a range of research perspectives from several countries by connecting mindfulness to prosocial behavior and to positive social and physical environments in order to enhance resilience. Theoretical aspects and recommendations for practice aimed at promoting mental health and healthy lifestyles in adolescents, such as school-based interventions, are presented. We would like to gain a broad understanding of the levels and variables which require attention in order to enhance resilience in adolescents. This includes shedding light on the role of biopsychosocial conditions as "breeding grounds" which may allow school-based interventions to flourish and be sustainable within the educational system.

The primary objective of this book is to describe what is needed to plan, develop, and implement peer-supported mindfulness-based interventions to prevent mental disorders in children and adolescents. Given the tremendous challenges posed by increasing rates of mental disorders and their associated costs and psychosocial problems for society, it is crucial to investigate possible early intervention programs aimed at children and adolescents that may help prevent the development of mental disorders in the future. We focus on interventions designed to maintain psychosocial health and prevent emotional and behavioral problems in children and adolescents around the globe. Our intercultural perspective will allow for the discussion of complex topics such as the influence of cultural differences and the generalizability of program effects. This transfer of knowledge and experience will facilitate the successful cross-cultural implementation of future interventions.

In sum, the objectives of this book are to (1) present theories and research on psychosocial mindfulness-based and peer-oriented prevention and intervention programs; (2) describe biological (e.g., epigenetics), individual (e.g., generosity), social (e.g., peer support), and intercultural (e.g., values, differences in educational systems) factors associated with program outcomes and feasibility; and (3) use an intercultural perspective to make recommendations for the implementation of interventions aimed at children and adolescents, seeking to reduce the existing psychosocial problems and the risks of developing other such problems or depression.

The articles will be grouped into four major parts. The first part, with pieces by Catherine Andreu, Carlos García-Rubio, Álvaro I. Langer, Christoph Steinebach, Tri Thi Minh Thuy, and Leandro Torres-Díaz, provides an introduction to peer support and mindfulness. Both articles outline the ways in which interventions focusing on mindfulness, compassion, and social support in adolescence might be connected from a multilevel and culturally sensitive perspective. In doing, both articles give valuable insights into theoretical and conceptual aspects of mindfulness-based and peer-related interventions in adolescents. The second part provides a closer look at the basics of resilience and mindfulness. The articles follow the biopsychosocial model of development and therefore focus on different intrapersonal and interpersonal aspects: Perla Kalimann on the epigenetics of well-being; Christoph Steinebach, Marcel Schaer, and Imke Knafla on generosity, peer support, and resilience; Sabine Pirchio and Yelina Passiatore on the school environment; Volker Schulte and Larisa Zotova on the organizational aspects of resilience in the workplace; and finally, Giuseppe Carrus and Angelo Panno on sustainability and resilience in the community. In the third part, we examine the question of how mindfulness and peer support are combined in interventions aimed at promoting resilience. With a view to the multitude of serious behavioral problems that characterize school age, Matías Irarrázaval gives several recommendations for psychological interventions in educational contexts. As Catherine Andreu and Carlos García-Rubio point out in their chapter, it is important to enhance competencies to regulate one's emotions via an exploration of change mechanisms linked to mindfulness interventions in schools. In this regard, Marcel Schaer and Imke Knafla discuss how counseling can meet students' basic needs by creating positive relations. Sebastián Medeiros and Simón Guendelman discuss in which ways a socio-affective, developmentally informed perspective for contemplative practices in adolescence can promote resilient communities. Vanessa Nowak and Felix Fuders discuss the role that education should play in the development of a resilient society and advocate for a paradigm shift in economics. How might mindfulness-based and peer-oriented theory and practice evolve in the future? The fourth part discusses promising approaches for constructive development in mental health promotion: Roberto Arístegui and Claudio Araya-Véliz focus on relational mindfulness; Nathania Klauser and Philipp Steinebach on current developments in the psychotherapy of adolescence; and Adolfo J. Cangas, María José Fínez, Consuelo Morán, Noelia Navarro, and Petra Moldes on new technologies and well-being. Mariane Krause examines the significance of social transformations in mental health. And last but not least, Felix Fuders and Vanessa Nowak discuss how an economy based on love can promote allocative efficiency and happiness.

All in all, the chapters cover three main levels of interventions:

1. On an individual level, we enhance mindfulness in adolescence via education, counseling, and/or psychotherapy.
2. At the group level, interventions in adolescence seem to be more effective if they aim to enhance peer support. Based on these observations, we adopt a systemic perspective.
3. But peers are not the sole representatives of social systems. From the perspective of the biopsychosocial model, we must also explore the contribution of organizations, residential communities, or society as a whole when it comes to promoting mindfulness in helping relationships.

Connecting mindfulness-based and peer-related interventions opens up a new understanding of education and intervention. Our goal must be to develop interventions that involve individual adolescents, their friends, other social factors (e.g., the organizational environment), and the community. It should also be possible to think about society as a whole. Thus, the design of more positive change becomes an important task at all levels. And this goal must also include the design of the physical environments of young people. All things considered, it is clear that combining mindfulness promotion and positive peer relationships allows interventions to have a lasting effect in other areas of life as well.

We would like to thank all the authors for having opened up these perspectives for us and for their contributions which show us how we can further develop theory and practice in this field. This project was funded by the Millennium Science Initiative of the Ministry of Economy, Development and Tourism, grant "Millennium Nucleus to Improve the Mental Health of Adolescents and Youths, Imhay," and the Innovation Fund for Competitiveness [FIC], part of the Chilean Ministry of Economy, Development, and Tourism, through the Millennium Scientific Initiative, Project IS130005. We are very grateful for this support. Our special thanks go to Andrés Navarrete for his valuable work as a lecturer.

May you as readers take up the ideas and experiences of the various articles in this book and fill them with life. With this in mind, we hope you enjoy reading and experiencing this book!

Zürich, Switzerland
Valdivia, Chile
March 2019

Christoph Steinebach
Álvaro I. Langer

Contents

Contributors

Catherine I. Andreu Millennium Institute for Research in Depression and Personality (MIDAP), Santiago, Chile;
School of Psychology, Pontificia Universidad Católica de Chile, Santiago, Chile

Claudio Araya-Véliz Escuela de Psicología, Universidad Adolfo Ibáñez, Santiago de Chile, Chile

Roberto Arístegui Escuela de Psicología, Universidad Adolfo Ibáñez, Santiago de Chile, Chile

Adolfo J. Cangas University of Almería, Almería, Spain

Giuseppe Carrus Department of Education, Roma Tre University, Rome, Italy

María José Fínez University of León, León, Spain

Felix Fuders Faculty of Economics and Administration, Economics Institute, Universidad Austral de Chile, Valdivia, Chile

Carlos García-Rubio Department of Biological and Health Psychology, Faculty of Psychology, Universidad Autónoma de Madrid, Madrid, Spain

Simón Guendelman Centro Mindfulness y Medicina, Santiago, Chile;
Social Cognition Group, Berlin School of Mind and Brain, Humboldt Universität, Berlin, Germany

Matías Irarrázaval Department of Mental Health, Ministry of Health, Santiago, Chile;
Millennium Institute for Research in Depression and Personality, Santiago, Chile;
Department of Psychiatry, University of Chile, Santiago, Chile

Perla Kaliman Faculty of Health Sciences, Universitat Oberta de Catalunya, Barcelona, Spain;
Center for Healthy Minds, University of Wisconsin-Madison, Madison, US

Nathania Klauser Psychological Institute, University of Heidelberg, Heidelberg, Germany

Imke Knafla School of Applied Psychology, ZHAW Zürich University of Applied Sciences, Zürich, Switzerland

Mariane Krause School of Psychology, Pontificia Universidad Católica de Chile, Santiago, Chile;
Millennium Institute for Research in Depression and Personality, MIDAP, Santiago, Chile

Álvaro I. Langer Institute of Psychological Studies, Faculty of Medicine, Universidad Austral de Chile, Valdivia, Chile;
Millennium Nucleus to Improve the Mental Health of Adolescents and Youths, Imhay, Santiago, Chile;
Millennium Institute for Research in Depression and Personality (MIDAP), Santiago, Chile;
Center for Interdisciplinary Studies on the Nervous System (CISNe), Universidad Austral de Chile, Valdivia, Chile

Sebastián Medeiros Psychiatry Department, Pontificia Universidad Católica de Chile, Santiago, Chile;
Centro Mindfulness y Medicina, Santiago, Chile;
Millennium Institute for Research in Depression and Personality, Santiago, Chile

Petra Moldes University of Almería, Almería, Spain

Consuelo Morán University of León, León, Spain

Noelia Navarro University of Almería, Almería, Spain

Vanessa Nowak German Chilean Competency Center for Development, Valdivia, Chile;
Faculty of Engineering and Technology, Universidad San Sebastián, Valdivia, Chile

Angelo Panno Department of Education, Roma Tre University, Rome, Italy

Ylenia Passiatore Department of Education, Roma Tre University, Rome, Italy

Sabine Pirchio Department of Dynamic and Clinical Psychology, Sapienza University of Rome, Rome, Italy

Marcel Schaer School of Applied Psychology, ZHAW Zürich University of Applied Sciences, Zürich, Switzerland

Volker Schulte School of Business, FHNW University of Applied Sciences Northwestern Switzerland, Windisch, Switzerland

Christoph Steinebach School of Applied Psychology, ZHAW Zürich University of Applied Sciences, Zürich, Switzerland

Philipp Steinebach Department of Psychiatry and Psychotherapy, University Medical Center Göttingen, Göttingen, Germany

Tri Thi Minh Thuy Faculty of Psychology, University of Social Sciences and Humanities, HCMC Vietnam National University, Ho Chi Minh City, Vietnam

Leandro Torres-Díaz Instituto de Ciencias Naturales, Universidad de las Américas, Santiago, Chile;
Instituto de Investigación e Innovación en Salud, Universidad Central de Chile, Santiago, Chile

Larisa Zotova Moscow Region State University, Mytishchi, Russia

List of Figures

List of Tables

Part I
Introduction

Chapter 1
Enhancing Resilience in Youth: Sustainable Systemic Effects in Different Environments

Christoph Steinebach, Álvaro I. Langer and Tri Thi Minh Thuy

Abstract Nowadays, in order to promote psychological well-being and prevent diseases (mental and physical), several interventions have been developed and tested in school settings. These involve, for instance, mindfulness and compassion. Nevertheless, despite promising results attesting to the effectiveness of mindfulness in increasing well-being, there remain some open questions concerning how to implement mindfulness in a systematic way beyond research, incorporating it as a regular practice of the educational system which makes it possible to introduce a culture of resilience. In this chapter, we would like to give insights into the sustainability of psychosocial interventions considering a systemic approach in a variety of environments. To do this, we will revisit the concept of resilience (i.e. definition, resources) and how to enhance it (e.g. positive learning, positive peer culture, positive self-development). In summary, we wish to highlight that, to ensure the sustainability of psychosocial interventions in schools, a multilevel approach should be adopted. Specifically, we propose that a framework based on resilience may give rise to a pivotal concept through multiple novel interventions such as mindfulness and compassion, which should be integrated in more systemic and ecological view.

C. Steinebach (✉)
School of Applied Psychology, ZHAW Zürich University of Applied Sciences, Zürich, Switzerland
e-mail: Christoph.steinebach@zhaw.ch

Á. I. Langer
Institute of Psychological Studies, Faculty of Medicine, Universidad Austral de Chile, Valdivia, Chile

Millennium Nucleus to Improve the Mental Health of Adolescents and Youths, Imhay, Santiago, Chile

Millennium Institute for Research in Depression and Personality (MIDAP), Santiago, Chile

Center for Interdisciplinary Studies on the Nervous System (CISNe), Universidad Austral de Chile, Valdivia, Chile

T. T. M. Thuy
Faculty of Psychology, University of Social Sciences and Humanities, HCMC Vietnam National University, Ho Chi Minh City, Vietnam

C. Steinebach and Á. I. Langer (eds.), *Enhancing Resilience in Youth*,
https://doi.org/10.1007/978-3-030-25513-8_1

Keywords Peer group · Self-development · Resilience · Self-efficacy · Positive adaptation

1.1 Modeling Research and Practice

How can the different findings on mindfulness and positive peer relationships be integrated? Which models help us to classify the most important factors? We seek answers to this question from the perspective of psychology as an empirical science. This is associated with the claim that we must rely on evidence-based theories when discussing causes, interventions, and effects. Theory is thus closely related to practice. As current research shows, a meaningful model cannot be developed if it is not possible to incorporate the findings of other sciences. Integration is the result of a process of "consilience" whereby we bring together findings from different sciences (Wilson, 1998). Research on mindfulness and peer-related interventions is not yet complete. So, we need to develop theories and models that help us to better understand and positively develop practice. At the same time, our theories and models must be open and flexible enough to integrate new findings.

1.2 Basic Assumptions

We must certainly do everything we can to prevent behavioral problems such as depression or aggressive behavior. This must also be a central concern in adolescence, because psychological disorders occur more frequently during this time and can persist into adulthood. In addition, our aim must be to strengthen mental health and well-being, and to do so by means of services aimed at young people as well as their social environment. "Optimal (or desirable) well-being is characterized by (predominantly) positive feelings and attitude, positive relationships with other students and teachers, resilience, self-optimization, and high level of satisfaction with their learning experiences at school" (Noble, Wyatt, McGrath, Roffey, & Rowling, 2008, in Noble & McGrath, 2014, p. 137). Current research on interventions in childhood and adolescence emphasizes the importance of basic needs and strengths. Since peers are gaining greater importance in adolescence (e.g. Donlan, Lynch, & Lerner, 2015), attempts are being made to include peers in interventions in different ways: "Optimizing positive peer influence and protecting against negative peer influences are important to promote positive peer influence" (Donlan et al., 2015). Current research also makes it clear that every young person has strengths that can help himself or herself and others. Nowadays, in order to promote psychological well-being and prevent diseases (mental and physical), several interventions have been developed and tested in school settings, including mindfulness and compassion. Nevertheless, despite promising evidence of the effectiveness of mindfulness in increasing well-being (see Andreu & Garcia-Rubio in this book), there are open questions concerning how to implement it in a systematic way beyond research as a regular practice of the educational system aimed at introducing a culture of resilience. In this chapter, we would like to give insights into the sustainability of psychosocial interventions considering systemic approaches in a variety of environments. To do this, we will revisit the concept of resilience (i.e. definition, resources) and how to enhance it (e.g. positive learning, positive peer culture, positive self-development).

1.3 Resilience as a Touchstone for Positive Development

Theories of adolescence differ in focus, breadth, and degree of concretization (Newman & Newman, 2011). Even if we limit ourselves to questions about generosity, it becomes clear that we are compiling concepts and findings that have their place in various groups of theories. Ultimately, we are dealing with genetic foundations, hormonal influences, changes in the central nervous system and the brain, cognitive development, personality and identity development, development in social systems such as the family or peer group, and environmental and cultural psychological aspects (Sales & Irwin, 2013). "Dynamic Systems Theories" can then help us compile all these different concepts and findings in a meaningful way, as long as we succeed in mapping the diversity of internal system processes (Newman & Newman, 2011).

1.3.1 Defining Resilience

As a term from physics, resilience is the ability of an object to regain its original shape after being subjected to strong external forces. In psychology and pedagogy, however, we would not only wish that everything would remain as it was after stress. Rather, we would prefer that new challenges could be mastered more easily and better on the basis of the experience gained. We would also hope that overcoming difficult experiences would strengthen self-determination, self-development, and self-discipline. In the social sciences, the term "resilience revolution" (Brendtro & Larson, 2006) is often used. On the one hand, this may be due to the surprising finding of positive development even under adverse developmental conditions. Certainly, however, another factor that plays a role is that resilience is combined with pedagogical and psychological prevention and intervention aimed at boosting the strengths of children and young people. "Strengthening the strengths" becomes a pedagogical maxim. Resilience means the "resilience" of a person in their particular environment. It is about maintaining the ability to function, about a constant competence under acute stress conditions, about positive development in spite of a persistently high risk, about restoring the ability to function and rapid recovery after traumatic events, and finally about an improvement beyond the previous status. Several questions can now be derived from these considerations: (1) How can young people develop well in a "risky" environment (e.g. in a residential area that is considered a "social hotspot")? (2) Under stressful circumstances (e.g. after their parents' divorce), how can young people maintain their previously acquired skills (e.g. self-confidence, self-efficacy convictions)? (3) How can young people cope with traumatic experiences (e.g. war, accidents, abuse)? (4) How can young people restore their functional capacity (e.g. through impairments as a result of a chronic illness)? And finally: (5) How can we adequately support young people in these contexts (through education and therapy in formal or informal programs, e.g. open youth services)? At the same time, of course, we always have to ask which living conditions might weaken resilience by putting them at risk or more indirectly by reducing their strengths and resources.

1.3.2 Resources as Protective Factors

Crises and critical life events are important markers for the development and proof of resilience. Existing risk and protective factors affecting young people and their environment prove to be decisive factors in coping with them. Thus, individual vulnerability can be a risky weakness, for example, when it is due to neurological deficits or existing chronic diseases. The list of possible environmental risks is long: low social status, poverty, low educational level of the parents, family disharmony, mental illness of one or both parents, alcohol and drug abuse of the parents, criminality of the parents, separation and divorce of the parents, frequently changing partnership of the parents, residential areas with a high crime rate, educational deficits of the parents, very young parenthood, early and unwanted pregnancy, social isolation of the family, mobbing or rejection by peers… As can be seen, the occurrence of a random risk factor is relatively non-problematic. It is only when several factors come together that developmental problems become most probable. Protective factors are psychological characteristics of the child or positive characteristics of the social environment, which lower the probability of occurrence of durable disturbances. It is important to note that individual risk factors are not immediately seen as weaknesses but can be used as an opportunity to implement more personalized early interventions. Two groups of protective factors must be distinguished: (1) personal resources (positive temperament, above-average intelligence, positive self-concept) and (2) social resources (favorable family living conditions, person of trust, networks).

What resources are important in adolescence? And where should we focus on to enhance mindfulness while promoting a peer culture of mutual support and assistance? For young people, new competences based on physical development are an important resource. Neurophysiological development poses some risks that can be countered with mindfulness-related interventions. Good health is the basis for positive activities not only in sport, also promoting well-being and emotional balance. Performance motivation leads to the acceptance of challenges and the ability to withstand stress. With appropriate interventions, it is possible to promote endurance, concentration, and willingness to perform. Self-efficacy convictions and high self-esteem promote experiencing competence and self-compassion as important foundations for actively shaping one's development. Communicative skills are an important prerequisite for close social relationships and integration in groups. Group-related interventions promote social competences in a special way. Being able to fit in with others is an important factor for prosocial behavior. In addition to these individual resources, there are resources in the family. This is about communicating with each other, but it is also about structural aspects of proximity and distance and hierarchy in the family system. An actively supportive and, if necessary, orienting educational attitude makes it clear that one's family provides backing even in difficult situations. Educational closeness under parents' social commitment is a resource that promotes talents and interests. Friends of the same age are seen as resources, but they are also a model for social commitment. Because they are reliable in their support, they help establish an emotional balance. Permanent dialogue with each other helps develop positive identities. It might be important for family and friends to be on good terms with each other. The circle of friends should also be involved in activities in the community in which they live. The school or company is also part of the social environment. This is where positive relationships with teachers can be found, such as a good class- and school-climate or a positive working atmosphere, the matching of competences and requirements, positive role models, and good contact between family members, school, and/or company. These competences of the social environment enable people to deal with problems constructively, balance their emotional experience in everyday life, and promote personality development. In the residential community, special neighborly relations and the willingness of the living environment to assume responsibility are important resources. The availability of counseling services in the vicinity of the parents' home and good leisure activities for young people are also relevant. Likewise, society and culture provide useful resources. Other pros include the permeability of educational interventions, the availability of supplementary services and professional advice, and the competent networking of services (cf. Steinebach & Gharabaghi, 2018).

1.4 Enhancing Resilience

In the meantime, the idea of resilience has also been transferred to social groups and larger communities. Research and practice are devoted to the resilience of families, youth groups, teams, businesses, communities, and cities. So, if we want to define resilience, we must try to capture the crucial individual and social aspects. This is most likely to happen if we talk about systems and understand human beings as systems integrated into a complex structure of environmental systems. This makes sense if we consider the evidence for "a 'decentered' understanding of resilience in which changing the odds stacked against the individual contributes far more to changes in outcomes than the capacity of individuals themselves to change" (Ungar, Ghazinour, & Richter, 2013, p. 357). Keeping this in mind, resilience is "seen overall as the positive adaptation and sustainable development of a system to respond to short- or longer-term everyday challenges or severe stress. Based on internal system processes and through dealing with the environment, the system defines new reference values and develops required competencies, and the ability to cope with future stresses improves" (Steinebach, 2015, p. 557). In this definition, we must also bear in mind that all system elements and interactions change continuously. Today, in the 21st century, the everyday use of virtual media requires a variety of skills. At the same time, there are many opportunities to shape development in a new and different way. For young people, we can assume, the social environment today is new and different.

1.4.1 Positive Learning

The development of resilience can be understood as a learning process. Experiences in dealing with crises and critical life events lead at best to a permanent change in behavior and experience (see Steinebach, Süss, Kienbaum, & Kiegelmann, 2016). Learning must be regarded as a multifocal but integrated experience that influences cognitive, emotional, and physical processes (e.g. effects of mindfulness on cognitive functions and executive functions, Weare, 2014). For a better understanding, the most helpful learning theories are those which take into account the cognitive processes of learners in learning, especially those that see learning as an active construction process. In these theories, the individual makes an important contribution to learning. Without having to use the adjective "positive", we can assume that observational learning supports resilience when successful problem solving can be observed. Perceived similarity to the model, concentration, and attention etc. contribute as cognitive aspects. Cognitive learning theories cover learning in the sense of instruction, expertise, discovery learning, or learning using solution examples. We can easily imagine moments in which young people are guided, in which they develop expertise in a task area and thus the composure to deal with challenges. The confrontation with challenges and the constant effort in trying out different solutions may correspond to discovery learning. Lastly, examples of solutions may be seen as useful not only when it comes to helping e.g. with math homework, but also when it comes to more complex life questions. Such considerations are associated with the appeal to also understand the confrontation with the challenges of life as a learning process and thus to take learning seriously in everyday life, and especially outside school. This also includes the call to understand everyday pedagogical situations as learning opportunities (Gharabaghi, 2011). It is precisely here that the degrees of freedom of young people are very high. In order to understand learning in these unstructured and open situations, situated learning theories seem helpful. Here, learners are ascribed special responsibility in the learning process. They develop solutions in dealing with their concrete environment and at the same time in dialogue with others. The acquired action competences correspond to cognitive schemata, which are developed and stored in a highly situational way. And what does "positive learning" mean? The greater the individual's contribution to the learning process, the more the teacher's role changes. Moderation is required, along with coaching, support and motivation, empowerment, communication at eye level, and the effort to reflect together on the experiences and thus secure the knowledge gained.

In counseling young people, information should be conveyed or new behavior learned. Implicitly or explicitly, these interventions are therefore generally about learning. In most cases, however, this is not just about imparting knowledge alone. The actual aim is to allow students' personality to thrive as well. Following Mittelstraß (1989), we can assume that education is about more than just knowledge acquisition. Education, here likened to the concept of "Bildung", helps to mediate between one's knowledge and one's will. According to Mittelstraß (1989), education ("Bildung") is "the power of judgement that operates between what we know and what we want" (p. 56). Education thus has a great deal to do with ethics. The fundamentally available knowledge changes very quickly. That is why it is important to impart skills in educational processes that help students to orient themselves in a complex world that changes rapidly both professionally and ethically. Every intervention for young people can be understood as a teaching and learning opportunity. We know that surprises and possibly mistakes in the learning process are important, since they cause attention to be focused on learning outcomes, leading to new solutions. New experiences and experiments are important. Both, however, are much more likely to occur in socially secure relationships. This also makes it possible to focus and direct one's attention to the construction of new learning content (Steinebach et al., 2016). It is therefore becoming increasingly important for young people to make their own learning experiences. Education thus generally stands for self-education, in which adults have the task of accompanying young people, moderating learning processes, and not dominating them. This view has led authors to assert that "an investment in positive education at the school, system and national level, and in educational policies and practices for student well-being produce long-term benefits for individual students, for school communities and for the whole society" (Noble & McGrath, 2014, 149).

1.4.2 Positive Peer Culture

Collaborating in a group brings performance advantages, especially if the group norms are formulated positively. A group structure appropriate to the task can help to avoid conflicts or contribute to solving problems constructively and achieving the objectives set in good cooperation. Depending on the type of group and the task to be solved, observing self-organization, offering moderation, or leading the group might be helpful. In the workplace, it is usual to ask how teamwork can be conducted in order to achieve the set goals as effectively and efficiently as possible. Similarly, we also try to foster social and emotional skills in adolescence by using group processes. Young people live in formal and informal groups. In schools or sports clubs, we expect mostly formal groups. In the area of self-determined leisure time or in open youth services, young people often come together in informal groups. Goals and rules must then be negotiated through informal processes. This also includes norms and rules for mutual assistance. In appropriate programs working with formal groups, the organization's vision, mission, goals, processes, and composition are formalized. All these aspects are also the subject of the evaluation of the program (Brown & Braun, 2013). The pedagogical demands of the program refer to different developmental tasks or to existing behavioral problems: changes in social systems, upcoming challenges at school, or later career paths, the selection of a profession, the formulation of a sustainable personal identity, or the challenges of sexuality.

But what are the arguments in favor of including peers into interventions? Following Brown and Larson (2009), we can assert that, overall, relationships with friends of the same age become more important in adolescence. Adolescence is characterized by very fundamental physical, emotional, and cognitive changes. At the same time, however, the social environments of young people are also changing. It is important to spend time with others, learn more about their expectations, and align oneself with the group in one's own identity and behavior in order to orient oneself in these changing worlds. Another argument may be that the complexity of relationships in the groups of young people increases. We find informal groups that may also have the character of cliques, we find closer friendships, but also the first romantic relationships. Individual groups can understand themselves as parts of larger groups or specific youth cultures. This is about identity, but also about one's own status and the desire to experience satisfying relationships in a group of like-minded people. It is noticeable that, in friendships and peer groups, young people are more similar to each other. On the one hand, this can be seen as the result of a common learning and development process. On the other hand, of course, group members are also selected for membership in the group based on their fit. Status and prestige are important, not only for the group as a whole, but also for one's own role within the group. The formulation of a positive and stable identity is an important developmental task for young people. Group membership in a socially recognized group and personal status within the group make an important contribution (Steinebach & Steinebach, 2013). Social skills are important in order to survive within the group. The recognition that a young person receives from his or her friends thus becomes an important indicator of the adaptation of the individual to the group. There may be at least three reasons why friends of the same age become more important:

(1) Integration into the group meets the need for belonging.
(2) Young people like to choose their friends in groups according to similarities in behavior. This can increase development risks, but can also create opportunities.
(3) Young people also experience social support in groups. Groups offer the opportunity to develop solutions to problems together. The competences thus gained by coping with problems ensure a sustainable positive development (Steinebach, Steinebach, & Brendtro, 2012; Steinebach, Schrenk, Steinebach, & Brendtro, 2018).

1.4.3 Positive Self-development and Health Actions

Today, human development and health appear to be influenced to a large extent by human beings themselves. Behavior, attitudes, and competencies determine whether health can be developed and maintained in interaction with external difficulties or resources. Both health and positive development are reflected in the successful interplay of personal and environmental conditions (Ungar & Lerner, 2008). This is also reflected in the Ottawa Charter of 1986, which has played a key role in shaping the current understanding of health promotion. With its focus on health and the contribution of the individual to positive development, it overcame the purely biomedical model common at the time (World Health Organization, 1986, 2009). The work of Antonovsky (1987) also specified which factors are important for coping with stress and thus for maintaining health. The Bangkok Charter of the WHO follows suit by stating that health promotion stands for "a positive and inclusive concept of health as a determinant of the quality of life and encompassing mental and spiritual well-being" (World Health Organization, 2009, 24). In addition to the individual aspect of well-being, various environmental levels and systems are taken into account, such as direct social relations, the community in which one lives, superordinate political systems, and society.

The gap between knowledge and attitudes on the one hand and concrete action on the other is proving to be a central problem in health promotion. Many people know what would be healthy, but they do not act accordingly. In principle, the question arises when people are prepared to follow their wishes in a concentrated and consistent manner and implement the decisions they have made. According to the self-determination theory of Ryan and Deci (2000), people are particularly motivated when the action in question serves the fulfillment of their basic needs: belonging, experiencing competence, and autonomy.

In this context, it becomes clear why peer groups are so important for young people. Belonging not only offers social-emotional support: it is also an essential part of one's own identity. In joint activities, young people experience themselves as competent and this promotes well-being (Bandura, 1997; Sternberg & Spear-Swerling, 1998). And this well-being is regarded as a protective factor in the struggle for health and resilience (Steptoe, Dockray, & Wardle, 2009). Belonging is important, but so is the possibility to distinguish oneself and live autonomously. Thus, the peer group helps to differentiate oneself from one's family, while the first romantic relationships promote differentiation from one's peer group. By striving to balance belonging and autonomy, young people learn to live their needs in a socially appropriate way.

1.5 Outlook: Creating Cultures of Mutual Support

Even though we already have some reliable findings, a few unanswered questions remain. These concern preventive interventions, counseling and therapy, and finally future research.

1.5.1 Everyday Life

Following Luthar (2006), we can assume that interventions are most effective when they (a) are tailored to a specific high-risk group (see also Rutter, 2013; Steinebach, 2012), (b) address aspects of behavior and experience that can be easily changed, (c) are readily available and reliable, (d) last longer, and (e) aim to develop new environmental resources such as personal strengths and competences. In addition, it makes sense to (f) align the interventions with risk factors present in the person and their environment and (e) simultaneously address the interventions at different levels (e.g. physical, emotional, cognitive, social with family, peers, school, community; Ungar et al., 2013; "Multidimensional Treatment Foster Care"; Leve, Fisher, & Chamberlain, 2009: 1869). All of this must be done as early as possible so that problems do not solidify, thus enabling the early strengthening of the five "Cs" (competence, confidence, connection, character, and caring for; Lerner, Almerigi, Theokas, & Lerner, 2005: 12) to support positive development in childhood and adolescence. In this regard, it has been pointed out that "Such programs are most likely to result in the development of these Cs when they involve sustained positive adult-youth relationships, youth skill building activities, and opportunities for youth participation in and leadership of community based activities" (Lerner et al., 2005: 12).

Emotional competence is a key competence. Learning is not only associated with surprises, but also with disappointments such as self-doubt or even social conflicts. This is why emotional competence is so important. It is regarded as a key competence for teaching and learning processes. Many interventions based on peer counseling and training appeal to the helpfulness of young people. However, especially in helping situations, it is necessary to deal with very different and sometimes contradictory feelings. The perception of the situation in which another person needs help, the evaluation of one's own abilities, and the weighting of different norms require not only mental consideration, but also coping with feelings, with contradictions between compassion and the spontaneous desire to distance oneself from the unpleasant demands of the situation. Interventions that involve peers aim to make young people more compassionate, to notice social situations in a more nuanced way, to be able to classify their perceptions better, to process complex and contradictory information more appropriately, and to be able to evaluate the effects of their actions. It is to be assumed that self-assessment changes as part of this process. Those who are helped receive social support and see themselves as valued members of the social system. The result is appreciation of one's own identity and self-esteem. In this context, willingness to help is an important social motive. If young people help each other, they come closer to their own self-ideal. At the same time, there is the possibility of questioning exaggerated ideals and coming to a realistic assessment in the group (Steinebach & Steinebach, 2013). These processes, information, and feelings ultimately form the basis for concrete action. The group offers a good training field to implement actions, to give each other feedback, and ultimately to decide on the basis of perceived results whether the action was good and right. Therefore, effective intervention focuses not only on obtaining experiences, but also on encouraging reflection and securing the results obtained. This also makes it clear that cognitive, emotional, and social skills are promoted by interventions for peers. Such interventions can then also focus on certain topics, e.g. career choice and career entry (cf. Petermann & Schultheiß, 2013).

1.5.2 Counseling and Therapy

It seems that professionals are particularly challenged when working with young people. The recommended counseling is different from the one we would choose when talking to children. A dialogue at eye level that avoids dominance is also recommended. At the same time, young people should be treated with spontaneity and openness, with a language that is appropriate for them. According to Geldard and Geldard (2010), this is most successful when counselors are still aware of their "inner adolescent". In addition, it is helpful to know about adolescent development. However, self-congruence and unconditional appreciation in dealing with young people as well as the development of a good professional relationship with empathy are also important. This again offers points of contact with the model of general factors of successful counseling and therapy (see chapter by Schaer & Knafla). Irrespective of whether one wants to follow the thoughts of one's own inner adolescent, it will certainly be important for young people that the counselor "meets them at eye level". Likewise, appreciation, openness, and creativity offer many opportunities for surprising learning experiences. On the basis of their own conditional model, counselors will then have to make decisions about their strategies and methods.

In supporting peers, many different ways to intervene come into question. From the point of view of learning theory, positive affirmation, asking for solutions, and transferring responsibility can be important for the development of desired behavior. In order to reduce unwanted behavior, it can be helpful to focus attention on the injured person, accompany conversations during conflicts with peers, and seek solutions together. Active listening or ego-messages, strategies, and methods, as used in humanistic counseling, are helpful in these situations. Working with groups offers the opportunity to clarify individual schemata from the here and now of the group, reflect feelings, and discuss possible behaviors from the perspective of other group members. What happens in the group can be a chance to reflect on individual behavior patterns. However, the group itself can also provide important support for this reflection process to succeed. When working with groups, experience-activating methods such as dream travel or role-playing can be helpful. In addition, mutual support and help can be an important experience for countering previous negative relationship experiences.

1.5.3 Research and Theory Development

The evaluation of interventions to promote resilience is not easy. In complex quasi-experimental designs, large samples would have to be monitored in longitudinal sections in order to arrive at reliable conclusions (Ungar et al., 2013). Ideally, evaluations should be regarded as a self-evident contribution to a learning process in which interventions are designed on the basis of available knowledge, while at the same time theories and practical knowledge about the documented results are further developed (Leve et al., 2009). Resilience has many facets and, accordingly, evaluation is at best implemented on an interdisciplinary basis, so that fields such as medicine, psychology, pedagogy, and sociology can be included depending on the issue being examined. What do we know so far? Following Rutter (2006) we can say: (1) Resilience helps, especially when we succeed in eliminating risk factors. (2) If there are no dangers or demands, protective facts often prove to be neutral. Sometimes, however, they can also turn out to be risks. (3) Efforts to deal with stress can actually lead to the development of protective factors. (4) However, the development of such protective factors can only become apparent long after the negative event has been dealt with. Evaluations should therefore be multifocal and multi-methodological.

The demands on good research in this area are many: theoretically, a clearer definition of the core concepts should be called for. Research should focus more closely on peer relationships (Brown & Braun, 2013), with not only friendships, but also other relationships, such as sibling relationships or various types of "friendships", becoming a topic (Padilla-Walker, Dyer, Yorgason, Fraser, & Coyne, 2015). The interrelationships between the different relationship systems should be taken into account (Dijkstra & Veenstra, 2011). The importance of regional and culture differences should be examined (Greater Goods Science Centre, n.d.). Measurement instruments should be optimized. The positive should be given the importance it deserves, because the primarily negative focus of peer research is still proving to be a problem (Brown & Bran, 2013). The course of development in adolescence itself should be examined more closely (Carlo, Hausmann, Christiansen, & Randall, 2003). Longitudinal studies should then show whether short, medium, or long-term effects can be proven (Leve et al., 2009). Finally, the many theories on adolescence should be examined for similarities and, if possible, integrated (Newman & Newman, 2011).

In summary, we sought to highlight that, in order to ensure the sustainability of psychosocial interventions in schools, a multilevel approach should be adopted. Specifically, we proposed that a framework based on resilience may prove to be pivotal, yielding several novel interventions—such as mindfulness and compassion—that may be integrated into a more systemic and ecological perspective.

Acknowledgements This study was partially supported by the Millennium Science Initiative of the Ministry of Economy, Development and Tourism, grant "Millennium Nucleus to Improve the Mental Health of Adolescents and Youths, Imhay" and the Fund for Innovation and Competitiveness (FIC) of the Chilean Ministry of Economy, Development, and Tourism, through the Millennium Scientific Initiative, Grant N° IS130005.

References

Antonovsky, A. (1987). *Unraveling the mystery of health—How people manage stress and stay well.* San Francisco: Jossey-Bass Publishers.

Bandura, A. (1997). *Self-efficacy: The exercise of control.* New York: Freeman.

Brendtro, L. K., & Larson, S. J. (2006). *The resilience revolution.* Bloomington: Solution-tree.

Brown, B. B., & Braun, M. T. (2013). Peer relations. In C. Proctor & P. A. Linley (Eds.), *Research, applications, and interventions for children and adolescents: A positive psychology perspective* (pp. 149–164). Dordrecht: Springer.

Brown, B. B., & Larson, J. (2009). Peer relationships in adolescence. In R. M. Lerner & L. Steinberg (Eds.), *Handbook of adolescent psychology, Vol 2: Contextual influences on adolescent development* (3rd ed., pp. 74–103). Hoboken, NJ: Wiley.

Carlo, G., Hausmann, A., Christiansen, S., & Randall, B. A. (2003). Sociocognitive and behavioral correlates of a measure of prosocial tendencies for adolescents. *Journal of Early Adolescence, 23*(1), 107–134.

Dijkstra, J. K., & Veenstra, R. (2011). Peer Relations. In B. B. Brown & M. Prinstein (Eds.), *Encyclopedia of adolescence* (Vol. 2, pp. 255–259). New York: Academic.

Donlan, A. E., Lynch, A. D., & Lerner, R. M. (2015). Peer relationships and positive youth development. In E. P. Bowers, G. J. Geldhof, S. K. Johnson, L. J. Hilliard, R. M. Hershberg, J. V. Lerner, & R. M. Lerner (Eds.), *Promoting positive youth development, advancing responsible adolescent development* (pp. 121–136). New York: Springer International.

Geldard, K., & Geldard, D. (2010). *Counselling adolescents. The proactive approach for young people* (3rd ed.). Los Angeles: Sage.

Gharabaghi, K. (2011). A culture of education: Enhancing school performance of youth living in residential care in Ontario. *Child Welfare, 90*(1), 75–92.

Greater Goods Science Center. (n.d.). *The science of generosity.* White paper prepared for the John Templeton Foundation by the Greater Good Science Center at UC Berkeley. https://www.templeton.org/wp-content/uploads/2018/01/Generosity_White_Paper-FinalJTF.pdf. Accessed January 12, 2019.

Lerner, R. M., Almerigi, J. B., Theokas, C., & Lerner, J. V. (2005). Positive youth psychology. A view of the issues. *Journal of early adolescence, 25*(1), 10–16.

Leve, L. D., Fisher, P. A., & Chamberlain, P. (2009). Multidimensional foster care as a preventive intervention to promote resiliency among youth in the child welfare system. *Journal of Personality, 77,* 1869–1902.

Luthar, S. S. (2006). Resilience in development: A synthesis of research across five decades. In D. Cicchetti & D. J. Cohen (Eds.), *Developmental psychopathology. Vol. III, Risk, disorder, and adaptation* (pp. 739–795). Hoboken, NJ: Wiley.

Mittelstraß, J. (1989). *Der Flug der Eule. Von der Vernunft der Wissenschaft und der Aufgabe der Philosophie.* Frankfurt a. M.: Suhrkamp.

Newman, B. M., & Newman, P. R. (2011). Adolescence, theories of. In R. J. R. Levesque (Ed.), *Encyclopedia of adolescence* (Vol. 1, pp. 20–29). New York: Springer.

Noble, T., & McGrath, H. (2014). Well-being and resilience in school settings. In G. A. Fava & C. Ruini (Eds.), *Increasing psychological well-being in clinical and educational settings, Cross-cultural advancements in positive psychology* (Vol. 8, pp. 135–152). Dordrecht: Springer.

Noble, T., Wyatt, T., McGrath, H., Roffey, S., & Rowling, L. (2008). *Scoping study into approaches to student well-being: Final report*. Brisbane, Qld.: Australian Catholic University and Erebus International. https://docs.education.gov.au/documents/scoping-study-approaches-student-wellbeing-final-report. Accessed January 12, 2019.

Padilla-Walker, L. M., Dyer, W. J., Yorgason, J. B., Fraser, A. M., & Coyne, S. M. (2015). Adolescents' prosocial behavior toward family, friends, and strangers: A person-centered approach. *Journal of Research on Adolescence, 25*(1), 135–150.

Petermann, U., & Schultheiß, J. (2013): Übergänge: Beruf als Zukunft. In C. Steinebach & K. Gharabaghi (Eds.), *Resilienzförderung im Jugendalter. Praxis und Perspektiven* (pp. 147–163) Heidelberg: Springer.

Rutter, M. (2006). Implications of resilience concepts for scientific understanding. *Annals of the New York Academy of Sciences*, 1–12.

Rutter, M. (2013). Annual research review: Resilience—clinical implications. *Journal of Child Psychology and Psychiatry, 54*(4), 474–487.

Ryan, R. M., & Deci, E. L. (2000). Self-determination theory and the facilitation of intrinsic motivation, social development, and well-being. *American Psychologist, 55*, 68–78.

Sales, J. M., & Irwin, C. E. (2013). A biopsychosocial perspective of adolescenct health and disease. In W. T. O'Donohue, L. T. Benuto, & L. Woodward Tolle (Eds.), *Handbook of adolescent health psychology* (pp. 13–29). New-York: Springer.

Steinebach, C. (2012). Resilienz. In C. Steinebach, D. Jungo & R. Zihlmann (Eds.), *Positive Psychologie in der Praxis. Anwendung in Psychotherapie, Beratung und Coaching* (pp. 95–101). Weinheim: Beltz.

Steinebach, C. (2015). Resilience. In J. D. Wright (Ed.), *International encyclopedia of the social & behavioral sciences* (2nd ed., Vol. 20, pp. 555–560). Oxford: Elsevier.

Steinebach, C., & Gharabaghi, K. (2018). Resilienz. In B. Gniewosz & P. F. Titzmann (Eds.), *Handbuch Jugend* (pp. 508–525). Stuttgart: Kohlhammer.

Steinebach, C., Schrenk, A., Steinebach, U., & Brendtro, L. K. (2018). *Positive Peer Culture. Ein Manual für starke Gruppengespräche*. Weinheim: Beltz-Juventa.

Steinebach, C., & Steinebach, U. (2013). Gleichaltrige. Peers als Ressource In C. Steinebach & K. Gharabahi (Eds.), *Resilienzförderung im Jugendalter. Praxis und Perspektiven* (pp. 93–109). Heidelberg: Springer.

Steinebach, C., Steinebach, U., & Brendtro, L. K. (2012). Peerbeziehungen und Gesundheit im Jugendalter. In C. Steinebach, D. Jungo, & R. Zihlmann (Eds.), *Positive Psychologie in der Praxis. Anwendung in Psychotherapie, Beratung und Coaching* (pp. 153–161). Weinheim: Beltz.

Steinebach, C., Süss, D., Kienbaum, J., & Kiegelmann, M. (2016). *Basiswissen Pädagogische Psychologie*. Weinheim: Beltz.

Steptoe, A., Dockray, S., Wardle, J. (2009). Positive affect and psychobiological processes relevant to health. *Journal of Personality, 77*(6), 1747–1775.

Sternberg, R. J., & Spear-Swerling, L. (1998). Personal navigation. In M. Ferrari & R. J. Sternberg (Eds.), *Self- awareness: Its nature and development* (pp. 219–245). New York: Guilford Press.

Ungar, M., Ghazinour, M., & Richter, J. (2013). Annual research review: What is resilience within the social ecology of human development? *Journal of Child Psychology and Psychiatry, 54*(4), 348–366.

Ungar, M., & Lerner, R. M. (2008). Introduction to a special issue of research in human development: Resilience and positive development across the life span: A View of the Issues. *Research in Human Development, 5*(3), 135–138.

Weare, K. (2014). Mindfulness in schools. Where are we and where might we go next? In A. Ie, C. T. Ngnoumen, & E. J. Langer (Eds.), *The Wiley Blackwell handbook of mindfulness* (pp. 1037–1053). Hoboken, NJ: Wiley.

Wilson, E. O. (1998). *Consilience: The unity of knowledge*. New York: Alfred A. Knopf.

World Health Organization. (1986). *Ottawa-Charta*. http://www.euro.who.int/__data/assets/pdf_file/0004/129532/Ottawa_Charter.pdf. Accessed September 10, 2011.

World Health Organization. (2009). *Milestones in health promotion: Statements from global conferences*. Geneva: World Health Organization.

Chapter 2
Looking for a Broad Framework for the Integration of Mindfulness-Based Interventions in the Educational System

Álvaro I. Langer, Christoph Steinebach, Carlos García-Rubio, Catherine I. Andreu and Leandro Torres-Díaz

Abstract Today, there is a crucial need for well-being to be a priority in the educational curriculum. 21st-century schools not only provide a broad set of academic skills, but they also promote the healthy development and mental health of children and adolescents through strengths-based education and the cultivation of socio-emotional and behavioral skills. Some of the evidence-based interventions that may address these requirements include mindfulness- and compassion-based programs (MBIs and CBIs). Nevertheless, there are still several open questions concerning the implementation of mindfulness in the educational system. In this chapter, our concern is how mindfulness may be integrated in a more comprehensive way in order to help ensure its sustainability in schools as well as in institutions embedded in specific socio-cultural contexts. Particularly, we suggest that a common, shared meaning in

Á. I. Langer (✉)
Institute of Psychological Studies, Faculty of Medicine, Universidad Austral de Chile, Valdivia, Chile
e-mail: Alvaro.langer@uach.cl

Millennium Nucleus to Improve the Mental Health of Adolescents and Youths, Imhay, Santiago, Chile

Center for Interdisciplinary Studies on the Nervous System (CISNe), Universidad Austral de Chile, Valdivia, Chile

Á. I. Langer · C. I. Andreu
Millennium Institute for Research in Depression and Personality (MIDAP), Santiago, Chile

C. Steinebach
School of Applied Psychology, ZHAW Zürich University of Applied Sciences, Zürich, Switzerland

C. García-Rubio
Department of Biological and Health Psychology, Faculty of Psychology, Universidad Autónoma de Madrid, Madrid, Spain

C. I. Andreu
School of Psychology, Pontificia Universidad Católica de Chile, Santiago, Chile

L. Torres-Díaz
Instituto de Ciencias Naturales, Universidad de las Américas, Santiago, Chile

Instituto de Investigación e Innovación en Salud, Universidad Central de Chile, Santiago, Chile

C. Steinebach and Á. I. Langer (eds.), *Enhancing Resilience in Youth*,
https://doi.org/10.1007/978-3-030-25513-8_2

the educational system (i.e. individual and institutional level) may result in a network where mindfulness could be supported more sustainably. A shared meaning about why and for what ends adolescents should practice mindfulness may consider not solely a personal perspective but also a social and ecological one. In this context, MBIs would play a relevant role by mediating the multiple requirements introduced by a new mental health promotion paradigm in schools.

Keywords Compassion · Mental problems · Community development · Mindfulness · Educational curriculum

2.1 The Current State of Mental Health in Children and Adolescents

During the last decade, the mental health of young people has continued to worsen. From 2007 to 2017, the number of young people who persistently feel sadness or despair, and who consider suicide, has increased. In addition, the percentage of young people who attempt suicide has remained stable (Kann et al., 2018).

Although these are USA data, the worldwide prevalence of mental disorders during childhood and adolescence is high, with the most common issues being depression, anxiety, attention deficit hyperactivity disorder (ADHD), and behavioral problems (Polanczyk, Salum, Sugaya, Caye, & Rohde, 2015). It is noteworthy that 50% of the mental problems in a person's life emerge before the age of 15, and that 75% do so before the age of 24 (Kessler, Amminger, et al., 2007). In fact, most of the serious mental problems in adulthood are usually secondary conditions to mental problems that emerged early in childhood and adolescence, and these are usually not treated until years after their first appearance (Kessler, Angermeyer, et al., 2007). In addition, a large part of the mental problems that emerge in childhood and adolescence are treated mainly with pharmacological treatment, as evidenced by the increased use of antidepressants and antipsychotics in childhood and adolescence (Bachmann et al., 2016; Hálfdánarson et al., 2017), despite the fact that some recent meta-analyses point to the need to use them with caution due to an increase in adverse effects (Sharma, Guski, Freund, & Gøtzsche, 2016).

The development of mental health problems entails a high personal, social, and economic cost. For example, at a social level, in the United Kingdom, the annual economic cost of mental health problems has been estimated at £105 billion (Centre for Mental Health, 2010; Collins et al., 2011). At the individual level, children and adolescents experience a reduction in their quality of life and worse levels of social and occupational functioning (e.g., worse academic performance, more family and school problems, worse physical health) (Goodyer, Herbert, Tamplin, Secher, & Pearson, 1997). Unfortunately, the increase in early mental problems could continue following the same trend in the next few years, or at least remain unchanged, if, as some authors point out, current lifestyles may be favoring their early appearance and diminishing the psychological well-being of children and young people

(Twenge et al., 2018a). Young people's increased engagement in activities involving electronic devices with screens may be related to the greater occurrence of mental problems (Suchert, Hanewinkel, & Isensee, 2015). In addition, non-screen activities are becoming less common among young people (e.g. in-person social interaction) (Twenge et al., 2018a) and trust in others has dropped (Twenge, Campbell, & Carter, 2014). Some studies point out that the current social model that prioritizes extrinsic goals, such as wealth, materialism, or status, to the detriment of more intrinsic goals, such as life meaning, affiliation, or community development, may account for the early increase in mental problems in adolescence (Twenge et al., 2018b; Twenge, 2013). For all these reasons, the need for evidence-based programs that promote mental health during childhood and adolescence is absolutely critical.

2.2 Development and Mental Health in School

Childhood and adolescence are periods characterized by constant and profound changes in development (Giedd et al., 1999). Neuroplasticity during childhood and adolescence is greater than at any later stage of life (Paus, 2005). Therefore, from a neurodevelopmental perspective, these vital stages can be seen as a window of opportunity to implement interventions that support the development of brain regions involved in psychological processes and behavioral skills that are central to healthy development (Fuhrmann, Knoll, & Blakemore, 2015; Spear, 2013). Since the difficulties in attentional and emotional regulation, as well as those affecting social skills, underlie many childhood and adolescent mental health problems (Ehrenreich-May & Chu, 2013; White, Jarrett, & Ollendick, 2013), carrying out interventions that promote cognitive, emotional, and social development can help prevent the early onset of mental health problems and enhance well-being (Hawkins, Catalano, Kosterman, Abbott, & Hill, 1999; Werner-Seidler, Perry, Calear, Newby, & Christensen, 2017).

During childhood and adolescence, schools are active agents of development (Vygotsky, 1978). Children and adolescents spend much of their time at school, and the experiences they have there are crucial for their mental health and development (Waenerlund et al., 2016). Due to their wide scope and central role in family life, schools are presented as a primary context in which to conduct universal interventions for the prevention of mental health and promotion of well-being (Durlak & Wells, 1997). Although selective school interventions (i.e. only delivered to adolescents considered at risk of later mental health problems) and targeted school interventions (i.e. provided only to students identified as having mental health problems) have been shown to be effective in reducing mental health problems (Sanchez et al., 2018), universal school-based interventions reduce the stigma that children and adolescents attach to mental health treatment (Bulanda, Bruhn, Byro-Johnson, & Zentmyer, 2014) and are a more cost-effective alternative since they involve no screening costs. In addition, universal school-based interventions are accessible to all students, including those who have lower risk profiles at the time of intervention but whose risk profile may change later. Numerous recent studies show that, compared to control groups, universal school-based interventions are effective in reducing depressive symptoms, internalizing problems, externalizing problems, and general psychological distress (Dray et al., 2017). Interestingly, in addition to improving mental health, universal school-based interventions have been found to be effective in promoting well-being and improving relevant outcomes for healthy development, such as self-efficacy, optimism, or self-esteem (Shoshani & Steinmetz, 2014). Therefore, universal school-based interventions are suited to the competencies of 21st-century schools (Skills, 2017).

Today, there is a crucial need for well-being to be a priority in the educational curriculum (Langford et al., 2014). 21st-century schools not only provide a broad set of academic skills (e.g. math, reading, writing, and science), but they also promote the healthy development and mental health of children and adolescents through strengths-based education and the cultivation of socio-emotional and behavioral skills. In addition, 21st century schools are making a transition in their conception of human beings and well-being, moving from a deficit-based model to a strength-based model (Climie & Henley, 2016), and thus aligning with the definition of health issued by the World Health Organization (WHO, 2004), according to which health is "*a state of complete physical, mental and social well-being and not merely the absence of disease or infirmity*". In this regard, Greenberg et al. (2003, p., 466) states that "*a comprehensive mission for schools is to educate students to be knowledgeable, responsible, socially skilled, healthy, caring, and contributing citizens*", while the Mind & Life Education Research Network (2012) point out that the schools of this century are responsible for cultivating a set of mental skills and socio-emotional dispositions that underlie positive development. Specifically, they refer to attentional and emotional self-regulation skills, the ability to handle stress, self-awareness to be able to transcend habits and self-representations understood as fixed, and the acquisition of prosocial dispositions such as empathy and compassion. Already in the 3rd century B.C., Aristotle pointed out that "*educating the mind without educating the heart is not to educate at all*".

In this context, as previously noted, it is crucial to devote all our efforts to implement evidence-based interventions at schools, which fit students' new skills and especially the new paradigm of mental health promotion that is required. Some of the evidence-based interventions that may address these requirements include mindfulness- and compassion-based programs (MBIs and CBIs). MBIs in school settings have been extensively studied in the last decade. Nowadays, it is clearer that mindfulness is feasible to applied in school settings and MBIs are valued by pupils and educational staff (e.g. Dariotis et al., 2016). Recent meta-analyses and systematic reviews have shown small to moderate significant results in the cognitive, emotional, and behavioral domains (Carsley, Khoury, & Heath, 2018; Felver, Celis-de Hoyos, Tezanos, & Singh, 2016) (Additionally see Chaps. 8 and 9 in this book). Nevertheless, there are still several open questions concerning the implementation of mindfulness in the educational system beyond limited research studies. In this chapter, our concern is how mindfulness may be integrated in a more comprehensive way, in order to help ensure its sustainability in schools as well as in institutions embedded in specific socio-cultural contexts. Thus, we would like to highlight some elements which may support the implementation of MBIs in a fluid and ecological way.

2.3 Basic Elements of Mindfulness

Mindfulness can be understood as a trait (dispositional mindfulness) and as a practice, which is cultivated through a variety of programs (MBIs). Mindfulness is a 2500-year-old Buddhist practice traditionally understood as part of the process of "awakening" (Gethin, 1998, 2011). Many teachers describe mindfulness as a process that involves an increase in bodily awareness of internal or external stimuli and emotional states (Davis and Thompson, 2015). According to Kabat-Zinn (1996), Mindfulness is based on two canonical source texts of the Theravāda Buddhist tradition (Pāli Nikāyas.), the Ānāpanasati-sutta and the Mahāsatipaṭṭhāna-sutta. Both of them consist in a discourse attributed to the Buddha.

Commonly, the scientific literature indicates that "mindfulness" is a translation of the Pāli term sati. The Pāli texts employ sati to refer to everything from "minding" one's livestock (MN.I.117) to "minding" one's meditation object in practices such as loving-kindness (Sn.26) (Davis & Thompson, 2015). Tibetan Buddhists usually complement this practice with ethical ones such as reflecting on the inevitability of death (maraṇasati), lovingkindness, or literally friendliness (mettā), practices aimed simply at cultivating a settled and unified state of mind (samādhi) through concentration on a sensory or mental object. In these forms of meditation, practitioners counteract mind-wandering by repeatedly bringing the mind back to the object of meditation. Mindfulness in this sense consists in certain practices and attitudes that practitioners put into play in the social world.

The most common definition of mindfulness found in psychology and mental health literature is: "*the practice of paying attention in a particular way: on purpose, in the present moment, and non-judgmentally*" (Kabat-Zinn, 1994: p. 4) or more recently: "*Mindfulness can be thought of as moment-to-moment, non-judgmental awareness, cultivated by paying attention in a specific way, that is, in the present moment, and as non-reactively, as non-judgmentally, and as openheartedly as possible. When it is cultivated intentionally, it is sometimes referred to as deliberate mindfulness*" (Kabat-Zinn, 2005).

Based on all the proposed definitions (see Chaps. 8 and 9), it is possible to note at least two aspects of mindfulness: attentive orientation towards what is present and openness, curiosity, and acceptance as an expression of a particularly successful instance of current emotional regulation. What are the determinants of mindfulness? Attention to inner and outer processes, action based on this very consciousness, openness for experiences, accepting and non-judgmental attitude, intention not to react and not to focus, empathetic understanding, and relative calmness towards current thoughts (Bergomi, Tschacher, & Kupper, 2013).

Scientific investigation of Mindfulness training has thus far focused on how various forms of attention training alter cognitive and affective processes (see Lutz,

Slagter, Dunne, & Davidson, 2008 for a review). According to this, attentional skills can change the quality of our own behavior and promote an improvement in the practitioner's health and well-being (Chiesa and Malinowski, 2011; Malinowski, 2013; Wallace and Shapiro, 2006). Moreover, an often overlooked aspect is that Buddhist teachings include many other mind training methods. For example, moral discussion can be seen as a means for protecting oneself from unhealthy states, such as greed or hatred. Thus, some Buddhist schools consider this not only a complement but rather an essential element of the practice.

Several models of how mindfulness works have been proposed. One of the most integrative is the *Liverpool Mindfulness Model*, whose aims are to determine and integrate the more prominent events and structures involved in mindfulness practice and provide a framework for directing future research (Malinowski, 2013). Accordingly, and in line with the conceptualizations advanced above, the model is based on the predominance of attentional skills (Hölzel et al., 2011; Lutz et al., 2008; Tang and Posner, 2009; Slagter, Davidson, & Lutz, 2011; Wallace and Shapiro, 2006).

The model comprises the following interrelated levels:

(1) Driving motivational factors.
(2) If and how the individual engages in mind training.
(3) Regularity in the engagement in mindfulness practice based on the refinement of attentional capacities that facilitate regulatory processes of emotions.
(4) Changed and more balanced mental stance or attitude.
(5) Positive outcome in terms of physical and mental well-being and behavior quality.

Roughly speaking, the practice of Mindfulness meditation starts with a meditator focusing on a relevant meditation object (usually the bodily sensation of breathing). After a variable time period (dependent on the ability of the practitioner), the mind loses the focus on the object and mind wandering occurs. Sooner or later the practitioner will identify the mind wandering and lets go of the distracting train of thought by means of attentional disengagement. Finally, the meditator returns to the meditation object by shifting back his or her focus. All the timing in this process depends on the expertise of the practitioner (Wallace, 2006). Two forms of training are usually described in the literature: Focused Attention (FA) and Open Monitoring (OM) meditation practices (Lutz et al., 2008). They can be considered interdependent to some extent because a practitioner will initially engage in FA to develop attentional stability, clarity, and awareness of the present moment (mental state); only then will he or she be able to deploy moment-by-moment attentiveness to anything that occurs in his/her experience, to finally be able to maintain the OM state even without focusing on an explicit object with a non-judgmental attitude (Bishop et al., 2004; Chiesa & Malinowski, 2011; Malinowski, 2013; Shapiro, Carlson, Astin, & Freedman, 2006).

As the discussion about basic approaches in mindfulness research shows, effects are mostly interpreted as the result of a top-down process whereby the cognitive system is able to control the emotional system through practice and routine. So far, little attention has been paid to the fact that, especially in mindfulness promotion exercises, the bottom-up process might be important: physical processes influence the emotional system and thus also affect cognitive processes (Guendelman, Medeiros, & Rampes, 2017, cf. also the contribution by Steinebach and colleagues in this volume). Mindfulness has a variety of positive effects on human behavior and experience. It is connected with increased empathy and a differentiated perception of one's own experience and the environment. Non-judgmental perception leads to greater well-being and resilience (e.g. Tan & Martin, 2016), a benefit mostly resulting from the fact that it facilitates dealing with stress. Greater empathy promotes helpfulness, self-esteem, and self-efficacy. Mindful people perceive their social environment in a more differentiated way and can thus also better activate social resources. For their part, social resources strengthen self-esteem and self-efficacy regarding one's sense of attitude to mindfulness and skills for acting mindfulness.

2.4 Framework for Mindfulness-Based Interventions

2.4.1 Institutional Level: Toward a Shared Meaning of Mindfulness

Interventions to promote mindfulness have long since gained a foothold in counseling and therapy services for young people as well as in schools. These interventions are recommended to prevent stress disorders and increase pupils' ability to concentrate, but also to encourage teachers to be mindful when there is a threat of burnout. Mindfulness should thus also become a characteristic of the organizational culture of a "mindful school". Mindfulness becomes a strength of the young people, the professionals, and the organization itself. If we distinguish between neurochemical, neuromuscular, emotional, and cognitive systems in the bio-psycho-social model of human development, this offers us the possibility of making more a differentiated assessment of the effects of mindfulness-related interventions (Steinebach, Schrenk, Steinebach, & Brendtro, 2018). We can also assume that mindful attitudes are reflected in the social system of the organization and in characteristics of its physical environment. Therefore, any intervention to promote mindfulness in schools should include team development, a revision of the curriculum, parent education, and a redesign of classrooms and the school building (Willard, 2014). In addition, considering that MBIs may appear threatening in some way, it is crucial to incorporate the evaluation of the socio-cultural features of both the territory where the school is located and its students. For instance, a recent study by Langer et al. (under review) shows that some adolescents from a school with a low-mid percentage of social vulnerability, after the first sessions of a MBI, were uncomfortable with the resulting sensation of relaxation and therefore decided to withdraw from the intervention. Probably, these students interpreted feeling relaxed as a sign of personal vulnerability ("If I relax I am less alert, and therefore more vulnerable to others"). Thus, it is relevant to consider the function that some behaviors could have for adolescents in specific contexts; however, establishing how to change these behaviors requires a systemic program capable of providing understanding and meaning beyond the mindfulness workshop itself. Special attention should be paid to ethnic minorities, sexual diversity, migrant populations, and socially vulnerable students in general. Tailoring the narrative associated to MBIs may help overcome barriers for their implementation.

In this regard, one of the barriers reported in the implementation of mindfulness training (MT) across seven high schools in UK was *perceptions*, "highlighting the importance of members of the school community, sharing an understanding of what MT is and why it is being introduced in school context" (Wilde et al., 2019). We argued that, as a new field, mindfulness should be able to define how it will be integrated with the other school subjects. In other words, how will this subject *talk* with the others? For instance, this concerns how body awareness may be related to physical education, how a non-judgmental approach could be introduced as an excellent way to learn about different religions or cultures, or how the economy could be understood from a collaborative perspective (see Chap. 17). In this way, the practice of mindfulness could be embodied in a network of shared meaning for both students and staff of each school, thus enabling them to shift from individual to social resilience (for more details see Chap. 1).

2.4.2 Individual Level: How to Improve the Continuity of Mindfulness Practice

Young people are often not interested in taking special courses or doing exercises. How can we motivate them to get involved? We can assume that young people deem a given intervention to be attractive if they consider that it addresses their basic needs. This is first and foremost about autonomy, belonging, and experiencing competence (Ryan & Deci, 2000). But how do we bring basic needs and mindfulness together? Compassion appears to be key in this regard. Compassion has been proposed as a working mechanism that underlies the MBIs on youths (Van der Gucht, Takano, Raes, & Kuppens, 2018). This is what we call feelings of concern or compassion and willingness to improve the well-being of others (Singer & Klimecki, 2014). As current neurophysiological research shows, compassion activates specific areas of the brain. Compassion means empathy connected to the desire to reduce the suffering of others, which is linked to the fact that the suffering of others is perceived consciously. Emotionally compassionate empathy supports a person's intent to reduce this suffering and, on the behavioral level, strengthens his or her willingness to actually do something to help those suffering (Jinpa, 2010; Miller, 2018; Roeser & Eccles, 2015). Current neurophysiological research shows that compassion results in the activation of areas of the brain different from those that become active as a result of sympathetic empathy. "Empathic distress" is connected with clear negative feelings and can lead to avoidance and the renunciation of prosocial behavior (Singer & Klimecki, 2014). Compassion is closely related to generosity. Empathy, generosity, and compassion are demanded wherever young people are called upon to stand up for their peers in the classroom or other people in the community. Therefore, it seems obvious to enhance empathy, generosity, and compassion when doing "service learning" or when promoting a positive peer culture (PPC) (Steinebach et al., 2018).

PPC is an intervention model for strengthening resilience in children and adolescents and could help answer another relevant question: How to improve the continuity of mindfulness practice over time, considering that its effects are linked to the practice (Kuyken et al., 2013), which tends to decrease over time (Worthen & Luiselli, 2017). Specifically, PPC is based on peer-managed group dynamics in which adults participate as facilitators, seeking to increase the group's ability to manage and solve its problems. One of the main elements of PPC is Generosity, which basically involves answering the question "how can I help solve someone else's problem in the best way that I can?". This is quite close to compassion, but based on a socio-cognitive paradigm where relational rather that individual practices are encouraged (for a proposal of relational mindfulness see Chap. 13). Thus, PPC could strengthen the implementation of more stable mindfulness practices thanks to peer management. For instance, after a MBI, peers could lead the mindfulness practices and help others if they struggle with them.

This would also be conceivable within the framework of teaching modules focused on social emotional learning (Felver et al., 2016). These interventions can be supplemented by exercises to promote social emotional skills (e.g. Petermann, Petermann, & Nitkowski, 2016). For children and adolescents in particular, there are multiple opportunities to promote social skills in order to boost self-worth and reduce aggressive behavior. It may be that all these interventions again follow the usual top-down arguments: cognitions help to control emotions; cognitions help to recognize and name emotions. Accordingly, for example, instructions on physical activities can promote self-awareness and well-being (cf. Springer, 2013). With these exercises, it becomes clear how physical activity can be connected with emotional experience and social interaction.

2.5 Connecting the Dots

In this context, the incorporation of a multilevel perspective for the generation of psychosocial interventions in school contexts—that is, one that considers not only individual and group variables, but also organizational and community-related ones—is strongly recommended. We argue for the inclusion of the specific socio-cultural characteristics of each educational establishment where MFIs would be implemented. Likewise, we consider that planning psychosocial interventions in school contexts from a multilevel perspective is highly relevant in heterogeneous sociocultural realities. Thus, a shared meaning of mindfulness in specific contexts could help overcome barriers to the implementation of mindfulness. As we have pointed out, mindfulness practice depends on driving motivational factors and on how the individual engages in the practice. According to the Husserlian idea of "Intentionality" (Husserl, 1999), our mind is always making sense (intending) of the world. In concordance with this idea, the shared intentionality between practitioners (mindfulness instructors/practitioners) yields a broad meaning of what mindfulness is.

A shared meaning about why and for what ends adolescents should practice mindfulness may consider not solely a personal perspective (e.g. improving concentration and reducing anxiety or stress) but also a social and ecological one. In this regard, we believe that mindfulness needs to be understood as a way to change not only how we relate to our own thoughts and reduce unhealthy feelings but also how we relate with our world. Specifically, we propose the following paths:

a. To connect mindfulness practice with a broad sense of benefits and implications. This means answering the questions *Does the practice of mindfulness have an impact beyond myself?* And if so, *what is it?* One of these potential external effects is the promotion of the satisfaction of non-material needs, which directly and indirectly influences the adoption of sustainable behaviors for protecting nature. In fact, being more aware of how my behavior impacts on others and on the environment could help self-regulation (e.g. Langer, Schmidt, & Krogh, 2017). In this regard, mindfulness practice may yield benefits from both an individual and an interconnected and relational perspective.
b. To connect mindfulness practice with the intention to help others and actions directed toward this goal. This could be done under the model of compassion-based interventions or specific compassion sessions in MBIs. Additionally, we suggest that strengthening a positive peer culture (PPC) in mindfulness practice may give room to explicitly resolve the problem of one member of the group and to feeling competent as a supportive group member. Thus, it may give a more interpersonal perspective where mindfulness practice may help with basic needs while also helping develop a sense of generosity by pondering the question *how can I give the best of me to contribute to well-being of my peers?*

MBIs could improve the socio-emotional and behavioral skills of young people by making sense of the education process and basically by making explicit through multiple methodologies (see for example Chap. 12) how this process could help them *learn to be* and *to live together* (Delors, 1996). In our view, new insights at an individual and institutional level may play a role in the sustainability of MBIs through a realistic integration of mindfulness in the educational curriculum as a whole. It is necessary for all the educational staff to attain an overall conceptual and practical understanding of mindfulness. In this vein, it is important to carry out studies with the purpose of identifying socio-demographical and cultural targets for the application of this approach. This requires the efforts of the whole educational system; however, there has been little systemic research on this topic so far. Figure 2.1 outlines the multiple variables and the assumed interactions which should be considered.

From which theoretical perspective do we select the most important elements of our model? We assume that the behavior of young people is determined not only by social conditions such as social norms, but also by individual factors such as needs. In addition to these "soft" factors, physical characteristics of the environment are also important. Characteristics of the physical and social environment can directly and indirectly influence human development. These influences can be positive or

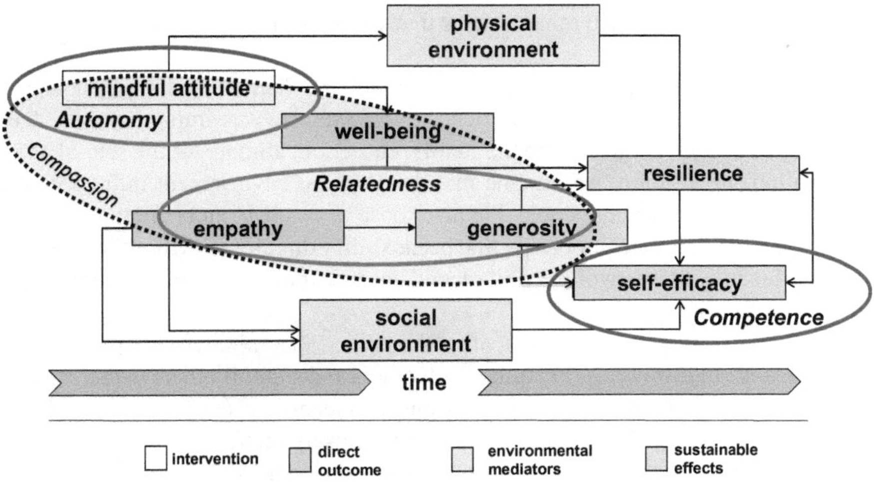

Fig. 2.1 Model of mindfulness-related interventions in positive environments

negative. We assume that early negative influences will show their effects directly or later in the life course. Negative developments can then be observed not only in the individual, but also in the social environment. Preventive measures are necessary to avert such negative developments. We also try to remedy disorders at an early stage with therapeutic interventions. Here, cognitions, emotions, and behaviors become the object of interventions. However, we also attempt to shape the physical environment in such a way that it has a positive influence on development. Interventions are particularly sustainable if the measures address basic human needs. In addition, it makes sense not only to target deficits but also to build up strengths. Individual environmental strengths and resources offer the opportunity to compensate for existing deficits. All this is intended to ensure that young people master their current problems through a learning and development process in which new and relevant competences are acquired.

The consideration of basic needs seems important to us because they help to bridge the gap between motivation and behavior (i.e. motivation for practicing mindfulness). Friends of the same age have a great influence on young people's behavior; therefore, it is necessary to involve peers when designing interventions. The circle of friends or peers thus becomes a place of mutual help. Mutual support can help to build self-efficacy and strengthen self-esteem. However, this requires that one can empathize with others. Mindfulness and empathy are therefore important prerequisites for a positive social togetherness.

Which basic needs have to be differentiated? With a view to current research on this topic, belonging, experiencing competence, and autonomy seem to be central basic needs. In the Circle of Courage (see the article on Generosity in this book), these three are supplemented by generosity. Generosity is an important need and a personal strength of character that ensures that young people will be inclined to help others selflessly.

Physical and social environment: In our model, we distinguish the physical and social environment. In adolescence, friends of the same age are important aspects of the social environment, and so are the family, classroom climate, or the school as an organization. In addition, we assume that the physical environment influences the attitudes not only of young people, but also those of teachers and parents. Environmental characteristics are important, first because they directly influence the behavior and experience of those involved, and second because they can indirectly support the effects of interventions.

Mindfulness, well-being, and empathy: We believe that mindfulness training programs enhance the ability to empathize with others and support others in their search for solutions to problems. There is now ample evidence of the positive effects of mindfulness on well-being, with the latter being closely related to resilience.

Compassion: In our model, the term "compassion" includes the concepts of generosity, empathy, and mindfulness, all of which are related to well-being. Here it also becomes clear that lived compassion "feels good" and thus contributes to well-being.

Resilience, generosity, and self-efficacy: The connections between self-efficacy and resilience are well documented. Experiencing generosity means having been able to feel what it is like to help others. These are experiences in which self-efficacy is the basis for help. But being able to help others also makes it possible to attribute positive results to oneself, which promotes self-efficacy as well. It is therefore necessary to create interventions in which young people experience generosity and in which they experience themselves to be self-effective, which will promote their resilience. Young people's willingness to be generous will depend to a large extent on their empathy. Therefore, we also expect the promotion of mindfulness to promote generosity and, ultimately, resilience.

Hypotheses: So, which central hypotheses can be based on this model?

1. We assume that mindfulness promotes individual well-being. Well-being is thus the cognitive and emotional bridge to resilience.
2. Strengthening mindfulness promotes the ability to empathize with others and thus the willingness to be generous toward others.
3. Acts of generosity and compassion strengthen self-esteem and self-efficacy.
4. Growing self-efficacy also strengthens resilience.
5. The physical environment (including nature) can promote mindfulness. This means that there are places where young people can meet, where they feel safe, and where they promote a positive togetherness.
6. Mindfulness-based interventions promote the positive aspects of the social environment in a special way. They support the growth of personality, especially in the sense of increasing generosity, self-efficacy, and resilience. In addition, they promote mutual helpfulness as a characteristic of school culture.

We expect that this model will help to highlight the relevance of promoting psychological well-being in children and young people through interventions that increase resilience, compassion, and emotional regulation, among other aspects. Particularly, we suggest that a common, shared meaning in the educational system (i.e. individual and institutional level) may result in a network where mindfulness could be supported more sustainably. In this context, MBIs would play a relevant role by mediating the multiple requirements introduced by a new mental health promotion paradigm in schools.

Acknowledgements This manuscript was supported by the Millennium Science Initiative of the Ministry of Economy, Development and Tourism, grant "Millennium Nucleus to Improve the Mental Health of Adolescents and Youths, Imhay" and the Fund for Innovation and Competitiveness (FIC) of the Chilean Ministry of Economy, Development, and Tourism, through the Millennium Scientific Initiative, Grant N° IS130005. Also, this manuscript was supported by a grant from the Spanish Ministry of Education, Culture, and Sport (FPU13/01677).

References

Bachmann, C. J., Aagaard, L., Burcu, M., Glaeske, G., Kalverdijk, L. J., Petersen, I., et al. (2016). Trends and patterns of antidepressant use in children and adolescents from five western countries, 2005–2012. *European Neuropsychopharmacology, 26*(3), 411–419.

Bergomi, C., Tschacher, W., & Kupper, Z. (2013). The assessment of mindfulness with self-report measures: Existing scales and open issues. *Mindfulness, 4*(3), 191–202.

Bishop, S. R., Lau, M., Shapiro, S., Carlson, L., Anderson, N. D., Carmody, J., et al. (2004). Mindfulness: A proposed operational definition. *Clinical Psychology: Science and Practice, 11*(3), 230–242.

Bulanda, J. J., Bruhn, C., Byro-Johnson, T., & Zentmyer, M. (2014). Addressing mental health stigma among young adolescents: Evaluation of a youth-led approach. *Health and Social Work, 39*(2), 73–80.

Carsley, D., Khoury, B., & Heath, N. L. (2018). Effectiveness of mindfulness interventions for mental health in schools: A comprehensive meta-analysis. *Mindfulness, 9*(3), 693–707. https://doi.org/10.1007/s12671-017-0839-2.

Centre for Mental Health. (2010). *The economic and social costs of mental health problems in 2009/2010*. London: Centre for Mental Health.

Chiesa, A., & Malinowski, P. (2011). Mindfulness-based approaches: Are they all the same? *Journal of Clinical Psychology, 67*(4), 404–424.

Climie, E., & Henley, L. (2016). A renewed focus on strengths-based assessment in schools. *British Journal of Special Education, 43*(2), 108–121. https://doi.org/10.1111/1467-8578.12131.

Collins, P. Y., Patel, V., Joestl, S. S., March, D., Insel, T. R., Daar, A. S., et al. (2011). Grand challenges in global mental health. *Nature, 475*(7354), 27–30.

Dariotis, J. K., Mirabal-Beltran, R., Cluxton-Keller, F., Gould, L. F., Greenberg, M. T., & Mendelson, T. (2016). A qualitative evaluation of student learning and skills use in a school-based mindfulness and yoga program. *Mindfulness, 7*(1), 76–89.

Davis, J. H., & Thompson, E. (2015). Developing attention and decreasing affective bias: Toward a cross-cultural cognitive science of mindfulness. In J. D. Creswell & K. W. Brown (Eds.), *Handbook of mindfulness: Theory and research*. Nueva York: Guilford Press.

Delors, J. (1996). International Commission on Education for the Twenty-first Century. Learning, the treasure within: Report to UNESCO of the International Commission on Education for the Twenty-first Century.

Dray, J., Bowman, J., Campbell, E., Freund, M., Wolfenden, L., Hodder, R. K., et al. (2017). Systematic review of universal resilience-focused interventions targeting child and adolescent

mental health in the school setting. *American Academy of Child & Adolescent Psychiatry, 56*(10), 813–824. https://doi.org/10.1016/j.jaac.2017.07.780.
Durlak, J. A., & Wells, A. M. (1997). Primary prevention mental health programs for children and adolescents: A meta-analytic review. *American Journal of Community Psychology, 25*(2), 115–152.
Ehrenreich-May, J., & Chu, B. C. (2013). *Transdiagnostic treatments for children and adolescents: Principles and practice*. New York, NY: Guilford Press.
Felver, J. C., Celis-de Hoyos, C. E., Tezanos, K., & Singh, N. N. (2016). A systematic review of mindfulness-based interventions for youth in school settings. *Mindfulness, 7*(1), 34–45.
Fuhrmann, D., Knoll, L. J., & Blakemore, S. J. (2015). Adolescence as a sensitive period of brain development. *Trends in Cognitive Sciences, 19*(10), 558–566. https://doi.org/10.1016/j.tics.2015.07.008.
Gethin, R. (1998). *The foundations of Buddhism*. Oxford University Press.
Gethin, R. (2011). On some definitions of mindfulness. *Contemporary Buddhism, 12*(01), 263–279.
Giedd, J. N., Blumenthal, J., Jeffries, N. O., Castellanos, F. X., Liu, H., Zijdenbos, A., et al. (1999). Brain development during childhood and adolescence: A longitudinal MRI study. *Nature Neuroscience, 2,* 861. https://doi.org/10.1038/13158.
Goodyer, I. M., Herbert, J., Tamplin, A., Secher, S. M., & Pearson, J. (1997). Short-term outcome of major depression. 2. Life events, family dysfunction, and friendship difficulties as predictors of persistent disorder. *Journal of the American Academy of Child & Adolescent Psychiatry, 36*(4), 474–480.
Greenberg, M. T., Weissberg, R. P., O'Brien, M. U., Zins, J. E., Fredericks, L., Resnik, H., & Elias, M. J. (2003). Enhancing school-based prevention and youth development through coordinated social, emotional, and academic learning. *American Psychologist, 58*(6–7), 466–474.
Guendelman, S., Medeiros, S., & Rampes, H. (2017). Mindfulness and emotion regulation: Insights from neurobiological, psychological, and clinical studies. *Frontiers in Psychology, 8*(220), 1–23.
Hálfdánarson, Ó., Zoëga, H., Aagaard, L., Bernardo, M., Brandt, L., Fusté, A. C., et al. (2017). International trends in antipsychotic use: A study in 16 countries, 2005–2014. *European Neuropsychopharmacology, 27*(10), 1064–1076.
Hawkins, J. D., Catalano, R. F., Kosterman, R., Abbott, R., & Hill, K. G. (1999). Preventing adolescent health-risk behaviors by strengthening protection during childhood. *Archives of Pediatrics and Adolescent Medicine, 153*(3), 226–234.
Hölzel, B. K., Lazar, S. W., Gard, T., Schuman-Olivier, Z., Vago, D. R., & Ott, U. (2011). How does mindfulness meditation work? Proposing mechanisms of action from a conceptual and neural perspective. *Perspectives on psychological science, 6*(6), 537–559.
Husserl, E. (1999). *The essential Husserl: Basic writings in transcendental phenomenology*. Indiana University Press.
Jinpa, G. T. (2010). *Compassion cultivation training (CCT): Instructor's manual.* Unpublished manuscript, Stanford: Stanford University.
Kabat-Zinn, J. (1994). *Wherever you go, there you are: Mindfulness meditation in everyday life.* New York: Hyperion.
Kabat-Zinn, J. (1996). Mindfulness meditation: What it is, what it isn't, and it's role in health care and medicine. In Y. Haruki, Y. Ishii, & M. Suzuki (Eds.), *Comparative and psychological study on meditation* (pp. 161–170). Netherlands: Eburon.
Kabat-Zinn, J. (2005). *Coming to our senses: Healing ourselves and the world through mindfulness*. New York: Hyperion.
Kann, L., McManus, T., Harris, W. A., Shanklin, S. L., Flint, K. H., Queen, B., et al. (2018). Youth risk behavior surveillance—United States, 2017. *MMWR Surveill Summaries, 67*(8), 1–114.
Kessler, R. C., Amminger, G. P., Aguilar-Gaxiola, S., Alonso, J., Lee, S., & Ustun, T. B. (2007a). Age of onset of mental disorders: A review of recent literature. *Current Opinion in Psychiatry, 20*(4), 359.

Kessler, R. C., Angermeyer, M., Anthony, J. C., De Graaf, R. O. N., Demyttenaere, K., Gasquet, I., et al. (2007b). Lifetime prevalence and age-of-onset distributions of mental disorders in the World Health Organization's World Mental Health Survey Initiative. *World Psychiatry, 6*(3), 168.
Kuyken, W., Weare, K., Ukoumunne, O. C., Vicary, R., Motton, N., Burnett, R., et al. (2013). Effectiveness of the mindfulness in schools programme: Non-randomised controlled feasibility study. *The British Journal of Psychiatry, 203*(2), 126–131.
Langer, A. I., Medeiros, S., Valdés, N., Cid-Parra, C., Magni, A., & Krause, M. (under review). Exploring mindfulness-based interventions in educational contexts: Experiences from Chilean adolescents. Manuscript submitted.
Langer, A. I., Schmidt, C., & Krogh, E. (2017). Mindfulness meditation and the perception of beauty: Implications for an ecological well-being. In M. Levine (Ed.), *Perception of beauty*. IntechOpen. https://doi.org/10.5772/intechopen.69529.
Langford, R., Bonell, C. P., Jones, H. E., Pouliou, T., Murphy, S. M., Waters, E., et al. (2014). The WHO Health Promoting School framework for improving the health and well-being of students and their academic achievement. *Cochrane Database Systematic Review, 4,* CD008958. https://doi.org/10.1002/14651858.cd008958.pub2.
Lutz, A., Slagter, H. A., Dunne, J. D., & Davidson, R. J. (2008). Attention regulation and monitoring in meditation. *Trends in Cognitive Sciences, 12*(4), 163–169.
Malinowski, P. (2013). Neural mechanisms of attentional control in mindfulness meditation. *Frontiers in Neuroscience, 7,* 8. https://doi.org/10.3389/fnins.2013.00008.
Miller, C. B. (2018). Generosity. A preliminary account of a surprisingly neglected virtue. *Metaphilosophy, 49*(3), 216–245.
Mind & Life Education Research Network. (2012). Contemplative practices and mental training: Prospects for American education. *Child Development Perspectives, 6*(2), 146–153. https://doi.org/10.1111/j.1750-8606.2012.00240.x.
Paus, T. (2005). Mapping brain maturation and cognitive development during adolescence. *Trends in Cognitive Sciences, 9*(2), 60–68. https://doi.org/10.1016/j.tics.2004.12.008.
Petermann, F., Petermann, U., & Nitkowski, D. (2016). *Das Emotionstraining in der Schule. Ein Programm zur Förderung der emotionalen Kompetenz.* Göttingen: Hogrefe.
Polanczyk, G. V., Salum, G. A., Sugaya, L. S., Caye, A., & Rohde, L. A. (2015). Annual Research Review: A meta-analysis of the worldwide prevalence of mental disorders in children and adolescents. *Journal of Child Psychology and Psychiatry, 56*(3), 345–365.
Roeser, R. W., & Eccles, J. S. (2015). Mindfulness and compassion in human development: Introduction to the special section. *Developmental Psychology, 51*(1), 1–6.
Ryan, R. M., & Deci, E. L. (2000). Self-determination theory and the facilitation of intrinsic motivation, social development, and well-being. *American Psychologist, 55*(1), 68–78.
Sanchez, A. L., Cornacchio, D., Poznanski, B., Golik, A. M., Chou, T., & Comer, J. S. (2018). The effectiveness of school-based mental health services for elementary-aged children: A meta-analysis. *Journal of the American Academy of Child and Adolescent Psychiatry, 57*(3), 153–165. https://doi.org/10.1016/j.jaac.2017.11.022.
Shapiro, S. L., Carlson, L. E., Astin, J. A., & Freedman, B. (2006). Mechanisms of mindfulness. *Journal of Clinical Psychology, 62,* 373–386. https://doi.org/10.1002/jclp.20237.
Sharma, T., Guski, L. S., Freund, N., & Gøtzsche, P. C. (2016). Suicidality and aggression during antidepressant treatment: Systematic review and meta-analyses based on clinical study reports. *BMJ, 352,* i65.
Shoshani, A., & Steinmetz, S. (2014). Positive psychology at school: A school-based intervention to promote adolescents' mental health and well-being. *Journal of Happiness Studies, 15*(6), 1289–1311. https://doi.org/10.1007/s10902-013-9476-1.
Singer, T., & Klimecki, O. M. (2014). Empathy and compassion. *Current Biology, 24*(18), 875–878.
Skills, P. f. C. (2017). Homepage. Retrieved July 24, 2017, from http://www.p21.org.
Slagter, H., Davidson, R., & Lutz, A. (2011). Mental training as a tool in the neuroscientific study of brain and cognitive plasticity. *Frontiers in Human Neuroscience, 5*(17). https://doi.org/10.3389/fnhum.2011.00017.

Spear, L. P. (2013). Adolescent neurodevelopment. *Journal of Adolescent Health, 52*(2), S7–13. https://doi.org/10.1016/j.jadohealth.2012.05.006.

Springer, J. B. (2013). "I am very, very proud of myself": Improving youth activity levels using self-determination theory in program development. *Frontiers in Public Health, 46*(1), 1–9.

Steinebach, C., Schrenk, A., Steinebach, U., & Brendtro, L. K. (2018). *Positive peer culture. Ein Manual für starke Gruppengespräche*. Weinheim: Beltz-Juventa.

Suchert, V., Hanewinkel, R., & Isensee, B. (2015). Sedentary behavior and indicators of mental health in school-aged children and adolescents: A systematic review. *Preventive Medicine, 76,* 48–57.

Tan, L. B. G., & Martin, G. (2016). Mind full or mindful: A report on mindfulness and psychological health in healthy adolescents. *International Journal of Adolescence and Youth, 21*(1), 64–74.

Tang, Y. Y., & Posner, M. I. (2009). Attention training and attention state training. *Trends in Cognitive Sciences, 13*(5), 222–227.

Twenge, J. M. (2013). The evidence for generation me and against generation we. *Emerging Adulthood, 1*(1), 11–16.

Twenge, J. M., Campbell, W. K., & Carter, N. T. (2014). Declines in trust in others and confidence in institutions among American adults and late adolescents, 1972–2012. *Psychological Science, 25*(10), 1914–1923.

Twenge, J. M., Joiner, T. E., Rogers, M. L., & Martin, G. N. (2018a). Increases in depressive symptoms, suicide-related outcomes, and suicide rates among US adolescents after 2010 and links to increased new media screen time. *Clinical Psychological Science, 6*(1), 3–17.

Twenge, J. M., Martin, G. N., & Campbell, W. K. (2018b). Decreases in psychological well-being among American adolescents after 2012 and links to screen time during the rise of smartphone technology. *Emotion, 18*(6), 765–780.

Van der Gucht, K., Takano, K., Raes, F., & Kuppens, P. (2018). Processes of change in a school-based mindfulness programme: Cognitive reactivity and self-coldness as mediators. *Cognition and Emotion, 32*(3), 658–665.

Vygotsky, L. S. (1978). Interaction between learning and development. In M. Cole, V. John-Steiner, S. Scribner, & E. Souber-Man (Eds.), *Mind in society: The development of higher psychological processes* (pp. 79–91). Cambridge, MA: Harvard University Press.

Waenerlund, A. K., Stenmark, H., Bergstrom, E., Hagglof, B., Ohman, A., & Petersen, S. (2016). School experiences may be important determinants of mental health problems in middle childhood—A Swedish longitudinal population-based study. *Acta Paediatrica, 105*(4), 407–415. https://doi.org/10.1111/apa.13326.

Wallace, B. A. (2006). *The attention revolution: Unlocking the power of the focused mind.* Somerville, MA: Wisdom Books.

Wallace, B. A., & Shapiro, S. L. (2006). Mental balance and well-being: Building bridges between Buddhism and Western psychology. *American Psychologist, 61*(7), 690–701.

Werner-Seidler, A., Perry, Y., Calear, A. L., Newby, J. M., & Christensen, H. (2017). School-based depression and anxiety prevention programs for young people: A systematic review and meta-analysis. *Clinical Psychology Review, 51,* 30–47. https://doi.org/10.1016/j.cpr.2016.10.005.

White, B. A., Jarrett, M. A., & Ollendick, T. H. (2013). Self-regulation deficits explain the link between reactive aggression and internalizing and externalizing behavior problems in children. *Journal of Psychopathology and Behavioral Assessment, 35*(1), 1–9. https://doi.org/10.1007/s10862-012-9310-9.

Wilde, S., Sonley, A., Crane, C., Ford, T., Raja, A., Robson, J., et al. (2019). Mindfulness training in UK secondary schools: A multiple case study approach to identification of cornerstones of implementation. *Mindfulness, 10*(2), 376–389.

Willard, C. (2014). Mindfulness with youth. Sowing the seeds of a mindful society. In A. Ie, C. T. Ngnoumen, & E. J. Langer (Eds.), *The Wiley Blackwell handbook of mindfulness* (pp. 1071–1084). Hoboken, NJ: Wiley.

World Health Organization. (2004). Promoting mental health: Concepts, emerging evidence, practice: Summary report.

Worthen, D., & Luiselli, J. K. (2017). Social validity assessment and intervention evaluation of mindfulness education and practices with high school students. *Mindfulness, 8*(4), 903–910.

Part II
Resilience in Youth: A General Framework of Understanding

Chapter 3
Lifestyle and Well-Being: Potential Epigenetic Benefits of Mindfulness Training, Healthy Eating and Physical Activity

Perla Kaliman

Abstract Epigenetics is acquiring a central role in twenty-first century medicine, revealing the relationships between individual genetic background and the environment. The somatic inheritability of epigenetic marks through cell division can often explain the long-lasting effects of environmental exposures at the individual level. Moreover, there is increasing evidence in plants, animal models, and humans for the transmission of epigenetic information across several generations, which has developmental and health implications. Importantly for the topic of this book, said epigenetic mechanisms play pivotal roles in the long-lasting consequences of chronic stress and trauma. Specifically, studies on early adversity, early experiences and aging, mindfulness-based interventions, and the impact of nutrition and physical activity on well-being will be revisited in light of new findings in the domain of epigenetics. We are currently starting to discover the intricate networks through which environmental factors and lifestyle can reshape the information contained in our genes, leaving imprints on physical and mental health which, in some circumstances, can be passed through gametes to subsequent generations. Future epigenetic studies involving Mindfulness Based Interventions will require a validation of molecular changes and bioinformatic predictions by exploring associations with specific neurophysiological outcomes in health and disease. Recent advances in epigenetics highlight the need to sensitize medicine and society to the impact of adverse experiences and unhealthy lifestyles on the physical, cognitive, and emotional health of present and future generations. The potential reversibility of acquired biological information and the possibility of modulating the epigenome towards healthier states should guide future research on epigenetics and well-being.

Keywords Genetic code · Self-development · Epigenetic information · Epigenetic clock · Lifestyle

---

P. Kaliman (✉)
Faculty of Health Sciences, Universitat Oberta de Catalunya, Barcelona, Spain
e-mail: pkaliman@uoc.edu

Center for Healthy Minds, University of Wisconsin-Madison, Madison, US

C. Steinebach and Á. I. Langer (eds.), *Enhancing Resilience in Youth*,
https://doi.org/10.1007/978-3-030-25513-8_3

Decades ago it was believed that, excluding mutations or other alterations in the primary DNA sequence, the inherited genetic code determined the biological destiny of an organism. Nowadays, we know that the genetic information is strongly modulated by a broad range of internal and external environmental factors, including experiences and lifestyle. This phenomena occurs through epigenetic mechanisms ("epi", from the Greek, means "around"), which generate layers of acquired molecular data that modulate the information contained in the genetic code. Epigenetic information regulates gene expression in a stable although potentially reversible manner, without modifying the DNA nucleotide sequence (Berger, Kouzarides, Shiekhattar, & Shilatifard, 2009). Epigenetics is acquiring a central role in twenty-first century medicine, revealing the relationships between individual genetic background and the environment. The somatic inheritability of epigenetic marks through cell division can often explain the long-lasting effects of environmental exposures at the individual level. Moreover, there is increasing evidence in plants, animal models, and humans for the transmission of epigenetic information across several generations, which has developmental and health implications (Radford, 2018).

The best-characterized epigenetic mechanisms include DNA methylation, post-translational modifications of histones and small non-coding RNAs. These processes influence each other, revealing the complexity of epigenetic regulation (Soshnev, Josefowicz, & Allis, 2016). DNA methylation is crucial for cell development, differentiation, and response to physiological and environmental stimuli. In mammals, most DNA methylation events occur in regions on the genome known as CpG islands (CpGI), which contain a C (cytosine) base immediately followed by a G (guanine) base at high frequency. DNA methylation at CpGIs is principally associated with transcriptional silencing of genes. In addition to DNA methylation, a broad collection of chemical groups can be bound to the histones, proteins located in nucleus of eukaryotic cells, around which DNA is wrapped to make up the chromatin (Bannister & Kouzarides, 2011). Histone modifications regulate gene expression in ways that depend on the type of chemical group attached to the histone and its location. Some of them activate genes while others have the effect of shutting down genes. A third increasingly characterized epigenetic mechanism involves small non-coding RNAs (sRNAs), short molecules that are not translated into protein but frequently mediate gene silencing either by hampering specific mRNA translation into protein and/or by promoting their degradation (Kapranov et al., 2007). There is increasing evidence of the impact of environmental exposures in the regulation of different types of small ncRNA (sRNA) such as microRNAs (miRNAs), tRNA fragments (tRFs), and PIWI-interacting RNAs (piRNAs, mainly expressed in the germline). Recent research suggests that piRNAs play an important role in the transgenerational transmission of epigenetic information (Donkin & Barrès, 2018; Luteijn & Ketting, 2013). Importantly for the topic of this book, said epigenetic mechanisms play pivotal roles in the long-lasting consequences of chronic stress and trauma. Among them, the methylation level of genes involved in the regulation of the hypothalamic-pituitary-adrenal (HPA) axis seems to be one of the molecular pathways through which childhood adversity can have long-lived effects (Tyrka, Ridout, & Parade, 2016). Increasing evidence has been found that stress adaptation and stress-related psychopathologies are linked to changes in the activity of histone deacetylases (HDACs), a family of enzymes that remove acetyl groups from histones (Misztak, Pańczyszyn-Trzewik, & Sowa-Kućma, 2018). Notably, different types of small non-coding RNAs have been associated with depression and childhood trauma (Hu et al., 2017; Yuan, Mischoulon, Fava, & Otto, 2018) and seem to be implicated in epigenetic transgenerational inheritance (Donkin & Barrès, 2018; Rassoulzadegan et al., 2006). Although the epigenetics of resilience is still in its infancy, it holds great promise in the prevention and treatment of anxiety-related disorders. In particular, both negative and positive environmental factors can modulate the DNA methylation of genes involved in anxiety and related phenotypes, such as brain-derived neurotrophic factor, oxytocin receptor, corticotropin releasing hormone receptor, glucocorticoid receptor, norepinephrine transporter, monoamine oxidase A, and glutamate decarboxylase 1 (Schiele & Domschke, 2018; Zannas & West, 2014).

3.1 Epigenetics of Early Adversity

Many diseases in adults should be seen as disorders that begin early in life. Numerous environmental factors can stably modify gene transcription and influence development and health (e.g. nutrition, environmental chemicals, drugs, infections), including exposure to early life adverse experiences (e.g. lack of adult care, poor stimulation, harm, or threat) (Párrizas, Gasa, & Kaliman, 2012).

A growing body of scientific evidence suggests that the toxic and in some cases cumulative effects of early life negative experiences can manifest themselves in young people and adults as increased risk of addictive behaviors, psychiatric conditions, cardiovascular, metabolic, autoimmune, and inflammatory disorders, chronic pain, and alterations in brain areas related to stress response, emotions, and cognition (Felitti et al., 1998; Hughes et al., 2017; Johnson, Riley, Granger, & Riis, 2013; Suglia et al., 2018). Epigenetic programming is emerging as one of the mechanisms responsible for the long-lasting, and sometimes multigenerational, effects of chronic stress and adverse experiences on physical and mental health. Although the first evidence of stress-induced epigenetic programming was obtained in animal models (Turecki & Meaney, 2016; Weaver et al., 2004), epigenetic vestiges such as DNA methylation alterations have also been described in humans. Essex et al. (2013) examined DNA methylation patterns in fifteen-year-old adolescents ($N = 109$) in relation to adversity during childhood. Both maternal and paternal stressors were predictive of methylation changes, in particular the methylation of the glucocorticoid receptor gene. Adverse experiences at an early age and methylation of the glucocorticoid receptor gene have both been associated with a greater likelihood of developing psychopathologies during adolescence, especially symptoms of borderline personality disorder (Radtke et al., 2015). These findings add to increasing evidence that subjects exposed to early adversity can display alterations in the DNA methylation of HPA axis-related genes, such as the glucocorticoid receptor (NR3C1) and the FK506 binding protein 51 (FKBP5) genes (Tyrka et al., 2016). Moreover, multigenerational epigenetic studies in animal models as well as evidence from epidemiological research in humans show that epigenetic information acquired through parental environmental exposures during preconceptional and prenatal periods (e.g. stress, trauma, nutrition) may account for the susceptibility of the offspring to certain diseases that cannot be explained by genetic inheritance (Bowers & Yehuda, 2016; Yehuda & Meaney, 2018).

3.2 Early Experiences and Epigenetic Aging

Many environmental and lifestyle-related factors can modulate the aging rate of cells and tissues from an early age, strongly influencing health span. Childhood adversity and stressful and traumatic events have been linked to telomere shortening, a biomarker of cellular aging which correlates with many medical and psychiatric conditions (Epel & Prather, 2018; Li, He, Wang, Tang, & Tang, 2017). In addition to telomere biology, the combination of the DNA methylation patterns at specific sites of the genome is another accurate predictor of the rate of cell aging (Horvath, 2013). In healthy conditions, this "epigenetic clock" highly correlates with the chronological age of an individual, and the level of deviation between the DNA methylation age and the chronological age indicates the epigenetic aging rate (Chen et al., 2016; Hannum et al., 2013). When the ticking of this clock is too fast, the risk of developing many chronic diseases increases. Indeed, an accelerated epigenetic clock has been found to be associated with obesity, cardiovascular disease, cancer, Alzheimer's disease, frailty, and all-cause mortality risk (Breitling et al., 2016; Horvath et al., 2014; Levine, Lu, Bennett, & Horvath, 2015; Levine et al., 2015; Marioni, Shah, McRae, Chen, et al., 2015; Marioni, Shah, McRae, Ritchie, et al. 2015; Perna et al., 2016).

Cumulative lifetime stress and trauma are among the environmental factors described as epigenetic clock accelerators (Boks et al., 2015; Zannas et al., 2015), while a diet with lean meats, the physical activity, and education correlate with slower epigenetic clocks (Quach et al., 2017). Semi-supercentenarians (subjects between 105 and 109 years old) and their offspring display decreased epigenetic age in blood cells (Horvath et al., 2015). Slower epigenetic clocks also predict better cognitive and physical fitness in the elderly (Marioni, Shah, McRae, Chen, et al. 2015; Marioni, Shah, McRae, Ritchie, et al., 2015).

The rhythm of the epigenetic clock seems to be regulated from an early age Recent findings show that growing up in a psychologically adverse or violent environment accelerates the epigenetic clock in young people The study of a cohort of 399 African American families (parents and their 11-year-old children) during 9 years revealed that elevated parental depressive symptoms predicted emotional distress and accelerated epigenetic aging among offspring at age 20 (Brody, Yu, Chen, Beach, & Miller, 2016). Epigenetic age acceleration was also detected in saliva samples from children aged 6–13 ($N = 101$) exposed to neighborhood violence (Jovanovic et al., 2017). In this context, it is encouraging that a family-oriented preventive intervention to reduce harsh parenting was able to efficiently mitigate the epigenetic aging acceleration among offspring from parents reporting high depressive symptoms (Brody et al., 2016).

3.3 Mindfulness-Based Interventions: From Brain to Genes

Over the last two decades, there has been an increasing interest in characterizing mindfulness-based interventions (MBIs) aimed at preventing and treating many conditions caused or aggravated by stress (Ludwig & Kabat-Zinn, 2008). A growing body of scientific research describes the beneficial influence of MBIs on processes related to cognition, emotional regulation, and brain aging (several recent reviews have summarized these topics: Acevedo et al., 2016; Dahl, Lutz, & Davidson, 2015; Kurth et al., 2017; Lutz, Jha, Dunne, & Saron, 2015; Segal & Walsh, 2016; Vago & Zeidan, 2016).

Recently, the accumulation of data about the negative impact of prenatal and early postnatal stress has led to the design of interventions aimed at preventing depression during pregnancy or postnatal periods (Dimidjian et al., 2016; Potharst, Aktar, Rexwinkel, Rigterink, & Bögels, 2017) and promoting mindful childbirth and parenting (Braeken et al., 2017; Duncan et al., 2017). Considering the potential transgenerational implications of parental prenatal stress, trauma, and depression (Bowers & Yehuda, 2016; Yehuda & Meaney, 2018), these interventions may prove helpful not only for parents but for the mental and physical health of future generations. In this context, there is also accumulating evidence of the beneficial effects of MBIs on stress coping and emotion regulation in children and adolescents (e.g. Flook, Goldberg, Pinger, & Davidson, 2015; Perry-Parrish, Copeland-Linder, Webb, & Sibinga, 2016). Describing this type of interventions is beyond the scope of this chapter and the few studies cited here are just representative of an emerging and extremely relevant field in mindfulness research.

3.3.1 Gene Expression Changes in Response to MBIs

The first screening of whole-genome expression in practitioners of mindfulness-based techniques was published by Dusek et al. (2008). The study showed that practices aimed at reducing stress can increase the activity of some genes and decrease the activity of others in blood cells. More than 2209 changes were detected when comparing the genome expression of experienced practitioners of the relaxation response with that of inexperienced controls. The latter, after an 8-week attentional training program, also showed changes in the expression of 1561 genes compared with their own pre-training condition. Notably, 433 of the genes modulated by the practice were the same in beginners and experts. These data suggested that (i) some effects of these practices on gene expression might be long-lasting (those detected in experts) and (ii) some of these changes might be acquired after short interventions, however, no data exist on the stability of such dynamic outcomes in the absence of a sustained practice. The molecular pathways that changed with the mindfulness-based practices included oxidative stress, cell metabolism, and inflammation, highlighting the potential of these techniques to help in the treatment of pathologies such as cardiovascular, metabolic, immune disorders and other chronic conditions. In the same year, scientists from New Delhi published the analysis of the expression of genes involved in the regulation of oxidative stress in lymphocyte cells from 42 practitioners of a type of meditative breathing control technique known as Sudarsan Kriya (Sharma et al., 2008). The study compared the group of meditators with a control group composed of 42 individuals without any experience in this type of practice. Significantly higher levels of antioxidant gene expression were observed in cells of meditators compared to those of controls, providing new clues to understand how mental training may be converted into peripheral cell signals. These studies, together with more recent ones (Im, Kim, Kim, Kim, & Son, 2015; Pal et al., 2015; Rima, Shiv, Bhavna, Shilpa, & Saima, 2016; Tolahunase, Sagar, & Dada, 2017), indicate that mindfulness-based body-mind practices may contribute to reducing oxidative stress and inflammatory processes which, when excessive, promote cell and tissue damage and increase the risk of developing a broad range of chronic diseases, such as diabetes, depression, and Alzheimer's.

The modulation of inflammatory pathways is an increasingly reported outcome of MBIs. In the last 10 years, several studies have further explored the impact of MBIs on gene expression through genome-wide microarray techniques, bioinformatic analysis, quantification of gene expression (RtqPCR), and protein level analysis. A recent review analyzed data from transcriptional studies involving MBIs (i.e. mindfulness, meditation, yoga, Tai Chi, Qigong, relaxation response, and breath regulation) in clinical and non-clinical populations (Buric, Farias, Jong, Mee, & Brazil, 2017), revealing consistent findings on the downregulation of proinflammatory genes and pathways, in particular those dependent on the transcription factor NF-κB, a key mediator of inflammation which is upregulated by psychosocial stress (Kuebler et al., 2015; Wolf, Rohleder, Bierhaus, Nawroth, & Kirschbaum, 2009). Less evidence exists regarding genes that modulate the activity of the HPA axis. Through promoter-based bioinformatic analyses of leukocyte genome-wide transcriptional data, two studies predicted an increase in glucocorticoid receptor activity in response to MBIs. One of them analyzed the impact of a yoga intervention for breast cancer survivors and found reduced activity of NF-κB and increased activity of the glucocorticoid receptor in blood cells (Bower et al., 2014). The other study described that a 10-week cognitive-behavioral program to improve stress management seemed to decrease the activity of NF-κB/Rel and GATA family transcription factors (a type of DNA-binding proteins that play crucial roles in various biological processes, including hematopoiesis), and increased the activity of interferon response factors and the glucocorticoid receptor (Antoni et al., 2012). However, these bioinformatic predictions still require validation using specific gene and protein expression quantification methods.

To date, our molecular understanding of how MBIs influence neuroendocrine and neuroprotective processes remains limited and the available data mostly refer to adult samples. However, stress-sensitive pro-inflammatory pathways are also toxic for brain development and health in children and adolescents (Belem da Silva et al., 2017; Danese & Baldwin, 2017). Establishing whether MBIs could prevent or counterbalance such effects in vulnerable young people by downregulating pro-inflammatory pathways warrants further investigation.

3.3.2 Epigenetic Modifications in Meditators

We cannot assume that the MBI-induced gene expression changes so far described are the product of epigenetic regulation because they have not been causally associated with specific DNA methylation changes, histone modification, or any other epigenetic mechanism. To start exploring the potential epigenetic impact of meditation, we analyzed histone modifications and the expression of a set of chromatin modulatory genes in immune cells from experienced meditators after a day-long retreat (Kaliman et al., 2014). Epigenetic events can be extremely dynamic. In animal models and human peripheral tissues, DNA methylation and histone modifications can be detected just a few hours after exposure to environmental factors such as acute stress, diet, or physical exercise (Barrès et al., 2012; Myzak, Tong, Dashwood, Dashwood, & Ho, 2007; Papale et al., 2016; Rodrigues et al., 2015). In our study, we analyzed cells from a group of subjects with no meditation experience who engaged in leisure activities in the same environment as an active control. After the short intervention, we detected lower expression levels of several histone deacetylase genes in peripheral blood mononuclear cells (PBMCs) from meditators compared with controls, as well as an increase in the global acetylation level of histone H4 in meditator's cells. The downregulation of HDAC2 significantly correlated with a better cortisol recovery after a test of acute psychosocial stress. The meditation group also displayed a significant downregulation of the proinflammatory genes RIPK2 and COX2. The pharmacological inhibition of HDACs has gradually come to be regarded as a therapeutic avenue for depression (Misztak et al., 2018; Penney & Tsai, 2014), stress adaptation and recovery (Weaver et al., 2004), and inflammatory-related disorders (Sweet, Shakespear, Kamal, & Fairlie, 2012). A recent cross-sectional study (García-Campayo et al., 2018) supports these preliminary evidences of an epigenetic-mediated anti-inflammatory impact of meditation training. The authors compared the methylome of long-term meditators with a control group of non-meditators in PBMCs. Bioinformatic analysis of the methylation data suggested that the differentially methylated regions (DMRs) identified in meditators versus controls were involved in lipid metabolism, the cellular response to unfolded protein, glucose homeostasis, neurotransmission and inflammation through tumor necrosis factor alpha and NF-κB signaling.

Chaix et al. analyzed the epigenetic aging rate in long-term meditators compared with non-meditators (Chaix et al., 2017). Notably, the epigenetic clock in blood cells from expert meditators was not accelerated after midlife (age $\geq$ 52), in contrast with controls. Furthermore, the epigenetic aging rate significantly decreased with the number of years of regular meditation practice, which suggests that integrating meditation practice into daily routine as early in life as possible may have increasing protective effects on the epigenetic aging rate in the long run. Taking into account the reported acceleration of the epigenetic clock among young people exposed to adverse or violent environments (Brody et al., 2016; Jovanovic et al., 2017), the potential impact of MBIs on the epigenetic aging rate in children and adolescents is a relevant topic for future research.

Recently, Bishop et al. described that the eight week mindfulness-based stress reduction (MBSR) program induced changes in the DNA methylation of *FKBP15*, a gene involved in the modulation of the activity of the glucocorticoid receptor in response to stressors (Bishop et al., 2018). Participants were veterans with long-standing PTSD, classified as responders or non-responders based on PTSD symptom severity reduction post-MBSR. Responders showed decreased and non-responders showed increased methylation of a *FKBP5* region containing a glucocorticoid response element. These data indicate that the methylation of the FKBP5 gene is a potential biomarker of response to MBSR in PTSD.

There are still many questions that remain to be addressed, and it is important to avoid drawing too many conclusions from these few pilot studies that need to be reproduced and expanded through larger and randomized longitudinal trials. Moreover, the actual impact of MBI-induced epigenetic regulation in improving well-being and health care needs to be characterized. In this context, future epigenetic studies involving MBIs will require a validation of molecular changes and bioinformatic predictions by exploring associations with specific neurophysiological outcomes in health and disease.

3.4 Epigenetic Impact of Nutrition and Physical Activity on Well-Being

Advances in epigenetics are currently offering mechanisms to explain relationships between lifestyle and most noncommunicable diseases. In this context, two of the most relevant modifiable behaviors are nutrition and physical activity. In young people, the devastating outcomes of sedentary lifestyles and Western diets (i.e. based on highly processed foods, high intakes of red and processed meat, fried foods, excess of saturated fat, refined grains, and soft drinks) are widely documented. Currently, overweight and obesity in young people represent a major public health challenge. Worldwide, they affect around one person in 10 between 5 and 17 years old (Gupta, Goel, Shah, & Misra, 2012; World Health Organization, 2017). The main contributors to the overweight and obesity epidemic among children and adolescents are the increased consumption of fast food and soft drinks along with a decrease in meals shared with family (Duffey et al., 2012). A large proportion of adolescents do not eat the recommended five fruit and vegetable portions per day (Vereecken et al., 2015). This is aggravated by a decline in physical activity through adolescence. In this regard, the "Healthy Lifestyle in Europe by Nutrition in Adolescence Study" revealed that children and adolescents spend around 70% of their waking time involved in sedentary activities (Owen, Salmon, Koohsari, Turrell, & Giles-Corti, 2014).

The short- and long-term consequences of sedentarism, overweight, and obesity in young people include cognitive, behavioral, and emotional problems, as well as increased risk of non-communicable diseases in adulthood (World Health Organization, 2017). As described below, a healthy diet and an active lifestyle are critical health determinants to well-being as they significantly modulate metabolic, transcriptional, and epigenetic profiles.

3.4.1 *Food for Thought*

Resilience depends on many factors, among which we cannot ignore the "biochemical fertilizer" that the brain requires: nutrients. The current scientific literature highlights the role of micronutrients such as B vitamins (B12, folate, B6), choline, omega-3 fatty acids, zinc, and magnesium in the one-carbon metabolism. This cycle of biochemical reactions exerts a significant influence on the epigenetic programming of most brain, cardiovascular, and metabolic functions (Alachkar et al., 2018; Baek, Bernstein, & Nierenberg, 2013; Dhobale, 2017; Frankenburg, 2007; Gatta et al., 2017; Muskiet & Kemperman, 2006; Tomioka et al., 2018). The above mentioned nutrients are intermediates or cofactors for enzymes involved in the production of the main cellular donor of methyl groups, S-adenosylmethionine (SAM). SAM is required to generate cell membrane phospholipids, to methylate DNA and histones, and to synthesize neurotransmitters such as melatonin and epinephrine. In addition to its key role in the generation of SAM, folate is also required to form tetrahydrobiopterin (BH4), an essential cofactor to the synthesis of the monoamine neurotransmitters serotonin, dopamine, norepinephrine, and epinephrine. Vitamin C is also involved in monoamine neurotransmitter synthesis as a cofactor and stabilizer of BH4 (Miller, 2008). Deficient or excessive levels of said nutrients are risk factors for developing psychoemotional, cognitive, and psychiatric conditions (Bahous et al., 2017, 2018; Papakostas, Cassiello, & Iovieno, 2012; Sugden, 2006).

A large body of research also demonstrates that pre- and postnatal nutrition play a central role in most chronic diseases and all-cause mortality through the regulation of inflammatory pathways (Hodge et al., 2018; Micha et al., 2017; Moore et al., 2018). Recent data suggest that a pro-inflammatory diet is associated with higher incidence of depressive symptoms. A follow-up study over a period of 8 years, after adjusting for several potential confounders at baseline, revealed that individuals with the highest dietary inflammatory index score (e.g. high consumption of red meat, processed meat, cheese, sweets) had a 24% higher risk of depression compared with those with the lowest score (e.g. consuming a diet richer in vegetables, salad leaves, fruits, whole cereals rich in carbohydrates with a low glycaemic index, extra virgin olive-oil, spices, seeds and nuts, legumes, and fish) (Phillips, Shivappa, Hébert, & Perry, 2018). In particular, increasing evidence has been found that anti-inflammatory fatty acids from the omega-3 family are associated with emotional regulation. Epidemiological data reveal associations between omega-3 polyunsaturated fatty acid intake through fish consumption and decreased depressive symptoms in young adults (Smith et al., 2014); also, a 7-year longitudinal study concluded that raising the omega-3 to omega-6 ratio may help prevent mood disorders in young people with at-risk mental states (Berger et al., 2017). In a recent study, we observed that an increase in omega-3 intake correlated with decreased self-reported aggressiveness in healthy adults (Bègue et al., 2018). These and other findings (Adjibade et al., 2017; Akbaraly et al., 2016; Shivappa et al., 2018) suggest that adopting an anti-inflammatory diet may contribute to improving mental health.

Over the last decades, the population of microbes of the gut, which is heterogeneous between individuals, has been related to many pathological conditions, from obesity to mental health. The crosstalk between the central nervous system and the gastrointestinal tract, known as the gut-brain axis, is being increasingly characterized and the microbiota composition has been proposed as a potential tool to detect individual differences in depressed population (Horne & Foster, 2018). The composition of the microbiota is highly influenced by antenatal and postnatal dietary factors and contributes to the modulation of inflammatory, metabolic, and neurodevelopmental pathways through epigenetic mechanisms (Dawson, Dash, & Jacka, 2016; Tengeler, Kozicz, & Kiliaan, 2018). Notably, bacteria fermentation of fiber in the colon generates the short-chain fatty acid butyrate, a well-known HDAC inhibitor with neuroprotective properties. As described above, HDAC inhibitors have become therapeutic candidates for promoting brain health due to their capacity to increase the expression of genes involved in neuronal survival, regeneration, and plasticity (Bourassa, Alim, Bultman, & Ratan, 2016).

3.4.2 Neuroprotective and Epigenetic Effects of Physical Exercise

Sedentary behavior in young people (e.g. leisure time spent using screens) has been linked to adverse health outcomes, including depressive symptomatology and psychological distress (Hoare, Milton, Foster, & Allender, 2016). In contrast, the positive impact of physical exercise in brain remodeling, cognition, and mood (e.g. promotion of neuronal survival and proliferation, learning and memory enhancement, decrease in depression and cardiometabolic risk) has been increasingly documented in animal models and humans. The mechanisms responsible for said effects include the upregulation of neurotrophic factors such as vascular endothelial growth factor (VEGF), brain derived neurotrophic factor (BDNF), and insulin-like growth factor 1 (IGF-1) as well as increases in the peripheral concentrations of neurotransmitters such as epinephrine, norepinephrine, and dopamine (Basso & Suzuki, 2017; Kaliman et al., 2011).

Physical activity triggers epigenetic changes that regulate molecular pathways involved in most chronic diseases (Grazioli et al., 2017). In rodents, exercise has been reported to prevent brain changes in global DNA methylation in response to acute psychological stress (Rodrigues et al., 2015). The epigenetic regulation of the BDNF gene seems to mediate at least in part the opposite effects of stress and physical exercise on brain plasticity and behavioral functions (Ieraci, Mallei, Musazzi, & Popoli, 2015; Seo et al., 2016). Furthermore, lower levels of anxiety were observed in exercised versus sedentary rats when exposed to a novel environment (Collins et al., 2009) or social defeat (Patki et al., 2014), which correlated with significant changes in histone modifications in the hippocampus. Recent studies suggest that prenatal maternal exercise and preconceptional paternal exercise in humans may also account for neurodevelopment in the next generation (Ferrari et al., 2018; Ingerslev et al., 2018).

3.5 Concluding Remarks

In 1942, Conrad Waddington described epigenetics as "the interactions of genes with their environment, which bring the phenotype into being" (Waddington, 1942). We are currently starting to discover the intricate networks through which environmental factors and lifestyle can reshape the information contained in our genes, leaving imprints on physical and mental health which, in some circumstances, can be passed through gametes to subsequent generations.

Recent advances in epigenetics highlight the need to sensitize medicine and society about the impact of adverse experiences and unhealthy lifestyles on the physical, cognitive, and emotional health of present and future generations. The potential reversibility of acquired biological information and the possibility of modulating the epigenome towards healthier states should guide future research on epigenetics and well-being.

Acknowledgements The author thanks Marta Cosín-Tomás for helpful comments.

References

Acevedo, B. P., Pospos, S., & Lavretsky, H. (2016). The neural mechanisms of meditative practices: novel approaches for healthy aging. *Current Behavioral Neuroscience Reports, 3*(4), 328–339.

Adjibade, M., Andreeva, V. A., Lemogne, C., Touvier, M., Shivappa, N., Hébert, J. R., et al. (2017). The inflammatory potential of the diet is associated with depressive symptoms in different subgroups of the general population. *The Journal of Nutrition, 147*(5), 879–887.

Akbaraly, T. N., Kerleau, C., Wyart, M., Chevallier, N., Ndiaye, L., Shivappa, N., et al. (2016). Dietary inflammatory index and recurrence of depressive symptoms: Results from the Whitehall II study. *Clinical Psychological Science, 4*(6), 1125–1134.

Alachkar, A., Wang, L., Yoshimura, R., Hamzeh, A. R., Wang, Z., Sanathara, N., et al. (2018). Prenatal one-carbon metabolism dysregulation programs schizophrenia-like deficits. *Molecular Psychiatry, 23*(2), 282–294.

Antoni, M. H., Lutgendorf, S. K., Blomberg, B., Carver, C. S., Lechner, S., Diaz, A., et al. (2012). Cognitive-behavioral stress management reverses anxiety-related leukocyte transcriptional dynamics. *Biological Psychiatry, 71*(4), 366–372.

Baek, J. H., Bernstein, E. E., & Nierenberg, A. A. (2013). One-carbon metabolism and bipolar disorder. *The Australian and New Zealand Journal of Psychiatry, 47*(11), 1013–1018.

Bahous, R. H., Cosín-Tomás, M., Deng, L., Leclerc, D., Malysheva, O., Ho, M. K., et al. (2018). Early manifestations of brain aging in mice due to low dietary folate and mild MTHFR deficiency. *Molecular Neurobiology*, 1–17.

Bahous, R. H., Jadavji, N. M., Deng, L., Cosín-Tomás, M., Lu, J., Malysheva, O., & Rozen, R. (2017). High dietary folate in pregnant mice leads to pseudo-MTHFR deficiency and altered methyl metabolism, with embryonic growth delay and short-term memory impairment in offspring. *Human Molecular Genetics, 26*(5), 888–900.

Bannister, A. J., & Kouzarides, T. (2011). Regulation of chromatin by histone modifications. *Cell Research, 21*(3), 381–395.

Barrès, R., Yan, J., Egan, B., Treebak, J. T., Rasmussen, M., Fritz, T., et al. (2012). Acute exercise remodels promoter methylation in human skeletal muscle. *Cell Metabolism, 15*(3), 405–411.

Basso, J. C., & Suzuki, W. A. (2017). The effects of acute exercise on mood, cognition, neurophysiology, and neurochemical pathways: A review. *Brain Plasticity, 2*(2), 127–152.

Bègue, L., Zaalberg, A., Shankland, R., Duke, A., Jacquet, J., Kaliman, P., et al. (2018). Omega-3 supplements reduce self-reported physical aggression in healthy adults. *Psychiatry Research, 261,* 307–311.

Belem da Silva, C. T., de Abreu Costa, M., Kapczinski, F., de Aguiar, B. W., Salum, G. A., & Manfro, G. G. (2017). Inflammation and internalizing disorders in adolescents. *Progress in Neuro-Psychopharmacology and Biological Psychiatry, 77,* 133–137.

Berger, M. E., Smesny, S., Kim, S. W., Davey, C. G., Rice, S., Sarnyai, Z., et al. (2017). Omega-6 to omega-3 polyunsaturated fatty acid ratio and subsequent mood disorders in young people with at-risk mental states: A 7-year longitudinal study. *Translational Psychiatry, 7*(8), 1220.

Berger, S. L., Kouzarides, T., Shiekhattar, R., & Shilatifard, A. (2009). An operational definition of epigenetics. *Genes & Development, 23,* 781–783.

Bishop, J. R., Lee, A. M., Mills, L. J., Thuras, P. D., Eum, S., Clancy, D., et al. (2018). Methylation of FKBP5 and SLC6A4 in relation to treatment response to mindfulness based stress reduction for posttraumatic stress disorder. *Frontiers in Psychiatry, 9,* 1–11.

Boks, M. P., van Mierlo, H. C., Rutten, B. P. F., Radstake, T. R. D. J., De Witte, L., Geuze, E., et al. (2015). Longitudinal changes of telomere length and epigenetic age related to traumatic stress and post-traumatic stress disorder. *Psychoneuroendocrinology, 51,* 506–512.

Bourassa, M. W., Alim, I., Bultman, S. J., & Ratan, R. R. (2016). Butyrate, neuroepigenetics and the gut microbiome: Can a high fiber diet improve brain health? *Neuroscience Letters, 625,* 56–63.

Bower, J. E., Greendale, G., Crosswell, A. D., Garet, D., Sternlieb, B., Ganz, P. A., et al. (2014). Yoga reduces inflammatory signaling in fatigued breast cancer survivors: A randomized controlled trial. *Psychoneuroendocrinology, 43,* 20–29.

Bowers, M. E., & Yehuda, R. (2016). Intergenerational transmission of stress in humans. *Neuropsychopharmacology, 41*(1), 232–244.

Braeken, M. A. K. A., Jones, A., Otte, R. A., Nyklíček, I., & Van den Bergh, B. R. H. (2017). Potential benefits of mindfulness during pregnancy on maternal autonomic nervous system function and infant development. *Psychophysiology, 54*(2), 279–288.

Breitling, L. P., Saum, K. U., Perna, L., Schöttker, B., Holleczek, B., & Brenner, H. (2016). Frailty is associated with the epigenetic clock but not with telomere length in a German cohort. *Clinical Epigenetics, 8,* 21.

Brody, G. H., Yu, T., Chen, E., Beach, S. R. H., & Miller, G. E. (2016). Family-centered prevention ameliorates the longitudinal association between risky family processes and epigenetic aging. *Journal of Child Psychology and Psychiatry and Allied Disciplines, 57,* 566–574.

Buric, I., Farias, M., Jong, J., Mee, C., & Brazil, I. A. (2017). What is the molecular signature of mind-body interventions? A systematic review of gene expression changes induced by meditation and related practices. *Frontiers in Immunology, 8,* 670.

Chaix, R., Alvarez-López, M. J., Fagny, M., Lemee, L., Regnault, B., Davidson, R. J., et al. (2017). Epigenetic clock analysis in long-term meditators. *Psychoneuroendocrinology, 85,* 210–214.

Chen, B. H., Marioni, R. E., Colicino, E., Peters, M. J., Ward-Caviness, C. K., Tsai, P. C., et al. (2016). DNA methylation-based measures of biological age: Meta-analysis predicting time to death. *Aging, 8*, 1844–1865.

Collins, A., Hill, L. E., Chandramohan, Y., Whitcomb, D., Droste, S. K., & Reul, J. M. H. M. (2009). Exercise improves cognitive responses to psychological stress through enhancement of epigenetic mechanisms and gene expression in the dentate gyrus. *PLoS ONE, 4*(1), e4330.

Dahl, C. J., Lutz, A., & Davidson, R. J. (2015). Reconstructing and deconstructing the self: Cognitive mechanisms in meditation practice. *Trends in Cognitive Sciences, 19*(9), 515–523.

Danese, A., & Baldwin, J. R. (2017). Hidden wounds? Inflammatory links between childhood trauma and psychopathology. *Annual Review of Psychology, 68*, 517–544.

Dawson, S. L., Dash, S. R., & Jacka, F. N. (2016). The importance of diet and gut health to the treatment and prevention of mental disorders. *International Review of Neurobiology, 131*, 325–346.

Dhobale, M. (2017). Neurotrophic factors and maternal nutrition during pregnancy. *Vitamins and Hormones, 104*, 343–366.

Dimidjian, S., Goodman, S. H., Felder, J. N., Gallop, R., Brown, A. P., & Beck, A. (2016). Staying well during pregnancy and the postpartum: A pilot randomized trial of mindfulness-based cognitive therapy for the prevention of depressive relapse/recurrence. *Journal of Consulting and Clinical Psychology, 84*(2), 134–145.

Donkin, I., & Barrès, R. (2018). Sperm epigenetics and influence of environmental factors. *Molecular Metabolism, 14*, 1–11.

Duffey, K. J., Huybrechts, I., Mouratidou, T., Libuda, L., Kersting, M., De Vriendt, T., et al. (2012). Beverage consumption among European adolescents in the HELENA study. *European Journal of Clinical Nutrition, 66*(2), 244–252.

Duncan, L., Cohn, M., Chao, M., Cook, J., Riccobono, J., & Bardacke, N. (2017). Benefits of preparing for childbirth with mindfulness training: A RCT with active comparison. *BMC Pregnancy and Childbirth, 17*(1), 140.

Dusek, J. A., Otu, H. H., Wohlhueter, A. L., Bhasin, M., Zerbini, L. F., Joseph, M. G., et al. (2008). Genomic counter-stress changes induced by the relaxation response. *PLoS ONE, 3*(7), e2576.

Epel, E. S., & Prather, A. A. (2018). Stress, telomeres, and psychopathology: Toward a deeper understanding of a triad of early aging. *Annual Review of Clinical Psychology, 14*, 371–397.

Essex, M. J., Thomas Boyce, W., Hertzman, C., Lam, L. L., Armstrong, J. M., Neumann, S. M. A., & Kobor, M. S. (2013). Epigenetic vestiges of early developmental adversity: Childhood stress exposure and DNA methylation in adolescence. *Child Development, 84*(1), 58–75.

Felitti, V. J., Anda, R. F., Nordenberg, D., Williamson, D. F., Spitz, A. M., Edwards, V., et al. (1998). Relationship of childhood abuse and household dysfunction to many of the leading causes of death in adults: The adverse childhood experiences (ACE) study. *American Journal of Preventive Medicine, 14*(4), 245–258.

Ferrari, N., Bae-Gartz, I., Bauer, C., Janoschek, R., Koxholt, I., Mahabir, E., et al. (2018). Exercise during pregnancy and its impact on mothers and offspring in humans and mice. *Journal of Developmental Origins of Health and Disease, 9*(1), 63–76.

Flook, L., Goldberg, S. B., Pinger, L., & Davidson, R. J. (2015). Promoting prosocial behavior and self-regulatory skills in preschool children through a mindfulness-based kindness curriculum. *Developmental Psychology, 51*(1), 44–51.

Frankenburg, F. R. (2007). The role of one-carbon metabolism in schizophrenia and depression. *Harvard Review of Psychiatry, 15*(4), 146–160.

García-Campayo, J., Puebla-Guedea, M., Labarga, A., Urdánoz, A., Roldán, M., Pulido, L., et al. (2018). Epigenetic response to mindfulness in peripheral blood leukocytes involves genes linked to common human diseases. *Mindfulness, 9*(4), 1146–1159.

Gatta, E., Auta, J., Gavin, D. P., Bhaumik, D. K., Grayson, D. R., Pandey, S. C., & Guidotti, A. (2017). Emerging role of one-carbon metabolism and DNA methylation enrichment on δ-containing GABAA receptor expression in the cerebellum of subjects with Alcohol Use Disorders (AUD). *International Journal of Neuropsychopharmacology, 20*(12), 1013–1026.

Grazioli, E., Dimauro, I., Mercatelli, N., Wang, G., Pitsiladis, Y., Di Luigi, L., & Caporossi, D. (2017). Physical activity in the prevention of human diseases: Role of epigenetic modifications. *BMC Genomics, 18*(Suppl 8), 802.

Gupta, N., Goel, K., Shah, P., & Misra, A. (2012). Childhood obesity in developing countries: Epidemiology, determinants, and prevention. *Endocrine Reviews, 33*(1), 48–70.

Hannum, G., Guinney, J., Zhao, L., Zhang, L., Hughes, G., Sadda, S. V., et al. (2013). Genome-wide methylation profiles reveal quantitative views of human aging rates. *Molecular Cell, 49*, 359–367.

Hoare, E., Milton, K., Foster, C., & Allender, S. (2016). The associations between sedentary behaviour and mental health among adolescents: A systematic review. *International Journal of Behavioral Nutrition and Physical Activity, 13*(1), 108.

Hodge, A. M., Bassett, J. K., Dugué, P. A., Shivappa, N., Hébert, J. R., Milne, et al. (2018). Dietary inflammatory index or Mediterranean diet score as risk factors for total and cardiovascular mortality. *Nutrition, Metabolism and Cardiovascular Diseases, 28*(5), 461–469.

Horne, R., & Foster, J. A. (2018). Metabolic and microbiota measures as peripheral biomarkers in major depressive disorder. *Frontiers in Psychiatry, 9*, 513.

Horvath, S. (2013). DNA methylation age of human tissues and cell types. *Genome Biology, 14*, R115.

Horvath, S., Erhart, W., Brosch, M., Ammerpohl, O., von Schonfels, W., Ahrens, M., et al. (2014). Obesity accelerates epigenetic aging of human liver. *Proceedings of the National Academy of Sciences, 111*, 15538–15543.

Horvath, S., Pirazzini, C., Bacalini, M. G., Gentilini, D., Di Blasio, A. M., Delledonne, M., et al. (2015). Decreased epigenetic age of PBMCs from Italian semi-supercentenarians and their offspring. *Aging, 9*, 419–446.

Hu, Z., Jiang, Y., Huo, X., Yang, Y., Davies, H., Botchway, B. O. A., et al. (2017). Prospective role of microRNAs in depression. *Current Medicinal Chemistry, 24*(32), 3508–3521.

Hughes, K., Bellis, M. A., Hardcastle, K. A., Sethi, D., Butchart, A., Mikton, C., et al. (2017). The effect of multiple adverse childhood experiences on health: A systematic review and meta-analysis. *The Lancet Public Health, 2*(8), e356–e366.

Ieraci, A., Mallei, A., Musazzi, L., & Popoli, M. (2015). Physical exercise and acute restraint stress differentially modulate hippocampal brain-derived neurotrophic factor transcripts and epigenetic mechanisms in mice. *Hippocampus, 25*(11), 1380–1392.

Im, H. J., Kim, Y. J., Kim, H. G., Kim, H. S., & Son, C. G. (2015). Kouksundo, a traditional Korean mind-body practice, regulates oxidative stress profiles and stress hormones. *Physiology & Behavior, 141*, 9–16.

Ingerslev, L. R., Donkin, I., Fabre, O., Versteyhe, S., Mechta, M., Pattamaprapanont, P., et al. (2018). Endurance training remodels sperm-borne small RNA expression and methylation at neurological gene hotspots. *Clinical Epigenetics, 10*, 12.

Johnson, S. B., Riley, A. W., Granger, D. A., & Riis, J. (2013). The science of early life toxic stress for pediatric practice and advocacy. *Pediatrics, 131*(2), 319–327.

Jovanovic, T., Vance, L. A., Cross, D., Knight, A. K., Kilaru, V., Michopoulos, V., et al. (2017). Exposure to violence accelerates epigenetic aging in children. *Scientific Reports, 7*(1), 8962.

Kaliman, P., Álvarez-López, M. J., Cosín-Tomás, M., Rosenkranz, M. A., Lutz, A., & Davidson, R. J. (2014). Rapid changes in histone deacetylases and inflammatory gene expression in expert meditators. *Psychoneuroendocrinology, 40*, 96–107.

Kaliman, P., Párrizas, M., Lalanza, J. F., Camins, A., Escorihuela, R. M., & Pallàs, M. (2011). Neurophysiological and epigenetic effects of physical exercise on the aging process. *Ageing Research Reviews, 10*(4), 475–486.

Kapranov, P., Cheng, J., Dike, S., Nix, D. A., Duttagupta, R., Willingham, A. T., & Gingeras, T. R. (2007). RNA maps reveal new RNA classes and a possible function for pervasive transcription. *Science, 316*, 1484–1488.

Kuebler, U., Zuccarella-Hackl, C., Arpagaus, A., Wolf, J. M., Farahmand, F., von Kanel, R., et al. (2015). Stress-induced modulation of NF-κB activation, inflammation-associated gene expression, and cytokine levels in blood of healthy men. *Brain, Behavior, and Immunity, 46*, 87–95.

Kurth, F., Cherbuin, N., & Luders, E. (2017). Promising links between meditation and reduced (brain) aging: an attempt to bridge some gaps between the alleged fountain of youth and the youth of the field. *Frontiers in Psychology, 8*, 860.

Levine, M. E., Hosgood, H. D., Chen, B., Absher, D., Assimes, T., & Horvath, S. (2015). DNA methylation age of blood predicts future onset of lung cancer in the women's health initiative. *Aging, 7*, 690–700.

Levine, M. E., Lu, A. T., Bennett, D. A., & Horvath, S. (2015). Epigenetic age of the pre-frontal cortex is associated with neuritic plaques, amyloid load, and Alzheimer's disease related cognitive functioning. *Aging, 7*(12), 1198–1211.

Li, Z., He, Y., Wang, D., Tang, J., & Chen, X. (2017). Association between childhood trauma and accelerated telomere erosion in adulthood: A meta-analytic study. *Journal of Psychiatric Research, 93*, 64–71.

Ludwig, D. S., & Kabat-Zinn, J. (2008). Mindfulness in medicine. *Journal of the American Medical Association, 300*(11), 1350–1352.

Luteijn, M. J., & Ketting, R. F. (2013). PIWI-interacting RNAs: From generation to transgenerational epigenetics. *Nature Reviews Genetics, 14*(8), 523–534.

Lutz, A., Jha, A. P., Dunne, J. D., & Saron, C. D. (2015). Investigating the phenomenological matrix of mindfulness-related practices from a neurocognitive perspective. *American Psychologist, 70*(7), 632–658.

Marioni, R. E., Shah, S., McRae, A. F., Chen, B. H., Colicino, E., Harris, S. E., & Deary, I. J. (2015). DNA methylation age of blood predicts all-cause mortality in later life. *Genome Biology, 16*, 25.

Marioni, R. E., Shah, S., McRae, A. F., Ritchie, S. J., Muniz-Terrera, G., Harris, S. E., et al. (2015). The epigenetic clock is correlated with physical and cognitive fitness in the Lothian Birth Cohort 1936. *International Journal of Epidemiology, 44*, 1388–1396.

Micha, R., Peñalvo, J. L., Cudhea, F., Imamura, F., Rehm, C. D., & Mozaffarian, D. (2017). Association between dietary factors and mortality from heart disease, stroke, and type 2 diabetes in the United States. *Journal of the American Medical Association, 317*(9), 912–924.

Miller, A. L. (2008). The methylation, neurotransmitter, and antioxidant connections between folate and depression. *Alternative Medicine Review, 13*(3), 216–226.

Misztak, P., Pańczyszyn-Trzewik, P., & Sowa-Kućma, M. (2018). Histone deacetylases (HDACs) as therapeutic target for depressive disorders. *Pharmacological Reports, 70*(2), 398–408.

Moore, B. F., Sauder, K. A., Starling, A. P., Hébert, J. R., Shivappa, N., Ringham, B. M., et al. (2018). Proinflammatory diets during pregnancy and neonatal adiposity in the healthy start study. *Journal of Pediatrics, 195*, 121–127.e2.

Muskiet, F. A. J., & Kemperman, R. F. J. (2006). Folate and long-chain polyunsaturated fatty acids in psychiatric disease. *The Journal of Nutritional Biochemistry, 17*(11), 717–727.

Myzak, M. C., Tong, P., Dashwood, W.-M., Dashwood, R. H., & Ho, E. (2007). Sulforaphane retards the growth of human PC-3 xenografts and inhibits HDAC activity in human subjects. *Experimental Biology and Medicine, 232*(2), 227–234 (Maywood, N.J.).

Owen, N., Salmon, J., Koohsari, M. J., Turrell, G., & Giles-Corti, B. (2014). Sedentary behaviour and health: Mapping environmental and social contexts to underpin chronic disease prevention. *British Journal of Sports Medicine, 48*(3), 174–177.

Pal, R., Singh, S. N., Halder, K., Tomer, O. S., Mishra, A. B., & Saha, M. (2015). Effects of yogic practice on metabolism and antioxidant-redox status of physically active males. *Journal of Physical Activity and Health, 12*(4), 579–587.

Papakostas, G. I., Cassiello, C. F., & Iovieno, N. (2012). Folates and S-adenosylmethionine for major depressive disorder. *Canadian Journal of Psychiatry, 57*(7), 406–413.

Papale, L. A., Li, S., Madrid, A., Zhang, Q., Chen, L., Chopra, P., et al. (2016). Sex-specific hippocampal 5-hydroxymethylcytosine is disrupted in response to acute stress. *Neurobiology of Disease, 96*, 54–66.

Parrizas, M., Gasa, R., & Kaliman, P. (2012). Epigenetics of lifestyle: The plasticity of the genetic information. *Epigenetics of Lifestyle, 33*, 3–35.

Patki, G., Solanki, N., Atrooz, F., Ansari, A., Allam, F., Jannise, B., & Salim, S. (2014). Novel mechanistic insights into treadmill exercise based rescue of social defeat-induced anxiety-like behavior and memory impairment in rats. *Physiology and Behavior, 130*, 135–144.

Penney, J., & Tsai, L.-H. (2014). Histone deacetylases in memory and cognition. *Science Signaling, 7*(355), re12.

Perna, L., Zhang, Y., Mons, U., Holleczek, B., Saum, K. U., & Brenner, H. (2016). Epigenetic age acceleration predicts cancer, cardiovascular, and all-cause mortality in a German case cohort. *Clinical Epigenetics, 8*, 64.

Perry-Parrish, C., Copeland-Linder, N., Webb, L., & Sibinga, E. M. S. (2016). Mindfulness-based approaches for children and youth. *Current Problems in Pediatric and Adolescent Health Care, 46*(6), 172–178.

Phillips, C. M., Shivappa, N., Hébert, J. R., & Perry, I. J. (2018). Dietary inflammatory index and mental health: A cross-sectional analysis of the relationship with depressive symptoms, anxiety and well-being in adults. *Clinical Nutrition, 37*(5), 1485–1491.

Potharst, E. S., Aktar, E., Rexwinkel, M., Rigterink, M., & Bögels, S. M. (2017). Mindful with your baby: Feasibility, acceptability, and effects of a mindful parenting group training for mothers and their babies in a mental health context. *Mindfulness, 8*(5), 1236–1250.

Quach, A., Levine, M. E., Tanaka, T., Lu, A. T., Chen, B. H., Ferrucci, L., et al. (2017). Epigenetic clock analysis of diet, exercise, education, and lifestyle factors. *Aging, 9*, 419–446.

Radford, E. J. (2018). Exploring the extent and scope of epigenetic inheritance. *Nature Reviews Endocrinology, 14*(6), 345–355.

Radtke, K. M., Schauer, M., Gunter, H. M., Ruf-Leuschner, M., Sill, J., Meyer, A., & Elbert, T. (2015). Epigenetic modifications of the glucocorticoid receptor gene are associated with the vulnerability to psychopathology in childhood maltreatment. *Translational Psychiatry, 26*(5), 571.

Rassoulzadegan, M., Grandjean, V., Gounon, P., Vincent, S., Gillot, I., & Cuzin, F. (2006). RNA-mediated non-mendelian inheritance of an epigenetic change in the mouse. *Nature, 441*, 469–474.

Rima, D., Shiv, B. K., Bhavna, C., Shilpa, B., & Saima, K. (2016). Oxidative stress induced damage to paternal genome and impact of meditation and yoga—Can it reduce incidence of childhood cancer? *Asian Pacific Journal of Cancer Prevention, 17*(9), 4517–4525.

Rodrigues, G. M., Toffoli, L. V., Manfredo, M. H., Francis-Oliveira, J., Silva, A. S., Raquel, H. A., et al. (2015). Acute stress affects the global DNA methylation profile in rat brain: Modulation by physical exercise. *Behavioural Brain Research, 279*, 123–128.

Schiele, M. A., & Domschke, K. (2018). Epigenetics at the crossroads between genes, environment and resilience in anxiety disorders. *Genes, Brain and Behavior, 17*(3), e12423.

Segal, Z. V., & Walsh, K. M. (2016). Mindfulness-based cognitive therapy for residual depressive symptoms and relapse prophylaxis. *Current Opinion in Psychiatry*.

Seo, M. K., Ly, N. N., Lee, C. H., Cho, H. Y., Choi, C. M., Nhu, L. H., & Kim, Y. H. (2016). Early life stress increases stress vulnerability through BDNF gene epigenetic changes in the rat hippocampus. *Neuropharmacology, 105*, 388–397.

Sharma, H., Datta, P., Singh, A., Sen, S., Bhardwaj, N. K., Kochupillai, V., & Singh, N. (2008). Gene expression profiling in practitioners of Sudarshan Kriya. *Journal of Psychosomatic Research, 64*(2), 213–218.

Shivappa, N., Stubbs, B., Hébert, J. R., Cesari, M., Schofield, P., Soysal, P., et al. (2018). The relationship between the dietary inflammatory index and incident frailty: A longitudinal cohort study. *Journal of the American Medical Directors Association, 235*, 39–44.

Smith, K. J., Sanderson, K., McNaughton, S. A., Gall, S. L., Dwyer, T., & Venn, A. J. (2014). Longitudinal associations between fish consumption and depression in young adults. *American Journal of Epidemiology, 179*, 1228–1235.

Soshnev, A. A., Josefowicz, S. Z., & Allis, C. D. (2016). Greater than the sum of parts: Complexity of the dynamic epigenome. *Molecular Cell, 62*, 681–694.

Sugden, C. (2006). One-carbon metabolism in psychiatric illness. *Nutrition Research Reviews, 19*(1), 117–136.

Suglia, S. F., Koenen, K. C., Boynton-Jarrett, R., Chan, P. S., Clark, C. J., Danese, A., et al. (2018). Childhood and adolescent adversity and cardiometabolic outcomes: A scientific statement from the American Heart Association. *Circulation, 137*(5), e15–e28.

Sweet, M. J., Shakespear, M. R., Kamal, N. A., & Fairlie, D. P. (2012). HDAC inhibitors: Modulating leukocyte differentiation, survival, proliferation and inflammation. *Immunology and Cell Biology, 90*(1), 14–22.

Tengeler, A. C., Kozicz, T., & Kiliaan, A. J. (2018). Relationship between diet, the gut microbiota, and brain function. *Nutrition Reviews, 76*(8), 603–617.

Tolahunase, M., Sagar, R., & Dada, R. (2017). Impact of yoga and meditation on cellular aging in apparently healthy individuals: A prospective, open-label single-arm exploratory study. *Oxidative Medicine and Cellular Longevity, 2017*, ID 7928981.

Tomioka, Y., Numata, S., Kinoshita, M., Umehara, H., Watanabe, S., Nakataki, M., et al. (2018). Decreased serum pyridoxal levels in schizophrenia: Meta-analysis and Mendelian randomization analysis. *Journal of Psychiatry and Neuroscience, 43*(2), 170053.

Turecki, G., & Meaney, M. J. (2016). Effects of the social environment and stress on glucocorticoid receptor gene methylation: A systematic review. *Biological Psychiatry, 79*(2), 87–96.

Tyrka, A. R., Ridout, K. K., & Parade, S. H. (2016). Childhood adversity and epigenetic regulation of glucocorticoid signaling genes: Associations in children and adults. *Development and Psychopathology, 28*(4pt2), 1319–1331.

Vago, D. R., & Zeidan, F. (2016). The brain on silent: mind wandering, mindful awareness, and states of mental tranquility. *Annals of the New York Academy of Sciences, 1373*(1), 96–113.

Vereecken, C., Pedersen, T. P., Ojala, K., Krølner, R., Dzielska, A., Ahluwalia, N., et al. (2015). Fruit and vegetable consumption trends among adolescents from 2002 to 2010 in 33 countries. *European Journal of Public Health, 25*(2), 16–19.

Waddington, C. H. (2012). The epigenotype. 1942 Reprinted in *International Journal of Epidemiology, 41*(1), 10–13.

Weaver, I. C. G., Cervoni, N., Champagne, F. A., D'Alessio, A. C., Sharma, S., Seckl, J. R., et al. (2004). Epigenetic programming by maternal behavior. *Nature Neuroscience, 7*(8), 847–854.

Wolf, J. M., Rohleder, N., Bierhaus, A., Nawroth, P. P., & Kirschbaum, C. (2009). Determinants of the NF-κB response to acute psychosocial stress in humans. *Brain, Behavior, and Immunity, 23*(6), 742–749.

World Health Organization. (2017). Adolescent obesity and related behaviours: Trends and inequalities in the WHO European Region 2002–2014. http://www.euro.who.int/__data/assets/pdf_file/0019/339211/WHO_ObesityReport_2017. Accessed October 9, 2018.

Yehuda, R., & Meaney, M. J. (2018). Relevance of psychological symptoms in pregnancy to intergenerational effects of preconception trauma. *Biological Psychiatry, 83*(2), 94–96.

Yuan, H., Mischoulon, D., Fava, M., & Otto, M. W. (2018). Circulating microRNAs as biomarkers for depression: Many candidates, few finalists. *Journal of Affective Disorders, 233*, 68–78.

Zannas, A. S., Arloth, J., Carrillo-Roa, T., Iurato, S., Röh, S., Ressler, K. J., et al. (2015). Lifetime stress accelerates epigenetic aging in an urban, African American cohort: Relevance of glucocorticoid signaling. *Genome Biology, 16*, 266.

Zannas, A. S., & West, A. E. (2014). Epigenetics and the regulation of stress vulnerability and resilience. *Neuroscience, 264*, 157–170.

Chapter 4
Generosity, Peer-Support, and Positive Development in Youth

Christoph Steinebach, Marcel Schaer and Imke Knafla

Abstract In adolescence, many physical, emotional, and cognitive changes bring along their own problems and risks. But they also offer the chance to develop new skills, including those connected with mindfulness, compassion, or generosity. Social relationships can support positive developments. Even in adolescence, family remains important, contributing to the satisfaction of basic needs. Peers can also support positive development and become particularly important in adolescence. With them, young people's radius widens into a more comprehensive and differentiated social and physical environment. The newly acquired competences also promote the acceptance of responsibility. The social and physical environments become relevant learning fields for the integration of identity, values, and norms. Generosity as part of one's own identity becomes a touchstone for positive development. In this paper, we discuss several forms and conditions of prosocial behavior as well as of generosity. We assign different internal conditions to "prosocial personality", ranging from genetic or biological factors to self-efficacy. External factors for prosocial behavior and generosity are described. In everyday life, young people must feel needed and require places to show their new autonomous generosity skills. Being generous not only helps others: it also satisfies one's own basic needs and thus contributes to positive development and well-being.

Keywords Developmental tasks · Structures of peer relations · Environmental systems · Definition of generosity · Citizenship

4.1 Youth Development in Changing Environments

Young people face a variety of challenges. On the one hand, these challenges arise from social demands and expectations. But challenges also result from the many physical, emotional, and cognitive changes that they must deal with. These changes

C. Steinebach (✉) · M. Schaer · I. Knafla
School of Applied Psychology, ZHAW Zürich University of Applied Sciences, Zürich, Switzerland
e-mail: Christoph.steinebach@zhaw.ch

C. Steinebach and Á. I. Langer (eds.), *Enhancing Resilience in Youth*,
https://doi.org/10.1007/978-3-030-25513-8_4

are often contradictory and conflictual, which makes adolescence a difficult time not only for young people, but also for those who live with them.

In tackling the various developmental tasks and critical life events, the adolescent shows whether resilience has been acquired and positive development is possible (Steinebach, 2015). This becomes clear when young people skillfully use their own resources and strengths to solve problems and balance their emotions. It also becomes apparent, however, whether young people's social relationships provide them with sufficient resources to master developmental tasks. From the point of view of a resilience and a strength-oriented approach, we (Knafla, Schaer, & Steinebach, 2016; Steinebach, 2015) note that

- most young people are well prepared for the challenges of adolescence. During childhood, they have learned skills that help them master the challenges of adolescence,
- physical, emotional, cognitive and social changes ("second major growth", Knafla et al., 2016, p. 17) are the basis for new competences acquired in this stage of development,
- challenges that young people have to face are very diverse. On the one hand there are socially formulated expectations, but there are also personal wishes, goals, or unforeseen necessities that are understood as developmental tasks or critical life events (Silbereisen & Weichold, 2012),
- like all people, young people shape their development. They try to achieve goals with their actions. With what they do, they express their own values. They try to satisfy their own needs and solve the problems that arise. They evaluate their development. If necessary, they correct the course of development and see what is needed to achieve a goal (Knafla et al., 2016; Trommsdorff, 2015). But this does not necessarily happen solely through conscious processes of goal setting and goal pursuit ("conscious vs. unconscious goal striving", Gantman, Gollwitzer, & Oettingen, 2014, p. 249),
- often the tendency to risky behavior stands in the way of goal achievement. On the other hand, young people prove to be particularly healthy and resilient in many respects (Giedd, 2015),
- important developmental tasks include: the development of intellectual and social competencies, the development of one's own gender role and the ability to enter into an intimate relationship, the ability to use the commodity market competently, the development of an appropriate system of norms and values (Hurrelmann, 2012), a competent handling of the media, and finally the development of one's own positive identity, which provides a meaningful framework for old and new competencies,
- the pressure to prepare for adult roles no longer weighs so heavily on young people because their school years are prolonged, while developmental tasks such as marriage or starting a family lose their normative power and are postponed until later. Thus, a relatively new phase of development emerges after adolescence: the "period of emerging adulthood" (Anderman, 2012, p. 42; Knafla et al., 2016, p. 20),

- developmental tasks are often linked to ecological transitions, such as changing schools or starting work in a company. These transitions change activities, roles, and time structures (Silbereisen & Weichold, 2012).
- Young people have strong resistance to diseases and are usually highly resilient (Giedd, Raznahan, Alexander-Bloch, Schmitt, Gogtay, & Rapoport, 2015),
- young people receive support and help from their social environment to cope well with important challenges and strains of everyday life,
- young people also use virtual media to cope with upcoming problems and tasks (Uhls, Greenfield, Subrahmanyam, & Šmahel, 2011),
- parents remain important contacts in adolescence and thus are a resource for positive development,
- during this time, however, friends gain additional importance,
- peers are sometimes a danger, but often also an important resource, e.g. if they provide emotional support, positive social orientation and identity, and emotional stability,
- the everyday life of young people is not only determined by special social relationships. The physical characteristics of the environment and the opportunities it offers to become active and shape everyday life independently are also of particular importance for young people.

4.1.1 Biological, Emotional, Cognitive Changes

Biological changes: Biologically, adolescence begins with puberty. With puberty, hormonal and structural changes commence that extend into the third decade of life. The particularly problematic, risk-prone behavior of adolescents is today largely attributed to a lack of fit in the maturation processes of the networks of the limbic system and the frontal cortex. While the limbic system plays a major role in emotional control, the frontal cortex is the basis for rational decisions and impulse control (Giedd, 2015; Worthman, 2011). Limbic structures are expanded and show themselves in the enlargement of the amygdala with corresponding effects on emotional experience. In adolescence, a decrease in gray matter has been proven. Synapses decrease as superfluous neuronal connections are degraded. At the same time, a reduction and redistribution of dopamine receptors in the paralimbic and prefrontal cortical regions has been proven. Because dopamine is associated with the limbic reward system, these changes increase individuals' willingness to seek variety and take risks.

As Magnetic Resonance Imaging studies show, gray matter is partially broken down throughout adolescence and white matter is built up into adulthood (Blakemore & Mills, 2014). With increasing myelination, nerve fibers and neurophysiological connections become more effective. "Connectivity is a major determinant of how the brain operates, so processes that shape how cells and regions of the brain talk with each other comprise the most powerful determinants of mature brain function"

(Worthman, 2011, p. 181). While the reduction of gray matter begins earlier, the development of white matter begins later and continues into adulthood. In the course of development, connectivity between cortical and subcortical regions improves. This lays the foundations for better regulation of emotions and a better understanding of social processes (Steinberg, 2008; Steinebach & Steinebach, 2013). It is therefore not only hormonal changes (raging hormones, Anderman, 2012) that are responsible for the particularities of young people's behavior: "The dynamics of hormones and behavior in adolescence must be understood to operate within a network of interacting developmental, physiological, perceptual, and social forces" (Worthman, 2011, p. 178). However, hormones play a special role. Hormones promote the growth of the skeleton and muscle tissue as well as sexual maturation. This is also accompanied by the development of primary and secondary sexual characteristics. With a view to the processes of sexual maturation that begin earlier in generational terms, the question arises as to whether "the accelerated timing and pace of puberty fuel a growing mismatch between physical and psychosocial development" (Worthman, 2011, p. 178). This is especially relevant because these hormones (Gonadal Steroid Hormones, glucocorticoids) also influence the emotional experience of stress. In addition, growth hormones influence the protein, fat, and carbohydrate metabolism as well as the electrolyte balance. In the female body, the gradual enlargement of the ovaries begins with puberty. In the male body, hormonal changes lead to an enlargement of the prostate and seminal vesicles (Sales & Irwin, 2013).

In the course of puberty, the increase in sex hormones is decisive for physical development. Thyroid hormones, insulin, and cortisone are also particularly important. They all promote bone development and general growth. The production of sex hormones is activated by a regulatory cycle: as the sensitivity of the sensor located in the hypothalamus is reduced, a luteinizing hormone (LH) and a folic-stimulating hormone (FSH) are increasingly secreted by the pituitary gland to restore the regulatory balance. This stimulates the gonads to produce more sex hormones. In the female body, FSH and LH cause the formation of estrogen and progestin, whereas in the male body they lead to an increase in testosterone and androgen.

Emotional changes: It has already become clear that physical and emotional changes are closely related in adolescence. In this period, changes in the hypothalamic-pituitary-adrenal axis (HPA axis) are reflected in the basic level of cortisol as well as in sensitivity to stress (Worthman, 2011). Internal tensions and external conflicts are the rule. Especially in early adolescence, friends of the same age are a major source of support in this regard. Many internal changes are experienced as foreign. Sexual maturation influences peer selection as well as the shaping of the social relationships with them (Dijkstra & Veenstra, 2011). Due to the impact of deeply fundamental changes, it is necessary to develop a positive identity. High personal expectations go hand in hand with self-confidence, while emotional stability increases in late adolescence. Self-assurance and self-confidence also make it possible to distinguish oneself from others, which makes individual relationships more important. Social norms are adopted into one's own identity and integrated (Knafla et al., 2016). Developmental goals become clearer and more long-term. Perceived self-efficacy with regard to emotion regulation promotes psychosocial adaptation

(Gunzenhauser et al., 2013). However, cognitive changes also enable progress in moral development. Willingness to take responsibility for oneself and for others grows. Not least because of neurophysiological maturation processes (Giedd, 2015), young people are learning to perceive and manage internal changes better, while at the same time becoming more sensitive to the social environment with all its complexity (Blakemore & Mills, 2014, Knafla et al., 2016, p. 31).

Cognitive changes: Piaget (1973) describes cognitive development in adolescence as a phase of formal operations (12 years and older). During adolescence, cognitive processes can be related to multidimensional operations and integrations into complex mental structures are possible. This makes cognition more abstract as adolescents gain the ability to formulate hypotheses that are independent of concrete observations. Individuals' own predictions are tested through observations. Systematic combinations and permutations make the evaluation of variables and factors possible; for instance, the characteristics of an object can be varied systematically while maintaining other aspects. In principle, cognitive processes are reversible. For Piaget, the relationship between reality and possibility is an essential characteristic of young people's thinking (Dreher & Dreher, 2008). In this regard, he speaks of a "reversal of sense" between the real and the possible. Thus, according to Dreher and Dreher (2008), Piaget's constructivist perspective becomes clear once again.

The question of competence development focuses more on changes in cognitive abilities and their effects on thinking, emotion, motivation and behavior (cf. Dreher & Dreher, 2008). In a domain-specific approach, the acquisition of knowledge and skills in individual domains is decisive for cognitive development (Dreher & Dreher, 2008). Expertise is combined with a fundamental understanding of structures and processes. With process-related automation, cognitive performance is increased. Structures are differentiated and arranged more efficiently. In addition, adolescents gain the ability to reflect not only on processes and structures, but also on their changes: "conceptual coordination, conscious control of the acquisition processes and metacognitive awareness—collectively referred to as conscious coordination—represent the competences that guarantee a profound build-up of knowledge" (Dreher & Dreher, 2008, p. 66, translation by the authors).

Table 4.1 shows the effects of changes in cognition on emotion, motivation, and behaviour according to Dreher and Dreher (2008, Knafla et al., 2016). It can be assumed that different forms of prosocial behavior are associated with different social cognitive and social emotional competences and skills (Carlo, Hausmann, Christiansen, & Randall, 2003). The ability to adopt perspectives and make moral judgments still seems to be developing. Young people become increasingly successful in taking the social context into account in their decisions about prosocial behavior (Güroğlu, Woutervanden, & Crone, 2014). This also becomes clear when looking for the reasons for aggressive or prosocial behavior. In addition to social cognitive and social emotional factors, social ecology also plays a role (Carlo et al., 2003). Young people's ability to reflect on their own behavior gradually improves. Self-reflection is a major prerequisite for generosity. In this regard, authors have suggested that "there is another form of thinking that is not calculating but is certainly not spontaneous either. This form of thought is captured by the term self-reflection" (Raffel, 2001,

Table 4.1 Key competencies and prosocial behavior in adolescence

Key competencies				Competencies and skills	Prosocial behavior
Being able to control feelings better	Not being overwhelmed by feelings during an action	Being able to better reflect on reasons for action	Being able to implement actions appropriately		
Most relevant area					
Cognition		*Cognition*		Cognition shows possibilities instead of only reality	Possible necessities to help are evaluated
Cognition		*Cognition*		Information processing: Faster and more efficient	Emergencies are quickly identified and possibilities for helping are weighed up
Cognition		*Cognition*		Knowledge and skills in domains lead to expertise and new awareness	Cognitive processes accompany and correct own behavior if necessary. Missing knowledge and insufficient skills are recognized and corrected, so that in the long run it is possible to help

(continued)

Table 4.1 (continued)

Key competencies				Competencies and skills	Prosocial behavior
Being able to control feelings better	Not being overwhelmed by feelings during an action	Being able to better reflect on reasons for action	Being able to implement actions appropriately		
Most relevant area					
Emotion	*Emotion*			introspection	One's own behavior is critically reflected upon. One's own introspection is linked to one's own identity, self-esteem, and self-control
Emotion	*Emotion*			Self-confidence	One's own thoughts and motives are distinguished from those of others. One's own willingness to help is shielded from external distractions
Emotion	*Emotion*			Risk behavior is controlled by regulatory competence	The consequences of one's own actions are weighed up. Risks are evaluated critically and decisions for and against prosocial behavior can be discussed

(continued)

Table 4.1 (continued)

Key competencies				Competencies and skills	Prosocial behavior
Being able to control feelings better	Not being overwhelmed by feelings during an action	Being able to better reflect on reasons for action	Being able to implement actions appropriately		
Most relevant area					
		Motivation	*Motivation*	Abstract thinking also in social matters and convictions	Own motives are questioned
		Motivation	*Motivation*	Importance for moral decisions	Arguments for and against prosocial behavior are reflected upon
		Motivation	*Motivation*	Concentration and endurance increase	Own intentions to help are shielded against disturbances. Plans are designed and implemented
	Behavior		*Behavior*	Regulation of action through reflection	Demanding action goals and complex plans are reliably pursued. Errors are recognized and conditions are optimized

(continued)

Table 4.1 (continued)

Key competencies				Competencies and skills	Prosocial behavior
Being able to control feelings better	Not being overwhelmed by feelings during an action	Being able to better reflect on reasons for action	Being able to implement actions appropriately		
Most relevant area					
	Behavior		*Behavior*	Development and use of action-oriented knowledge	Plans, processes and results of one's own actions are evaluated and thus new competencies are acquired and consolidated
	Behavior		*Behavior*	Flexibility in perspectives, valuations and processes	Own actions are continuously reconsidered and, if necessary, adjusted in goals, means, and consequences

p. 118). It is important to highlight that help-related cognitions are not normatively bound; on the contrary, they are flexible and creative ("nonattachment, defined as a flexible way of relating to one's experiences without clinging to or suppressing them", Sahdra, Ciarrochi, Parker, Marshalland, & Heaven, 2015, p. 1).

4.1.2 Social Relations

If friends of the same age become more important for young people, this does not mean that parents or siblings lose importance. Often only the topics that young people want to discuss with their parents shift. In addition, it is necessary for adolescents to make arrangements appropriate to their age and level of development in order to be able to live out the newly gained independence and still maintain the family as an important living space and safe haven (Steinebach & Steinebach, 2013). Like young people, families are also confronted with certain developmental tasks. In adolescence, families must define free spaces for adolescents, reflect together on values and norms, and ensure that all family members get their rights according to their tasks, possibilities, and competences. Adolescents' relationships with parents depend on several factors: the temperament of the members of the family system, the quality of the relationship between the couple, the parenting style, or the extent to which parents take care of school matters (Anderman, 2012). And all these factors are subject to fundamental changes. In the interplay of autonomy and control, young people are given more freedom, even if conflicts arise in the debate about everyday routines. The topics discussed are homework, time management in everyday life, and pocket money, along with major problems or questions such as sexual behavior or drug use (Anderman, 2012). The big question for a family is: How can we preserve our relationship and at the same time promote the development of autonomy?

Family structures: Developmental tasks, but also unforeseen challenges, crises, and critical life events lead to burdens that have to be overcome. Very different factors influence dyadic relationships in families. Sibling relationships depend, for example, on the age and gender of the children, but also, of course, on parents' educational attitudes and behaviour as well as on the family culture as a whole (Brown & Braun, 2013). From the point of view of structural family therapy and family stress theory, proximity or distance along with power or mutual influence are important characteristics of family relationships. On an individual level, the dimension of closeness and distance is associated with the question of self-definition and identity, independence, and autonomy. Power and influence are associated with subjective freedom, but also with self-commitment to mutual support and help. As it turns out, families are particularly capable of dealing well not only with everyday challenges, but also with crises if both dimensions, proximity and distance as well as power or influence, are at a medium level. At least one of the two dimensions should be at an average level to compensate an extreme on the other dimension. It is problematic if the emotional bond among family members is too close or too loose.

But it is also problematic if the family system is not able to flexibly adapt roles and relationships to current needs (Schaer & Studer, 2013).

Structures of peer relations: In contrast to a focus on problems and deficits, positive youth development psychology not only emphasises the strengths of young people in general, but also the social resources of their peers. For this to happen, however, young people must shape their relationships with their peers well. This is because the system of social relationships is becoming increasingly complex. Two-person relationships are integrated into a wide circle of friends, some of whom overlap with larger groups such as the school class. And social systems have their own rules, norms, and processes. This makes it difficult for adolescents to meet the diverse expectations of others and at the same time to know who they are and who they want to be. It is in this area of tension that their own identity develops. This offers opportunities to try out and further develop new beliefs and behaviors (Brown & Braun, 2013): "Peers provide unique opportunities to establish and develop identity" (Dijkstra & Veenstra, 2011, p. 257). Comparisons provide information about appropriate behavior, norms and values, identity, one's own status in the group, and self-development. Of particular importance is also the focus on and sensitivity to the positive emotions of others, especially when it comes to building new relationships (Campos, Schoebi, Gonzaga, Gable, & Keltner, 2015).

Adolescence is a time of many and varied changes. Physical, emotional, and cognitive changes interact with environmental changes. Changes in the structures and functions of the peer system are already apparent at the beginning of adolescence (Brown & Braun, 2013). In a time of diverse social change, young people in particular, who are themselves undergoing a variety of changes, seem to be influenced by this change. Generations of youth are particularly challenged to redefine fundamental values and to make intensive and creative use of new opportunities. So, it is not surprising that new, sometimes very distinct youth cultures develop again and again over the generations.

In this field of tension, peers are often seen as a risk. On the one hand, the negative influence of peers is attributed to selection processes. Young people choose their friends according to their attitudes and thus strengthen any negative attitudes. On the other hand, young people learn negative attitudes in contact with others, which can then lead to problematic behavior. The selection and socialisation theses contradict each other only to a limited extent, because it is conceivable for both processes to lead to such negative effects (Brown & Braun, 2013; Dijkstra & Veenstra, 2011; Donlan, Lynch, & Lerner, 2015).

When young people are asked what is burdening them the most, they often mention school, social relationships, everyday family life, money worries, uncertainty about the future, and the need to take on more responsibility (Camara, Bacigalupe, & Padilla, 2014). It seems that the Storm and Stress ("Sturm und Drang") of adolescence is intensified by the problematic behavior of friends. It is therefore necessary that they successfully coordinate multiple relationships to build and maintain a positive identity and social recognition in these relationships (Brown & Braun, 2013).

4.1.3 Changing Settings

Environmental influences play a special role in cognition, motivation, learning, and development. First, the influence of social relations is obvious (Gifford, 2014; Oishi, 2014). However, there are many relevant environmental factors that change over the course of a person's life. An example might be the transition to secondary school or to vocational training for adolescents, which might also lead young people to look for groups in other places that are more likely to meet their needs (Dijkstra & Veenstra, 2011). The model developed by Bronfenbrenner (1917–2005; 1979, 1999) is helpful for classifying important factors. He distinguishes between different environmental systems that are assigned to each other in a nested structure. Bronfenbrenner describes the location- and time-specific activity and role-dependent relationship between person and environment as a microsystem. The mesosystem consists of the important settings in which a person finds himself or herself at a certain point in his or her life. Connectedness between the microsystems is beneficial for development. Changes in the course of development often correspond to transitions from one microsystem to the next. Bronfenbrenner sees such ecological transitions as a motor for development. Micro- and mesosystems are influenced by other formal and informal social structures, the exosystem. Superordinate patterns of culture are assigned to the macrosystem. Later on, Bronfenbrenner added the chronosystem by depicting special biographical transitions. From a pedagogical point of view, the design of settings is of particular importance. This concerns social relations as well as the physical and symbolic aspects of the environment. These characteristics of the setting should enable increasingly complex and demanding interactions and actions (Bronfenbrenner 1979, 1999). This systems model helps us to investigate how the school and extracurricular environments could be designed in a way that supports young people's positive learning and personality development. This applies to the design of interactive learning media as well as to the development of a positive school culture (Donlan et al., 2015) or the promotion of a "sense of community" (Albanesi, Cicognani, & Zani, 2007) as part of positive learning environment. In this regard, "Research indicates that adolescents are using interactive media to grapple with many normative offline developmental issues such as identity development, peer interaction, relationship building, and learning, potentially altering the shape of these developmental processes ... researchers must now take a constructivist approach, asking what kinds of environments adolescents construct for themselves. This is a consequence of the fact that popular interactive media ... are designed for active participation on the part of users" (Uhls et al., 2011, p. 160). Participation in sport, youth groups in the community, and similar activities have many positive effects on school development and personality development (Brown & Braun, 2013). Likewise, "Relations with peers form an important context in which adolescents acquire skills and exhibit behaviors that enable them to establish more mature relations with peers and achieve emotional independence from parents to prepare themselves to fully participate in life when moving toward adulthood" (Dijkstra & Veenstra, 2011, p. 255). But the wider social environment is also important, because it can have a significant influence on social relations. This notion is illustrated by the concept of "sense of community", "the belief that healthy communities exhibit an extra-individual equality of emotional interconnectedness of individuals played out in their collective lives" (Albanesi et al., 2007, p. 387). Concepts such as "livability", "environmental quality", "quality-of-life", and "sustainability" are then used to describe the quality of, for example, urban environments and their impact on well-being (van Kamp et al., 2003). Corresponding aspects are considered in particular in ecological developmental theories of adolescence (Newman & Newman, 2011). In addition, however, it is also important to combine socially relevant norms and values with one's own self-image and world view in order to find the best possible cultural fit (Trommsdorff, 2015): "Thus, adolescents regulate their individual development by integrating values, morals, and religious orientations in line with their self- and world-views by referring to individual and/or collective agency to achieve an optimal cultural fit" (Trommsdorff, 2015, p. 391). Ungar and colleagues name seven different aspects that ensure positive development even under stress: "relationships; a powerful identity; power and control; social justice; access to material resources; a sense of cohesion; belonging and spirituality; and cultural adherence" (Ungar, Ghazinour, & Richter, 2013, p. 351). In addition, there is evidence that singles out which characteristics of the physical environment make a decisive contribution to well-being (Vohs, Redden, & Rahinel, 2013 on physical order; Weinstein, Przybylski, & Ryan, 2009 on nature and motivation; Zhang, Piff, Iyer, Koleva, & Keltner, 2014 on nature and prosocial behavior).

4.2 Peer Support and Generosity

All in all, young people spend more than twice as much time with their peers as with their families (Dijkstra & Veenstra, 2011). Integration into the peer group is particularly important: "Most adolescents want to feel included and accepted in their peer groups. Feeling connected to the peer group brings several benefits, including social support, opportunities to practice social and cognitive skills, and a sense of belonging in school, which all predict academic achievement and well-being" (Donlan et al., 2015, p. 125). Peer relationships thus offer a good framework for satisfying basic needs such as belonging and experiencing competence and autonomy (Steinebach & Gharabaghi, 2018). However, social relations can also be a source of particular stresses (Camara et al., 2014). The expectations of adults and friends, for example, bring with them a variety of burdens. With all these tasks and demands, young people are often stressed. This can lead to behavioral problems or psychological disorders. There are also clear connections between young people's behavioral problems and the deviant behavior of their peers (Brown & Braun, 2013). Learning and performance problems, relationship problems at school (such as bullying, Donlan et al., 2015), and conflicts with parents and peers are seen as particularly stressful. Social relationships can thus be both a burden and an important resource in coping with problems. Young people appreciate social support if it is based on trust and reliability.

The prosocial behavior of peers thus becomes a protective factor (Brown & Braun, 2013). The value of the help is measured by the extent to which the offer fits young people's needs (Camara et al., 2014, "match hypothesis" vs. "principal effect model" or "buffering hypothesis", p. 3). Usually, social support can be classed as emotional support, instrumental or material support, informative support, or social accompaniment. Emotional support contributes to well-being: someone can be a good listener, express solidarity, and convey appreciation (Camara et al., 2014; Cohen & Wills, 1985). This is important because it is often easier for young people to talk about their problems with their peers than with their parents. The different forms of social support refer to the multiple ways in which one can contribute to someone else's problem-solving process. Social support thrives on the willingness of helpers to use their own resources and make them available to others: time and effort, material or immaterial support, without knowing whether this will pay off in the end. This shows "that adolescents' attachment to peers and participation with peers strongly facilitate being actively engaged in behaviors like taking part in fundraising activities, and supporting organizations that help disadvantaged people" (Albanesi et al., 2007, p. 389). In addition to orientation towards others, temperament and the ability to control oneself play an important role for generosity in adolescence (Güroğlu et al., 2014). At its core, therefore, it is about generosity as an individual strength in social relationships. For those who receive help, emotional support seems to be of particular importance because it conveys a sense of security and belonging, without interfering with their autonomy and competence. In this regard, emotional support is particularly oriented towards the basic needs of those seeking help (Camara et al., 2014).

4.2.1 Defining Generosity

Generosity is regarded as an underestimated and neglected virtue (Miller, 2018). This is all the more surprising since it is about actions in which one does good on one's own responsibility, which goes beyond what can be expected and benefits others, even if they are not suffering at all. It is therefore a matter of behavior that does no harm to anyone and benefits many: "The common underlying assumption seems to be that human generosity is a beneficial act that may be directed towards other human beings, the community or the society as such" (Komter, 2010, p. 443). Accordingly, the Notre Dame Center for the Study of Religion in Society defines generosity as "the disposition and practice of freely giving of one's financial resources, time, and talents, [including], for example, charitable financial giving, volunteering, and the dedication of one's gifts for the welfare of others or the common good" (Collett & Morrissey, 2007, p. 2).

Although the term is common, there is a lack of systematic description and research on generosity. Conceptual analysis makes it clear that altruism, helpfulness, and philanthropy are closely interwoven and that they stand for very similar but also very different forms of prosocial behavior, ranging from the willingness to cooperate to voluntary work, civic engagement, and the willingness to donate money or objects. It has also been observed that that such behavior can entail both very short-term actions and very long-term commitments.

Pro-social behavior appears to be the overarching category for all those actions that are intended to serve the welfare of the other person. As research shows, it is both internal and external factors that determine whether a person behaves prosocially. Internal factors include individual dispositional elements such as temperament, empathy, and emotionality, but also a willingness to think about the situation in which help is required by taking moral and ethical arguments into account. Finally, self-efficacy appears to be an important prerequisite for becoming active. Operant conditioning, modeling, and role identity are core concepts to explain the emergence of the willingness to act prosocially. With these approaches it becomes clear that the willingness to help others is also understood as the result of education and socialisation processes. Nevertheless, there are many references to evolutionary roots and biological foundations and correlates of prosocial behavior in general and of generosity in particular. Thus, for example, primates also show help behavior even if they do not get any reward for it and special efforts are required. On the other hand, certain forms of generosity are reserved for human beings: especially generous anonymous donations for those in need and who never will be met in person. The good feelings experienced when helping also seem to be rooted in evolution (c.f. brain structures, neurobiological cognitive systems such as the mesolimbic reward system, Greater Good Science Center, n.d.). In the meantime, there is a variety of evidence that both prosocial and anti-social behavior are associated with certain hormones (e.g. testosterone and oxytocin, Greater Good Science Center, n.d.). In addition, twin studies show that hereditary factors play an important role in prosocial personality traits. Of course, developmental and socialisation factors must be pointed out (Greater Good Science Center, n.d.). Even if children show prosocial behavior at a very early age (Warneken, 2016), this behavior must be further strengthened through education. Current research shows that "an individual child's propensity to behave more or less generously is dependent on both nature and nurture factors, as well as the complex interactions among these factors" (Greater Good Science Center, n.d., p. 18).

On the one hand, it feels good to help (cf. the evolutionary roots of this feeling, Greater Good Science Center, n.d.). On the other hand, social norms demand conformity and thus also prosocial behavior (Oarga, Stavrova, & Fetchenhauer, 2015). However, situational factors also play a role, e.g. the needs of those who need help. The emergency itself is important, but so is the availability of help (e.g. bystander effects).

"While inherent in most definitions of altruism is the tenet that the helper must not benefit from the altruistic act, helping lacks a similar precondition. Helping is any act that one does to assist another, regardless of whether the helper benefits from the act or not" (Collett & Morrissey, 2007, p. 6). This statement refers to the evidence that there is an altruism that is really altruistically motivated—in contrast to one that is at best egoistically motivated. Different models try to single out core factors influencing helping behavior. Relevant elements include emotional tension, the result of a cost-benefit analysis, an expected reward, imminent dangers and risks, the vic-

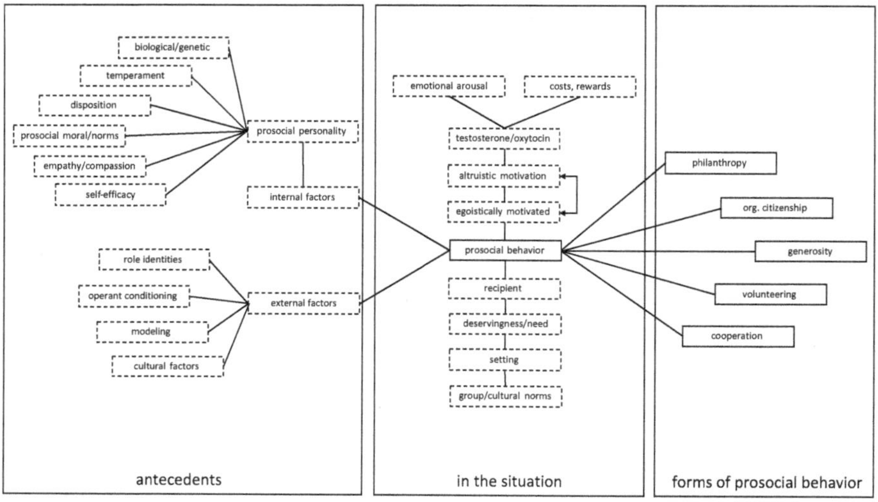

Fig. 4.1 Factors influencing prosocial behavior

tim's need for help, and willingness to assume responsibility in a given situation. In addition, a distinction must be made between short, medium, and long-term benefits for the helpers. For example, if one is generous, one is more likely to be viewed as trustworthy, which may pay off later when cooperating with others (Przepiorka & Liebe, 2016). However, Collett and Morrissey (2007) rightly point out that the social dimension, i.e. the group or organisation, is rarely taken into account in the relevant research. Figure 4.1 compiles forms and conditions of prosocial behaviour. In it, we assign very different conditions to "prosocial personality" as internal factors, ranging from genetic or biological factors to self-efficacy. Among the external factors we also include role identity, because this is defined essentially by being a member of a social group.

This confirms that "The development of prosocial behavior during adolescence is complex and multidimensional and may differ as a function of numerous individual and contextual factors" (Padilla-Walker, Dyer, Yorgason, Fraser, & Coyne, 2013, p. 135).

4.2.2 Emotions, Attitudes, and Identity

"Identity can be understood as that instance which enables one to give one's own life the right direction and to experience oneself as unique as well as to be perceived as unique by others" (cf. Kroger, 2015, p. 537, translation by the authors). The concept of identity is associated with the assumption that each person is unique with his or her strengths and weaknesses. The attribution of an identity is linked to the expectation that a person is capable of describing and understanding himself or herself in his or her particularity. Identity is therefore the result of a process of self-construction. However, this process does not take place on its own, but always in dialogue with others. Self-reflection makes it possible to distinguish between the real self and the ideal self, as well as between the image others have of one (external image) and how others would like one to be (external ideal). These characteristics and assumptions are integrated into an overall picture of oneself in the sense of an identity.

In adolescence, the generation of a positive identity is regarded as an important developmental task. The new possibilities of self-reflection, the increasing involvement in peer groups, and the tendency to try new behaviors offer many possibilities for developing an identity. In this process, being confronted with different expectations can prove to be particularly problematic for young people, even leading to identity diffusion. The task remains to overcome this diffusion and develop a sustainable positive identity.

Young people's desire and striving for a clear self-image leads to different results. A positive self-image is evident when it comes to new relationships, the willingness to learn, perform, and commit oneself, or the ability to deal step by step with the coming tasks of early adulthood. Factors such as emotions, personality, gender, and religion all have an impact on generosity. And they are also part of self-image and identity. Believing oneself to be a generous person is an important impulse to show more generosity (Greater Good Science Center, n.d.). This conviction also depends on whether one has already shown such behavior in the past, especially when it was costly. Such special commitment combined with higher costs also promotes a more sustainable self-attribution of this virtue. These cognitions and emotions, which are related to one's self-image, are influenced by different social and cultural factors. For example, it is important to assume that one will get something back later for your generosity. But generosity is also influenced by having information about how generous others have been. In addition, it can be of interest to promote one's reputation through generous behavior. Feeling connected to others, being involved in a group of friends, belonging to social networks and the community, and knowing that generosity is experienced in all these communities enhances one's generosity.

In this context, when it comes to enhancing generosity, arguments can be deduced as to why peer-related interventions are important in adolescence (e.g. in the Positive Peer Culture approach, Peer Group Counselling, Steinebach, Schrenk, Steinebach, & Brendtro, 2018). If it is possible to promote a culture of mutual help in a group, then a climate of generosity is created that can be contagious. Experiencing the ability to help others promotes a positive identity. Negative feelings of self-doubt are countered by the experience that one has helped promote togetherness, that one has made an important decision correctly, and that one has been able to implement it competently. This makes it clear how generous behavior in a group addresses the basic needs of young people while also promoting their resilience (Steinebach & Gharabaghi, 2018).

4.2.3 Social Engagement, Citizenship, and Volunteering

"The importance of civic engagement and community involvement to individuals, communities, and society has been widely acknowledged in research and political decision-making during the last decades. The benefits for young people are considered to be personal development, career opportunities, increased confidence as well as pro-social attitudes and behavior. Community involvement is also a means of promoting trust and cohesion in communities, as well as a psychological sense of community" (Grönlund et al., 2017, p. 5). With his pedagogical concepts, Kurt Hahn (1886–1974) is regarded as a pioneer of outdoor education and service learning. After fleeing from the National Socialists, he founded the British Salem School in Gordonstoun, Scotland, in 1934. In his course concept, he combined "service", physical "training", and care with personal initiative in different projects. "Outward Bound" thus became a forerunner of outdoor education and service learning. Hahn stresses the importance of personal motivation: "There are three ways of trying to capture the young; one is to preach at them—I'm afraid that is a hook without a worm; the second is to coerce them like the Fascists and the Communists do and to tell them 'You must volunteer'; that is of the devil; the third is an appeal which never fails, 'You are needed'" (Hahn, 1959, p. 6). In service learning projects, for example, young people now deal with the topic of "poverty" and offer homework assistance in socially deprived areas or spend afternoons playing with children from refugee families (Steinebach et al., 2018).

How can young people be motivated for such projects? Good initiatives try to meet the basic needs of young people with information and appeals:

(1) Present the project as a challenge to appeal to its strength: "This is important and will certainly be exhausting". "Mastery" is particularly addressed as a basic need here.
(2) Emphasize that the effort is a great help that is really needed by others. "These people need our help!" This is an appeal to one's own "generosity". The fact that generosity is required here also shows that the project makes sense.
(3) Promotion of short projects, from which a long-term commitment with special relationships can develop. Group projects are teamwork and therefore already offer opportunities for satisfying the basic need to "belong". Also, in the project itself, relationships can develop with those who are to be helped. This also addresses the basic need for belonging.
(4) Make the projects exciting and spontaneous so that participants are not suffocated by routine and rules. Unpredictability and flexibility demand that young people be involved in decisions and that the procedure depend on their decisions. This addresses the basic need for autonomy.

All these recommendations are associated with a model in which many factors are seen as conditions for civic engagement (cf. Fig. 4.2).

Altruistic action is also regarded as particularly satisfying because it can give life a meaning (Haidt, 2003). According to Damon (2008), it is a matter of achieving

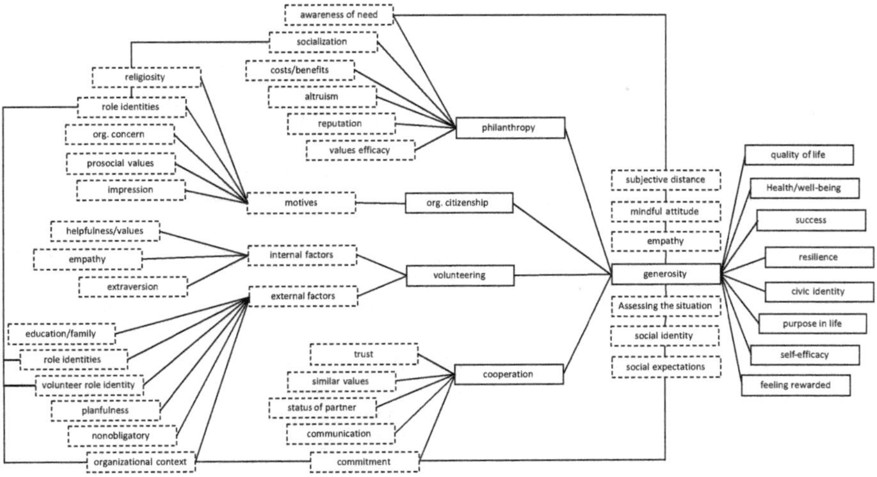

Fig. 4.2 Forms and effects of generosity

something that is regarded as meaningful from one's own point of view and which grows beyond oneself.

4.3 Conclusion

There are many challenges in adolescence, all of which have to be actively met. Physical, emotional, and cognitive changes bring along their own problems and risks. But they also offer the chance to develop new skills, including those connected with mindfulness, compassion, or generosity. Social relationships can support positive developments. Even in adolescence, family remains important, contributing to the satisfaction of basic needs. Peers can also support positive development and become particularly important in adolescence. With them, young people's radius widens into a more comprehensive and differentiated social and physical environment. The newly acquired competences also promote the acceptance of responsibility. The social and physical environments become relevant learning fields for the integration of identity, values, and norms. Generosity as part of one's own identity becomes a touchstone for positive development. Therefore, in everyday life, young people must feel needed and require places to show their new autonomous generosity skills. Being generous not only helps others: it also satisfies one's own basic needs and thus contributes to positive development and well-being. And this is especially relevant in adolescence, when all signs point to storms ahead.

References

Albanesi, C., Cicognani, E., & Zani, B. (2007). Sense of community, civic engagement and social well-being in Italian adolescents. *Journal of Community & Applied Social Psychology, 17*(5), 387–406.

Anderman, E. M. (2012). Adolescence. In K. R. Harris, S. Graham, & T. Urdan (Eds.), *APA educational psychology handbook: Vol. 3. Application to learning and teaching* (pp. 43–61). Washington: American Psychological Association.

Blakemore, S.-J., & Mills, K. L. (2014). Is Adolescence a sensitive period for sociocultural processing? *Annual Review of Psychology, 65,* 187–207.

Bronfenbrenner, U. (1979). *The ecology of human development*. Cambridge: Cambridge University Press.

Bronfenbrenner, U. (1999). Environments in developmental perspective: Theoretical and operational models. In S. L. Friedman & T. D. Wachs (Eds.), *Measuring environment across the life span* (pp. 3–28). Washington, D.C.: American Psychological Association.

Brown, B. B., & Braun, M. T. (2013). Peer relations. In C. Proctor & P. A. Linley (Eds.), *Research, applications, and interventions for children and adolescents: A positive psychology perspective* (pp. 149–164). Dordrecht: Springer.

Camara, M., Bacigalupe, G., & Padilla, P. (2014). The role of social support in adolescents: Are you helping me or stressing me out? *International Journal of Adolescence and Youth*, 1–14.

Campos, B., Schoebi, D., Gonzaga, G. C., Gable, S. L., & Keltner, D. (2015). Attuned to the positive? Awareness and responsiveness to others' positive emotion experience and display. *Motivation and Emotion, 39,* 780–794.

Carlo, G., Hausmann, A., Christiansen, S., & Randall, B. A. (2003). Sociocognitive and behavioral correlates of a measure of prosocial tendencies for adolescents. *Journal of Early Adolescence, 23,* 1.

Cohen, S., & Wills, T. (1985). Stress, social support, and the buffering hypothesis. *Psychological Bulletin, 98,* 310–357.

Collett, J. L., & Morrissey, C. A. (2007). *The social psychology of generosity: The state of current interdisciplinary research*. USA: University of Notre Dame. https://generosityresearch.nd.edu/assets/17634/social_psychology_of_generosity_final.pdf. Accessed January 12, 2019.

Damon, W. (2008). *The path to purpose: How young people find their calling in life*. New York, NY: Free Press.

Dijkstra, J. K., & Veenstra, R. (2011). Peer relations. In B. B. Brown & M. Prinstein (Eds.), *Encyclopedia of adolescence* (Vol. 2, pp. 255–259). New York: Academic.

Donlan, A. E., Lynch, A. D., & Lerner, R. M. (2015). Peer relationships and positive youth development. In E. P. Bowers, G. J. Geldhof, S. K. Johnson, L. J. Hilliard, R. M. Hershberg, J. V. Lerner, & R. M. Lerner (Eds.), *Promoting positive youth development. Advancing responsible adolescent development* (pp. 121–136). New York: Springer International.

Dreher, E., & Dreher, M. (2008). Kognitive Entwicklung im Jugendalter. In R. K. Silbereisen & M. Hasselhorn (Eds.), *Entwicklungspsychologie des Jugendalters. Enzyklopädie für Psychologie, Themenbereich C: Theorie und Forschung, Serie V: Entwicklungspsychologie* (pp. 55–107). Göttingen: Hogrefe.

Gantman, A. P., Gollwitzer, P. M., & Oettingen, G. (2014). Mindful Mindlessness in Goal Pursuit. In A. Ie, C. T. Ngnoumen, & E. J. Langer (Eds.), *The Wiley Blackwell handbook of mindfulness* (pp. 237–257). Oxford: Wiley.

Giedd, J. N. (2015). The "teen brain" is often ridiculed as an oxymoron—An example of biology gone wrong. *Scientific American, 312,* 32–37.

Giedd, J. N., Raznahan, A., Alexander-Bloch, A., Schmitt, E., Gogtay, N., & Rapoport, J. L. (2015). Child psychiatry branch of the National Institute of Mental Health longitudinal structural magnetic resonance imaging study of human brain development. *Neuropsychopharmacology, 40,* 43–49.

Gifford, R. (2014). Environmental psychology matters. *Annual Review of Psychology, 65,* 541–579.

Greater Goods Science Center. (o.J.). *The science of generosity. White paper prepared for the John Templeton Foundation by the Greater Good Science Center at UC Berkeley*. https://www.templeton.org/wp-content/uploads/2018/01/Generosity_White_Paper-FinalJTF.pdf. Accessed January 12, 2019.

Grönlund, H., Nortomaa, A., Aramburuzabala, P., McIlrath, L., Opazo, H., Altenburger, R., et al. (2017). *Guidelines for institutionalization of service-learning*. https://europeengagedotorg.files.wordpress.com/2015/10/guidelines-euengage-2.pdf. Accessed January 12, 2018.

Gunzenhauser, C., Heikamp, T., Gerbino, M., Alessandri, G., von Suchodoletz, A., Di Giunta, L., et al. (2013). Self-efficacy in regulating positive and negative emotions. A validation study in Germany. *European Journal of Psychological Assessment, 29*(3), 197–204.

Güroğlu, B., Woutervanden, B., & Crone, E. A. (2014). Sharing and giving across adolescence: An experimental study examining the development of prosocial behavior. *Frontiers in Psychology, 5*(291), 1–13.

Hahn, K. (1959). *Dr. Kurt Hahn at the forty-eighth annual dinner of Old Centralians*. http://www.kurthahn.org/wp-content/uploads/2017/02/2017-oldcentral.pdf. Accessed January 12, 2019.

Haidt, J. (2003). Elevation and the positive psychology of morality. In C. L. M. Keyes & J. E. Haidt (Eds.), *Flourishing: Positive psychology and the life well-lived* (pp. 275–289). Washington, D.C.: American Psychological Association.

Hurrelmann, K. (2012). Das Modell der produktiven Realitätsverarbeitung. *International Journal for the Advancement of Counselling, 33,* 127–138.

Komter, A. (2010). The evolutionary origins of human generosity. *International Sociology, 25*(3), 443–464.

Knafla, I., Schaer, M., & Steinebach, C. (2016). *Jugendliche stärken. Wirkfaktoren in Beratung und Therapie*. Weinheim: Beltz.

Kroger, J. (2015). Identity in childhood and adolescence. In J. D. Wright (Ed.), *International encyclopedia of the social & behavioral sciences* (2nd ed., Vol. 11, pp. 537–542). Bellingham, WA: Elsevier.

Miller, C. B. (2018). Generosity. A preliminary account of a surprisingly neglected virtue. *Metaphilosophy, 49*(3), 216–245.

Newman, B. M., & Newman, P. R. (2011). Theories of adolescence. In R. J. R. Levesque (Ed.), *Encyclopedia of adolescence* (Vol. 1, pp. 20–29). New York: Springer.

Oarga, C., Stavrova, O., & Fetchenhauer, D. (2015). When and why is helping others good for well-being? The role of belief in reciprocity and conformity to society's expectations. *European Journal of Social Psychology, 45,* 242–254.

Oishi, S. (2014). Socioecological psychology. *Annual Review Psychology, 65,* 581–609.

Padilla-Walker, L. M., Dyer, W. J., Yorgason, J. B., Fraser, A. M., & Coyne, S. M. (2013). Adolescents' prosocial behavior toward family, friends, and strangers: A person-centered approach. *Journal of Research on Adolescence, 25*(1), 135–150.

Piaget, J. (1973). *Einführung in die genetische Erkenntnistheorie*. Frankfurt. M.: Fischer.

Przepiorka, W., & Liebe, U. (2016). Generosity is a sign of trustworthiness—The punishment of selfishness is not. *Evolution and Human Behavior, 37,* 255–262.

Raffel, S. (2001). On generosity. *History of the Human Sciences, 14*(4), 111–128.

Sahdra, B. K., Ciarrochi, J., Parker, P. D., Marshalland, S., & Heaven, P. (2015). Empathy and non attachment independently predict peer nominations of prosocial behavior of adolescents. *Frontiers in Psychology, 6*(263), 1–12.

Sales, J. M., & Irwin, C. E. (2013). A biopsychosocial perspective of adolescent health and disease. In W. T. O'Donohue, L. T. Benuto, & L. Woodward Tolle (Eds.), *Handbook of adolescent health psychology* (pp. 13–29). New-York: Springer.

Schaer, M., & Studer, A. (2013). Familie. Gelungene Balance zwischen Nähe und Distanz. In C. Steinebach & K. Gharabaghi (Eds.), *Resilienzförderung im Jugendalter. Praxis und Perspektiven* (pp. 69–81). Heidelberg: Springer.

Silbereisen, R. K., & Weichold, K. (2012). Jugend (12–19 Jahre). In W. Schneider & U. Lindenberger (Eds.), *Entwicklungspsychologie* (7th ed., pp. 235–258). Weinheim: Beltz.

Steinberg, L. (2008). A social neuroscience perspective on adolescent risk-taking. *Developmental Review, 28,* 78–106.
Steinebach, C. (2015). Resilience. In J. D. Wright (Ed.), *International encyclopedia of the social & behavioral sciences* (2nd ed., Vol. 20, pp. 555–560). Oxford: Elsevier.
Steinebach, C., & Gharabaghi, K. (2018). Resilienz. In B. Gniewosz & P. F. Titzmann (Eds.), *Handbuch Jugend* (pp. 508–525). Stuttgart: Kohlhammer.
Steinebach, C., Schrenk, A., Steinebach, U., & Brendtro, L. K. (2018). *Positive Peer Culture. Ein Manual für starke Gruppengespräche.* Weinheim: Beltz-Juventa.
Steinebach, C., & Steinebach, U. (2013). Gleichaltrige. Peers als Ressource. In C. Steinebach & K. Gharabahi (Eds.), *Resilienzförderung im Jugendalter. Praxis und Perspektiven* (pp. 93–109). Heidelberg: Springer.
Trommsdorff, G. (2015). Cultural roots of values, morals, and religious orientations in adolescent development. In L. A. Jensen (Ed.), *The Oxford handbook of human development and culture: An interdisciplinary perspective* (pp. 377–395). Oxford: Oxford University Press.
Uhls, G. E., Greenfield, P., Subrahmanyam, K., & Šmahel, D. (2011). Internet and other interactive media. In R. J. R. Levesque (Ed.), *Encyclopedia of adolescence* (Vol. 2, pp. 160–168). New York: Springer.
Ungar, M., Ghazinour, M., & Richter, J. (2013). Annual research review: What is resilience within the social ecology of human development? *Journal of Child Psychology and Psychiatry, 54*(4), 348–366.
van Kamp, I., Leidelmeijer, K., Marsmana, G., & de Hollander, A. (2003). Urban environmental quality and human well-being. Towards a conceptual framework and demarcation of concepts; A literature study. *Landscape and Urban Planning, 65,* 5–18.
Vohs, K. D., Redden, J. P., & Rahinel, R. (2013). Physical order produces healthy choices, generosity, and conventionality, whereas disorder produces creativity. *Psychological Science, 24*(9), 1860–1867.
Warneken, F. (2016). Insights into the biological foundation of human altruistic sentiments. *Current Opinion in Psychology, 7,* 51–56.
Weinstein, N., Przybylski, A. K., & Ryan, R. M. (2009). Can nature make us more caring? Effects of immersion in nature on intrinsic aspirations and generosity. *Personality and Social Psychology Bulletin, 35*(10), 1315–1329.
Worthman, C. M. (2011). Hormones and behavior. In B. B. Brown & M. J. Prinstein (Eds.), *Encyclopedia of adolescence. Normative processes and development* (Vol. 1, pp. 177–186). Amsterdam: Elsevier.
Zhang, J. W., Piff, P. K., Iyer, R., Koleva, S., & Keltner, D. (2014). An occasion for unselfing: Beautiful nature leads to prosociality. *Journal of Environmental Psychology, 37,* 61–72.

Chapter 5
Schools as Positive Environments

Sabine Pirchio and Ylenia Passiatore

Abstract School environments can be regarded as the 'third educator', in addition to educators and peers. When focusing on the physical context of schools, we should consider environmental characteristics such as the presence of outdoor natural green spaces as well as indoor environmental quality, which includes classroom listening conditions or overcrowding. Natural environments have the capability to motivate and encourage child learning at school and are especially important for students with concentration problems or attention deficit. Natural environments can also reduce the stress affecting students' learning process. If outdoor spaces are relevant for shaping the students' learning and personal development, the importance of indoor settings, where students spend most of their day, is indisputable. When exploring the school as a developmental setting, one cannot avoid considering the role of interpersonal relationships in shaping the environment and, therefore, the experience that students derive from this process. The specific mechanisms linking environmental qualities, socio-relational processes, and behavioral and psychological outcomes need further investigation. First, it would be useful to identify which features of schools' physical settings influence relational processes and social interactions which, in turn, contribute to student development. Second, it would be important to identify the nature of the relationship between physical and social environments in order to design educational settings in a way that fosters positive relationships and an optimal learning experience.

Keywords School spaces · Environmental characteristics · Teacher-student relationship · Home-school relationship · Physical setting

When we close our eyes and think of our experience as schoolchildren, we certainly remember, more clearly than the contents of the books we studied, the smell and the light of our classroom, the colors of the walls, the shape of the garden, the

S. Pirchio (✉)
Department of Dynamic and Clinical Psychology, Sapienza University of Rome, Rome, Italy
e-mail: sabine.pirchio@uniroma1.it

Y. Passiatore
Department of Education, Roma Tre University, Rome, Italy

C. Steinebach and Á. I. Langer (eds.), *Enhancing Resilience in Youth*,
https://doi.org/10.1007/978-3-030-25513-8_5

arrangement of the desks where our classmates sat, the fun we had playing during the break, and the voice of our teacher explaining, helping, and maybe praising.

All these memories include physical aspects of the place we went to every day for years, together with the social relationships we established with significant peers and adults: they both contribute to characterizing students' experience at school. In this chapter, we summarize the literature about them in order to identify those features which make school a positive environment.

5.1 School Spaces as Positive Environments

Educators are, undisputedly, the most influential actors on the educational stage. However, in addition to their importance, the physical characteristics of the environments where the activities of children and educators/teachers take place represent a crucial factor for the quality of educational institutions. School environments can in fact be regarded as the 'third educator', in addition to educators and peers: studies in the field of environmental psychology have emphasized the role of the socio-physical environment in human psychological processes, behavior, and well-being (Bechtel & Tsertsman, 2002). When focusing on the physical context of schools, we should consider environmental characteristics such as the presence of outdoor natural green spaces as well as indoor environmental quality, which includes classroom listening conditions or overcrowding. Working in high quality environments improves students' and teachers' well-being and productivity. Teaching styles (Horne-Martin, 2002) and students' learning (Earthman, 2004; Schneider, 2002) are related to the physical environment of schools, which is able to shape teacher-child relationships and activities (Waters & Maynard, 2010). Therefore, is it worth examining the relationship between schools' environmental characteristics and their cognitive, physical, social-emotional, and personal benefits for children.

5.1.1 Outdoor Natural Environment

Natural environments have the capability to motivate and encourage child learning at school (Johnson, 2007) and are especially important for students with concentration problems or deficit of attention. Natural environments can also reduce the stress affecting students' learning process (Ozer, 2007). In fact, some environments—called restorative environments—are more able than others to promote physical and psychological benefits. Generally speaking, a restorative environment promotes recovery after a psychological or emotional breakdown due to a stressful day, allowing individuals to regenerate after a long activity requiring strong commitment. These events make individuals deplete their own resources to maintain and increase their adaptation to the environment. Problems in renewing these resources may lead to serious consequences for enacting planned actions and for subjective well-being and physical health (Hartig, 2004). Attention Restoration Theory (ART; Kaplan & Kaplan, 1989) and Stress Recovery Theory (SRT; Ulrich, 1983) explain how restorative environments work. ART assumes that four environmental characteristics—fascination, being away, extent, and compatibility—are involved in direct attention recovery. Natural environments more easily afford this experience. SRT focuses on the immediate emotional reaction to environmental stimuli. Psychological restoration should occur through viewing environmental scenes, fostering feelings of mild to moderate interest, pleasantness, and calm, thus reducing the surveillance level and parasympathetic nervous system stimulation. Viewing natural environments facilitates rapid recovery from stressful events by allowing the individual to replace negative with positive feelings. Psychological restoration is a crucial need for students at school because, in educational environments, children are usually exposed to many stressful factors (Shield & Dockrell, 2003) while needing attention to face important cognitive (Evans & Hygge, 2007) and relational demands (Abbas & Othman, 2010). Natural environments may moderate the impact of stressful life events for children (Carrus, Passiatore, Pirchio, & Scopelliti, 2015; Wells & Evans, 2003).

The use of natural environments to enrich the academic curriculum and integrate the standard teaching programs has a positive impact on students' learning outcomes in several subjects compared to traditional schools (Graham, Beall, Lussier, McLaughlin, & Zidenberg-Cherr, 2005; Ozer, 2007). Outdoor environments are an important factor in the improvement of students' learning: the school could use available green spaces not only for children's play activities but also to provide outdoor learning opportunities through learning by hearing, seeing, tasting, smelling, touching, and feeling (Dyment, 2005). In this way, teamwork with other students, inspiration to learn, behavioral engagement, responsibility, and self-esteem (Ozer, 2007) grow along with students' achievement. Also, given that movement has been described as one of the most natural and powerful modes of learning for young children, the presence of green spaces in the school setting is important because it gives them the possibility to move freely (Bilton, 2002). The Forest School movement is widespread in several North European countries, especially at the Primary School level. This is an educational approach where children engage in regular, repeated outdoor learning activities facilitated by a qualified forest school leader (Knight, 2009). Forest school practitioners find learning more enjoyable, motivating (Nundy, 2001), and memorable (Dillon et al., 2006; Peacock, 2006). This setting boosts students' personal, social, and emotional development (Harris, 2017; Mirrahimi, Tawil, Abdullah, Surat, & Usman, 2011). Also, other studies point out that green schools positively affect responsibility, patience, appreciation for relationships, self-esteem, and self-confidence (Bowker & Tearle, 2004). Students have the opportunity to learn significant social skills, cooperation, group work, and persistence (Bell & Dyment, 2008). Contact with nature promotes social relationships starting from infancy, improving emotional self-regulation and positive behaviors (Carrus et al., 2015; Taylor, Kuo, & Sullivan, 2002).

Experiences in green spaces are also important for effective environmental education—knowledge and attitudes—and consequently, for pro-environmental behaviors and sustainable lifestyle choices (Chawla, 2009; Pretty et al., 2009). Environmental knowledge and pro-environmental attitudes are highly interconnected and the use and management of outdoor spaces proposed at school by adults (most of all by teachers) influences children's environmental attitudes (Malone & Tranter, 2003). In fact, along with internal factors such as knowledge, values, and attitudes, stimuli arising from the immediate environment shape students' environmental behaviors (Asunta, 2004; Lukman, Lozano, Vamberger, & Krajnc, 2013). Environmental education at school could therefore help students change their behaviors, enhancing their environmental awareness and willingness to adopt pro-environmental behaviors (Boyes, Skamp, & Stanisstreet, 2009).

5.1.2 Indoor Environments

If outdoor spaces are relevant for shaping the students' learning and personal development, the importance of indoor settings, where students spend most of their day, is indisputable. Several studies have demonstrated that working or studying in good and comfortable indoor environmental conditions enhances well-being, satisfaction, productivity, and learning. The importance of improving the environmental conditions of educational buildings is related to the amount of time spent by children in school. Factors such as air quality, thermal comfort, and acoustic performance are often taken into account as parameters for assessing indoor conditions.

Appropriate ventilation can be guaranteed in naturally ventilated classrooms instead of using air conditioning systems. The importance of maintaining adequate indoor air quality in schools is recognized as a contributing factor in pupils' learning performance (Fisk, 2000). According to a recent study (De Giuli, Da Pos, & De Carli, 2012), windows are often not left open long enough to provide proper ventilation (the ventilation design should have the capability to deliver 8 l/s per person) and carbon dioxide (CO_2) concentration levels tend to be high (they should be lower than 1500 ppm while the classroom is being used). Mumovic et al. (2009) also collected data with semi-structured interviews with teachers and revealed that working in these conditions caused them persistent headaches. Usually, teachers open the windows only during breaks and not during lessons, which increases these risk conditions. Also, the temperature perceived by students during the lessons is important because it can impact performance. The number of hours the classroom is used per day, the classroom's crowding level, and students' behavior are factors to be considered as influencing ventilation condition.

Air quality, light conditions, acoustic performance, and thermal comfort are interrelated parameters to consider for students' well-being and performance.

Concerning light conditions, window size and lighting systems are often improperly designed, which makes it impossible to reach the minimum illuminance values (300 lx). Light conditions also vary according to the school's surroundings: houses, public parks, or traffic. In fact, teachers tend not to open the windows when there is heavy traffic because of the bad smells and noise. Acoustical conditions play a major role in learning process especially for younger pupils: in fact, their ability to perceive and understand spoken messages under adverse listening conditions is lower than in adolescents and adults. Exposure to noisy conditions may have harmful effects on children's learning and well-being at school. Experts recommend that reverberation times do not exceed 0.6 s for classrooms with a volume of about 250 m^3 and that ambient noise levels in empty rooms do not exceed 35 dB (Shield & Dockrell, 2003). In the presence of noise, children are more easily distracted by irrelevant sounds than adults and thus less able to focus their attention on the task (Gumenyuk, Korzyukov, Alho, Escera, & Naatanen, 2004). In these adverse listening conditions, more cognitive resources are required by children to decode speech signals and process information. In this regard, Klatte, Meis, Sukowski, and Schick (2007) show that primary school children exposed to long reverberation perform worse in a phonological processing task than children from classrooms with short reverberation. Chronic exposure to noise also has a negative impact on cognitive function, oral language acquisition (Maxwell & Evans, 2000), and reading development; later on, this hinders written language acquisition (Evans & Hygge, 2007).

In conclusion, it must be considered that both outdoor and indoor conditions affect teaching and child learning and well-being. Creating adequate conditions in the environment where instruction takes place also means improving students' learning and health in the long term.

5.2 Positive Relationships at School

A long tradition of psychology research confirms the importance of interpersonal relationships for human development and well-being. From an ecological perspective of individual development (Bronfenbrenner, 1979), relationships are components of the microsystem, the proximal ecological environment where individuals have a direct experience of the world, make mental representations of it, and act.

When exploring the school as a developmental setting, one cannot avoid considering the role of interpersonal relationships in shaping the environment and, therefore, the experience that students derive from this process. Even if relationships can be collectively created among all of the school's social actors (students, teachers, the principal, non-educational staff, volunteering parents, etc.), the psychological and educational literature looking for the basis of student's achievement, development, and well-being has focused on three particular types of relationships, located in students' microsystem and mesosystem, which we discuss in the following sections: the teacher-student and the teacher-parent relationships.

5.2.1 *The Teacher–Student Relationship*

In the learning process, the role of the teacher has always been an indisputable variable: the teacher's knowledge of the content, mastery of teaching strategies, and ability to translate them into activities are doubtlessly a fundamental part of the teaching/learning process.

Besides this, the psychological literature in the last 30 years has focused on a different aspect of the teaching process: the role of the teacher-student relationship. In fact, this relationship can be regarded as an ecological environment where the student develops knowledge, competences, and an image of him/herself as a student. This impacts on the student's academic success and psychological well-being.

A positive teacher-student relationship is defined as being warm and close, and having low levels of conflict (Driscoll, Wang, Mashburn, & Pianta, 2011). Such a relational experience since the beginning of the child's school life is linked with positive academic and social outcomes, both short- and long-term (e.g. Pianta et al., 2005), promoting the child's assumption of his/her role as a student and the fulfillment of the demands attached to this role (Hamre & Pianta, 2001).

In the framework of the ecological paradigm of human development, a positive relationship with the teacher provides the student with the scaffolding and the emotional support needed to acquire new abilities, while also affording a space to autonomously express and use the abilities that he/she already possesses, thus managing in a flexible way the balance of power between the expert and the novice (Bronfenbrenner, 1979). A clear example of this process is represented by the teacher's communicative behavior with young children and its role in fostering language learning (Girolametto, Hoaken, Weitzman, & van Lieshout, 2000; Taeschner, 2005).

This is an important topic for two main reasons: the increasing tendency to bring forward the child's first school experience at an early age—a critical or sensitive period for language learning—and the increasing number of non-native children in preschool and primary school who have poor second language competences.

Some research experiences involving the use of the narrative format approach (Taeschner, 2005) show the importance of the communicative relationship between teacher and students for language learning and social integration in various school contexts. The narrative format is a theoretical and practical language teaching model widely used in Europe for first, second, and foreign language learning. Its main theoretical stance is that, since language is a tool for communication and relationships, it is best learned and should be taught in an authentic and rich relational framework; consequently, teachers pay special attention to the use of positive verbal and non-verbal communication strategies to place students in an interactional structure characterized by mutual understanding and turn taking. This method has been shown to be effective in promoting foreign language learning in preschool and primary school. Importantly, in such settings, children's language performance has been found to depend on the teacher's communication (Taeschner, 2005): the teacher's sensitivity to the children's focus of attention, communicative turns, and emotional state, together with his/her use of nonverbal communication, create the best context for learning a foreign language. Significant outcomes were also found when using the narrative format to teach a second language to adolescent immigrant students: the program fostered language learning and also promoted positive feelings about the new country and was associated with better academic achievement at the end of the school year (Taeschner, Rinaldi, Tagliatatela, & Pirchio, 2008). The use of the narrative format in a framework of inclusive education in multicultural primary schools showed a positive effect on the social climate of the classroom: the native children who participated in the intervention program together with their immigrant classmates improved their level of interethnic relationships, while the opposite trend was observed in a comparable control classroom (Pirchio et al., 2017).

Promisingly, this line of research has also highlighted how the teacher-student relationship is grounded on specific communicative actions involving sensitivity to the child's needs and behaviors (Ansari & Pianta, 2018; Girolametto et al., 2000) and flexibility in using activities and verbal and non-verbal communication (Pirchio et al., 2017; Taeschner, Destino, & Pirchio, 2016).

5.2.2 The Home–School Relationship

The relationship between the two environments where children grow up and develop can be considered from the meso-system perspective: the ecological properties of the child's developmental environment depend on the quality of the relationships between two microsystems. In this framework, parental involvement in the child's school experience and its role in promoting adjustment and success is a major topic. In the literature, several types of parental involvement have been identified. For example, Hill and Tyson (2009) conceptualize three forms of parental involvement at school: a school-based involvement including participation in events occurring at school (meeting teachers, special events, volunteering); a home-based involvement including helping with homework, proposing cultural activities such as going to libraries or museums, and making books and newspapers available at home; and performing academic socialisation by making explicit their expectations about the child's education and how they value education, establishing connections with the job world, stimulating professional aspirations, discussing learning styles and strategies, and planning an educational program for the future. Of course, these types of involvement can be more influential in different developmental stages: for example, helping with homework may be useful in primary school, while establishing connections with the professional world and future jobs may make a difference in high school. Parental involvement has an impact on the child's school achievement, even in the long run (Arnold, Zeljo, Doctoroff, & Ortiz, 2008), and also on the child's socio-emotional adjustment (Mashburn & Serpell, 2011). The theme of parental engagement in children's education generally calls into consideration the role of school actors to involve them and create an actual partnership with the family. In the vast majority of cases, the teacher is the school actor committed to this task. Consequently, parental involvement is the outcome of parents' attitudes, values, and behaviors towards education and of the interaction between parents' and teachers' variables. A number of parental variables (e.g. socioeconomic level, status, education, parenting style, self-efficacy, stress) have been linked with the level of involvement. One of these variables is currently particularly relevant for European societies: belonging to an ethnic minority (e.g. Mendez, Waanders, & Downer, 2007) is associated with a lower level of parental engagement. This may be due to different causes: parents' lower SES and education, difficulties communicating with school staff and understanding school documents and the academic curriculum because of poor language knowledge, and cultural differences influencing parents' values toward education, expectations about schooling, and parenting (Crosnoe, 2010). These issues may create difficulties in encouraging teachers and parents to create an educational partnership that could be beneficial for the child's learning and socio-psychological adjustment.

Intervening in this process was the aim of a EU-funded project involving preschools and primary schools with multiethnic and multicultural classes in Italy, Scotland, Switzerland, and Spain. The project promoted the inclusion of children from an immigrant background through a multitarget model of intervention including a teacher training program, a class-based language learning activity that adopted the narrative format model, and an inventory of activities to be shared with parents that allowed for different levels and structures of participation. After the project's completion, benefits in terms of cognitive, language, and social outcomes were observed (Arcidiacono, Padiglia, & Miserez-Caperos, 2017; Pirchio, Passiatore, Carrus, & Taeschner, 2017; Robinson & Sorace, 2018).

5.3 Conclusion

The literature review conducted, together with our own research findings, showed how schools provide a wide range of challenges, limitations, and resources for human development.

Some of the first environmental psychology studies addressed the issue of the influence of the physical features of institutions on relationships and social variables and psychological outcomes. Importantly, in assessing the environmental factors influencing human behavior, the consideration of socio-environmental features instead of simple physical environmental features could make it possible to identify relevant psychological processes: for example, the level of crowding stress is better explained considering social density instead of spatial density (Evans, 2003; Stokols, 1972). Unfortunately, current psychological research addresses the role of the physical and social features of school settings on human development and well-being separately, with very few exceptions (Abbas & Othman, 2010; Cameron-Faulkner, Melville, & Gattis, 2018; Carrus et al., 2015; Legendre, 1999; Read, Sugawara, & Brandt, 1999).

The specific mechanisms linking environmental qualities, socio-relational processes, and behavioral and psychological outcomes need further investigation. Here, we envisage two possible directions for knowledge development in this area.

First, it would be useful to identify which features of schools' physical settings influence relational processes and social interactions which, in turn, contribute to student development. For instance, socio-relational processes may operate as mediating factors linking the physical environment and psychological development outcomes. Second, it would be important to identify the nature of the relationship between physical and social environments in order to design educational settings in a way that fosters positive relationships and an optimal learning experience.

References

Abbas, M. Y., & Othman, M. (2010). Social behavior of preschool children in relation to physical spatial definition. *Procedia-Social and Behavioral Sciences, 5,* 935–941.
Ansari, A., & Pianta, R. C. (2018). Teacher–child interaction quality as a function of classroom age diversity and teachers' beliefs and qualifications. *Applied Developmental Science*, 1–11. https://doi.org/10.1080/10888691.2018.1439749.
Arcidiacono, F., Padiglia, S., & Miserez-Caperos, C. (2017). Transitions in the representation and implementation of a language-learning project within a multicultural context. *European Journal of Psychology of Education*, 1–16. https://doi.org/10.1007/s10212-018-0367-z.
Arnold, D. H., Zeljo, A., Doctoroff, G. L., & Ortiz, C. (2008). Parent involvement in preschool: Predictors and the relation of involvement to preliteracy development. *School Psychology Review, 37*(1), 74–90.
Asunta, T. (2004). Knowledge sources, attitudes and self-reported behavior of secondary-level science students concerning environmental topics. In A. Laine, J. Lavonen, & V. Meisalo (Eds.), *Current research on mathematics and science education*. University of Helsinki, Research Report 253.
Bechtel, R. B., & Tsertsman, A. (2002). *Handbook of environmental psychology*. New York, NY: Wiley.
Bell, A. C., & Dyment, J. E. (2008). Grounds for health: The intersection of green school grounds and health promoting schools. *Environmental Education Research, 14*(1), 77–90.
Bilton, H. (2002). *Outdoor play in the early years*. London: David Fulton.
Boyes, E., Skamp, K., & Stanisstreet, M. (2009). Australian secondary students' views about global warming: Beliefs about actions, and willingness to act. *Research in Science Education, 39*(5), 661–680.
Bowker, R., & Tearle, P. (2004). Gardening as a learning environment: A study of children's perceptions and understanding of school garden as part of an international project. *Learning Environmental Research, 10,* 83–100.
Bronfenbrenner, U. (1979). *The ecology of human development*. Cambridge, MA: Harvard University Press.
Cameron-Faulkner, T., Melville, J., & Gattis, M. (2018). Responding to nature: Natural environments improve parent-child communication. *Journal of Environmental Psychology, 59,* 9–15.
Carrus, G., Passiatore, Y., Pirchio, S., & Scopelliti, M. (2015). Contact with nature in educational settings might help cognitive functioning and promote positive social behaviour. *Psyecology, 6*(2), 191–212.
Chawla, L. (2009). Growing up green: Becoming an agent of care for the natural world. *The Journal of Developmental Processes, 4*(1), 6–23.
Crosnoe, R. (2010). Two-Generation Strategies and Involving Immigrant Parents in Children's Education. *Urban Institute (NJ1).*
De Giuli, V., Da Pos, O., & De Carli, M. (2012). Indoor environmental quality and pupil perception in Italian primary schools. *Building and Environment, 56,* 335–345.
Dillon, J., Rickinson, M., Teamey, K., Morris, M., Choi, M. Y., Sanders, D., et al. (2006). The value of outdoor learning. *School Science Review, 87*(320), 107–111.
Driscoll, K. C., Wang, L., Mashburn, A. J., & Pianta, R. C. (2011). Fostering supportive teacher–child relationships: Intervention implementation in a state-funded preschool program. *Early Education & Development, 22*(4), 593–619.

Dyment, J. E. (2005). Green school grounds as sites for outdoor learning: Barriers and opportunities. *International Research in Geographical & Environmental Education, 14*(1), 28–45.

Earthman, G. I. (2004). *Prioritization of 31 criteria for school building adequacy*. Baltimore, MD: American Civil Liberties Union Foundation of Maryland.

Evans, G. W. (2003). The built environment and mental health. *Journal of Urban Health, 80*(4), 536–555.

Evans, G., & Hygge, S. (2007). Noise and cognitive performance in children and adults. In L. M. Luxon & D. Prasher (Eds.), *Noise and its effects* (pp. 549–566). New York: Wiley.

Fisk, W. J. (2000). Health and productivity gains from better indoor environments and their relationship with building energy efficiency. *Annual Review of Energy and the Environment, 25*(1), 537–566.

Girolametto, L., Hoaken, L., Weitzman, E., & van Lieshout, R. (2000). Patterns of adult-child linguistic interaction in integrated day care groups. *Language, Speech, and Hearing Services in Schools, 31*(2), 155–168.

Graham, H., Beall, D. L., Lussier, M., McLaughlin, P., & Zidenberg-Cherr, S. (2005). Use of school gardens in academic instruction. *Journal of Nutrition Education and Behavior, 37*(3), 147–151.

Gumenyuk, V., Korzyukov, O., Alho, K., Escera, C., & Naatanen, R. (2004). Effects of auditory distraction on electrophysiological brain activity and performance in children aged 8–13 years. *Psychophysiology, 41,* 30–36.

Hamre, B. K., & Pianta, R. C. (2001). Early teacher–child relationships and the trajectory of children's school outcomes through eighth grade. *Child Development, 72*(2), 625–638.

Harris, F. (2017). The nature of learning at forest school: Practitioners' perspectives. *Education 3–13, 45*(2), 272–291.

Hartig, T. (2004). Restorative environments. In C. Spielberger (Ed.), *Encyclopedia of applied psychology* (pp. 273–279). New York, NY: Academic Press/Elsevier.

Hill, N. E., & Tyson, D. F. (2009). Parental involvement in middle school: A meta-analytic assessment of the strategies that promote achievement. *Developmental Psychology, 45*(3), 740.

Horne-Martin, S. (2002). The classroom environment and its effects on the practice of teachers. *Journal of Environmental Psychology, 22*(1–2), 139–156.

Johnson, P. (2007). Growing physical, social and cognitive capacity: Engaging with natural environments. *International Education Journal, 8,* 293–303.

Kaplan, R., & Kaplan, S. (1989). *The experience of nature: A psychological perspective*. New York, NY: Cambridge University Press.

Klatte, M., Meis, M., Sukowski, H., & Schick, A. (2007). Effects of irrelevant speech and traffic noise on speech perception and cognitive performance in elementary school children. *Noise and Health, 9,* 64–74.

Knight, S. (2009). *Forest schools and outdoor learning the early years*. London: Sage.

Legendre, A. (1999). Interindividual relationships in groups of young children and susceptibility to an environmental constraint. *Environment and Behavior, 31*(4), 463–486.

Lukman, R., Lozano, R., Vamberger, T., & Krajnc, M. (2013). Addressing the attitudinal gap towards improving the environment: A case study from a primary school in Slovenia. *Journal of Cleaner Production, 48,* 93–100.

Malone, K., & Tranter, P. (2003). School grounds as sites for learning: Making the most of environmental opportunities. *Environmental Education Research, 9*(3), 283–303.

Mashburn, A. J., & Serpell, Z. N. (2011). Family-school connectedness and children's early social development. *Social Development, 21*(1), 21–46.

Maxwell, L. E., & Evans, G. W. (2000). The effects of noise on pre-school children's pre-reading skills. *Journal of Environmental Psychology, 20*(1), 91–98.

Mendez, J. L., Waanders, C., & Downer, J. T. (2007). Parent characteristics, economic stress and neighborhood context as predictors of parent involvement in preschool children's education. *Journal of School Psychology, 45,* 619–636.

Mirrahimi, S., Tawil, N. M., Abdullah, N. A. G., Surat, M., & Usman, I. M. S. (2011). Developing conducive sustainable outdoor learning: The impact of natural environment on learning, social and emotional intelligence. *Procedia Engineering, 20,* 389–396.

Mumovic, D., Palmer, J., Davies, M., Orme, M., Ridley, I., Oreszczyn, T., et al. (2009). Winter indoor air quality, thermal comfort and acoustic performance of newly built secondary schools in England. *Building and Environment, 44*(7), 1466–1477.

Nundy, S. (2001). *Raising achievement through the environment: The case for fieldwork and field centres*. Walsall: NAFSO.

Ozer, E. J. (2007). The effects of school gardens on students and schools: Conceptualization and considerations for maximizing healthy development. *Health Education & Behavior, 34*(6), 846–863.

Peacock, A. (2006). *Changing minds: The lasting impact of school trips*. Exeter: University of Exeter.

Pianta, R., Howes, C., Burchinal, M., Bryant, D., Clifford, R., Early, D., & Barbarin, O. (2005). Features of pre-kindergarten programs, classrooms, and teachers: Do they predict observed classroom quality and child-teacher interactions? *Applied Developmental Science, 9*(3), 144–159.

Pirchio, S., Passiatore, Y., Carrus, G., Maricchiolo, F., Taeschner, T., & Arcidiacono, F. (2017). Teachers and parents involvement for a good school experience of native and immigrant children. *Journal of Educational, Cultural and Psychological Studies, 15,* 73–94.

Pirchio, S., Passiatore, Y., Carrus, G., & Taeschner, T. (2017). Children's interethnic relationships in multiethnic primary school: Results of an inclusive language learning intervention on children with native and immigrant background in Italy. *European Journal of Psychology of Education,* 1–14. https://doi.org/10.1007/s10212-017-0363-8.

Pretty, J., Angus, C., Bain, M., Barton, J., Gladwell, V., Hine, R., et al. (2009). *Nature, childhood, health and life pathways*. ICES Occasional Paper 2009–02. Colchester: University of Essex.

Read, M. A., Sugawara, A. I., & Brandt, J. A. (1999). Impact of space and color in the physical environment on preschool children's cooperative behavior. *Environment and Behavior, 31*(3), 413–428.

Robinson, M. G., & Sorace, A. (2018). The influence of collaborative language learning on cognitive control in unbalanced multilingual migrant children. *European Journal of Psychology of Education*, 1–18. https://doi.org/10.1007/s10212-018-0377-x.

Schneider, M. (2002). Do school facilities affect academic outcomes? *ERIC Publications, National Clearinghouse for Educational Facilities*. http://www.edfacilities.org.

Shield, B., & Dockrell, J. E. (2003). The effects of noise on children at school: A review. *Building Acoustics, 10,* 97–116.

Stokols, D. (1972). On the distinction between density and crowding: Some implications for future research. *Psychological Review, 79*(3), 275.

Taeschner, T. (2005). *The magic teacher*. London: CILT.

Taeschner, T., Destino, K., & Pirchio, S. (2016). The onset of story comprehension and production in young Italian children learning English as a second language: or1495. *International Journal of Psychology, 51,* 814.

Taeschner, T., Rinaldi, P., Tagliatatela, D., & Pirchio, S. (2008). Le parole per raccontarmi. Una ricerca sull'apprendimento dell'italiano da parte di adolescenti figli di immigrati. *Psicologia dell'educazione e della formazione, 10*(1), 21–35.

Taylor, A. F., Kuo, F. E., & Sullivan, W. C. (2002). Views of nature and self-discipline: Evidence from inner city children. *Journal of Environmental Psychology*, 22(1–2), 49–63. (Licentiate thesis). Linköping University, Linköping.

Ulrich, R. S. (1983). Aesthetic and affective response to natural environment. In I. Altman & J. F. Wohlwill (Eds.), *Human behavior and environment: Advances in theory and research. Vol. 6: Behavior and the natural environment* (pp. 85–125). New York, NY: Plenum.

Waters, J., & Maynard, T. (2010). What's so interesting outside? A study of child-initiated interaction with teachers in the natural outdoor environment. *European Early Childhood Education Research Journal, 18*(4), 473–483.

Wells, N. M., & Evans, G. W. (2003). Nearby nature: A buffer of life stress among rural children. *Environment and Behavior, 35*(3), 311–330.

Chapter 6
Schools as Mindful, Supportive, and Healthy Workplaces at All Ages

Volker Schulte and Larisa Zotova

Abstract Many schools are only tentatively addressing the issue of health. They offer their employees and pupils fresh fruits, exercise over lunch or after work, or recreational opportunities such as yoga courses or wellness subscriptions. However, the possibilities for a school to influence the health of its employees, such as teachers, are much greater. The effect of measures can be increased if health can be promoted in the daily working life of each individual employee, which is why Corporate Health Management focuses on the work tasks of employees. In order to promote health, the company's mission statement and its management and cooperation culture must be geared toward this goal, while human resources management and work organization must be designed accordingly. Certification and labeling are good motivators for employers and employees to improve health-promoting structures. Better employee motivation significantly reduces absenteeism rates and increases productivity. The authors present several institutions, methods, awarding logos, and titles in the area of Workplace Health Promotion for companies at a European level.

Keywords Health promotion · Management of health · Organization · Organizational culture · Labeling

6.1 Introduction—How Is Health Produced?

Health is produced and created at all levels and settings of a society. To guarantee a life without harm, you need to organize proper health care, prevention, and health promotion programs. Our aim is not so much to describe the management of health care as to describe the management of health. This also changes the way we look at the system as a whole and at the objects of research. Everything that is available for the promotion and preservation or even restoration of health in terms of instruments

V. Schulte (✉)
School of Business, FHNW University of Applied Sciences Northwestern Switzerland, Windisch, Switzerland
e-mail: Volker.schulte@fhnw.ch

L. Zotova
Moscow Region State University, Mytishchi, Russia

C. Steinebach and Á. I. Langer (eds.), *Enhancing Resilience in Youth*,
https://doi.org/10.1007/978-3-030-25513-8_6

and methods is subsumed under the term "health management". With this system, we both limit and expand the term. The term is limited because our definition of health management always refers to people as individuals or collectively. The management of groups and organizations is thus solely focused on the goal of maintaining and promoting health. On the other hand, the term is extended through the multi-dimensionality of health fields of action, which we describe in the following sections (Schulte & Verkuil, 2016).

6.1.1 Micro Health Management

The first dimension of health management consists in individual planning and organization aimed at the preserving and improving personal health. We deal with health behavior and with methods to improve our own health competences through learning and experience. With this approach, we touch on the classic characteristics of health promotion, personal resource management, and the development of resilience. We describe this dimension with the term "micro-health management".

6.1.2 Meso Health Management

Let us turn to the second dimension the health management of groups and organizations such as schools. Health is also produced based on healthy management models, healthy processes, and healthy company cultures. In concrete terms, it deals with current requirements in the world of work and their effects on the health of employees. Here, too, we are concerned with the current effects of the burdens and resources of individuals, which are, however, significantly influenced by the organization and the company. For instance, a school must have the necessary knowledge to promote the performance and commitment of its teachers. At the so-called meso level of health management, we are therefore concerned with the models and goals of Corporate Health Management.

6.1.3 Macro Health Management

The third dimension deals with the political and social framework conditions that make it possible to generate health individually or collectively. Here we are at the political system level, Macro-Health Management, whose organization is decisive for the design of health and social determinants. These have an impact on the health of individuals, groups, and the population as a whole. At the macro level, economic, social, political, and cultural conditions are of particular importance, as are access to social, cultural, and medical facilities and services. Macro Health Management includes all aspects of health care, health economics, and health policy.

In this article, we focus on the Meso Level. We try to develop an answer to the question of how mindful, supportive, and healthy workplaces for all ages can be established.

6.2 Corporate Health Management in Schools

Talking about Corporate Health Management in schools means talking about Health Management for Organizations. There is no significant distinction between a company and a school organization. We can define both as bodies with a specific organizational culture. Therefore, Corporate Health Management Interventions also play a major role in schools. Employed people spend a large part of their lives working. Work is an important health resource: for many people, especially for teachers, work is a source of identity, meaning, and fulfillment in life. But working can also make people ill. Not everyone stays healthy until retirement. The reason for this is often to be found in working life itself. A considerable part of work-related illnesses result from specific working conditions. In fact, people who are exposed to several health risks at work have poorer health and more health problems (Scheil-Adlung & Kuhl, 2011). This not only has consequences for employees, but also results in high costs for companies and society.

Work is never solely responsible for health problems. The reasons are often to be found in the professional as well as in the private sphere. For example, the triggering factors of burnout often take place in the private sphere. Nevertheless, companies should not underestimate the potential of intervention in the business environment, because health problems can also lead to cost increases or losses. From this point of view, it is worthwhile for companies to strive to help keep their employees healthy.

Many schools are only tentatively addressing the issue of health. They offer their employees and pupils fresh fruit, exercise over lunch or after work, or recreational opportunities such as yoga courses or wellness subscriptions.

These are all praiseworthy offers. They ensure that individuals can do more for their health.

However, the possibilities for a school to influence the health of its employees, such as teachers, are much greater. The effect of measures can be increased if it is possible to promote health in the daily working life of each individual employee, which is why the central focus of Corporate Health Management is on the work tasks of the employees. In order to promote health, the company's mission statement and management and cooperation culture must be geared to this, while human resources management and work organization must be designed accordingly.

Corporate Health Management means the systematic optimization of health-relevant workplace factors. This refers to the design of company structures and processes with the aim of systematically optimizing the conditions for the health of employees and thus contributing to the success of the company. Corporate Health

Management requires the participation of all groups of people in the company, is integrated into corporate management, and is reflected in the corporate culture. Thus, it covers aspects of health promotion and prevention as well as health protection and the reintegration of sick employees (case management).

Teacher stress and the resulting frustration are serious problems that negatively impact the quality of teachers' health, their educational skills, and their general behavior when working with pupils (Jennings et al., 2017). The teaching profession is challenging, since practitioners must deal with migration processes, social problems, and the changing behavior of children in classrooms. With this situation in mind, the RADIX organization, a Swiss National competence center for the development and implementation of public health and sustainable development measures, runs comprehensive Health Promoting School Programs. In them, special attention is paid to stress prevention and teacher well-being (Radix, 2018).

The prevention of risks and diseases and thus the focus on risk groups in the company is only one aspect of our comprehensive understanding of Corporate Health Management. There is great potential in promoting the health of all employees; for instance, measures to improve motivation and performance are especially promising.

In the following, we would like to contrast the prevailing culture of carelessness with a culture of mindfulness for health, which is a central component of Corporate Health Management. In our opinion, a culture of mindfulness towards health consists of a high appreciation of health and its prerequisites, the continuous observation and reporting of the physical and mental condition of all workers, the mobilization of collective intelligence to promote the social and human assets of the company, and the consistent observance of data protection.

So, Corporate Health Management, as we understand it here, goes beyond basic legal requirements concerning occupational safety and health protection and thus represents a voluntary commitment of companies. Companies get involved because it pays off for them, not because they are forced to do so. Companies can actually promote the health of their employees and at the same time increase their competitiveness and corporate success.

In concrete terms, this means that Corporate Health Management is planned before its actual implementation on the basis of an explicit clarification of the initial situation, the definition of strategic and operational goals, and an optimal project organization (→ plan). The first step in the subsequent implementation is to ascertain the current situation and interpret the results. Based on this, the objectives and the target groups for the implementation of the measures are defined (→ do). The process flow and the achievement of objectives should be regularly evaluated in terms of effectiveness and efficiency (→ check) and reviewed by management at a higher level (→ act).

6.3 Corporate Health Management with System—Labeling

6.3.1 Preliminaries

Certification and labeling are good motivators for employers and employees to improve health promoting structures (Landstad, Hedlund, & Vinberg, 2017). Better employee motivation significantly reduces absenteeism rates and increases productivity (Mattig & Weber, 2016a). The variety of institutions, methods, awarding logos, and title names in the area of Workplace Health Promotion for valued companies is hardly to be overlooked at a European level. Therefore, the authors selected a set of countries based on the degree to which WHP certification is present in each. It should also be noted that labels are to be found mainly in Western European countries with high social standards. For countries in Eastern Europe and Eastern Central Europe, as well as for Southern European countries, only rudimentary activities can be identified.

A label for Corporate Health Management should encourage companies to invest in the health of their employees. The first research objective is to present an overview of the different types of labels for sustainable employability and occupational health that exist in Europe. The second is to compare the levels of Corporate Health Management labeling throughout the continent. The third objective is to describe a future scope of Corporate Health Management labeling.

We conducted a study that comprises an international comparison of labeling throughout Europe and an analysis of their development level. Mattig and Weber define Corporate Health Management as "systematic optimization of health-relevant factors in the company" (Mattig & Weber, 2016a, p. 154; Mattig & Weber, 2016b, p. 181).

Labeling is also a modern type of employer branding. The goal is to attract highly motivated and qualified employees given the ubiquitous, increasing demand for efficiency and the fast growing complexity of professional requirements. Due to the skills shortage in all industrial sectors, every company as well as public employers compete for well-trained staff. Any company wishing to be successful in personnel recruitment and human resources development must demonstrate its attractiveness as an employer. Thus, new studies reveal that job seekers are specifically looking for those employers who have more to offer to their employees than a well-paid job (Eichel, Dloughy, Schmitz, & Braun, 2013). In general, we notice the trend for companies to seek external assessment as a neutral confirmation of their well-being and health promotion programs, in addition to the measures already implemented. This is usually done by granting a seal of quality or an award.

A label allows the company to brand and advertise the quality of its management and working culture. In this context, we are focusing on the following aspects of Corporate Health Management:

- Its effectiveness: Is the health (and productivity) of the employees supported? Can absences be reduced?

- Its system integration: Is health management an integral part of strategic management and business processes?
- Its accessibility: Does it reach the employees and especially those in need?
- Its sustainability: Is Corporate Health Management designed to have long-term effects?

6.3.2 Acceptance in the Economy

In addition, labels have to be accepted in the economy and perceived as value added for the company in order to achieve higher market penetration. This depends on the cost of the investment in the label, a measurable benefit, and added value, as well as confidence in the label within the market. Corporate Health Management quality is measured via a criteria system that must be highly relevant and applicable. This requires measurability and comparability of the results of an assessment within an organization as well as between different organizations. Labels must be designed to be context-independent so that they can be applied to various businesses and industry settings. Also, the processes defined by the certifying agency must be clear and comprehensible. Finally, it needs a functioning scope of action in the agency as well as in the company to be certified. The label must be embedded in a functioning ecosystem. In particular, before starting the applying process, it must be clarified whether the label is embedded in organizational structures (including decision-making processes). The parties must be able to secure the necessary financial and human resources. Dissemination and marketing strategies must also be established and networking with stakeholders and politicians must be ensured.

Most quality seals are awarded by private institutions. These are often company networks, which, in cooperation with or sponsored by state institutions, usually with the relevant ministries, establish a corresponding service organization. In addition, there are also distributions and methods with strong public-law anchoring. At this point, the political debate should be led to the extent to which public-law bodies or government bodies must intervene in an evaluation structure with a quality seal. This is often also dependent on the political-traditional context in each country. Thus, the Austrian as well as the Scottish example show a stronger statist tendency than other countries, which work on an entirely private and commercial basis.

6.3.3 Quality Seal and Quality Criteria in a European Overview

Even in the relatively narrow area of Corporate Health Management, there already is a large number of quality seals, which are intended to prove the professionalism of employers in the promotion of workers' health. As many initiatives come and go, we tried to make a selection of quality labels that are already established and have achieved a sustainable level of national penetration.

The quality criteria of the European Network for Workplace Health Promotion (European Network of Workplace Health Promotion, 1996) is the reference system for any labeling. It is a comprehensive concept of occupational health management as a systematic, process-oriented approach that aims to make the company's operating environment healthier and to improve workers' health literacy. With these efforts, companies seek to reduce absenteeism, presentism, and fluctuation, in addition to the (already emphasized) steps to ensure the effective recruitment of employees. All these aspects have a direct impact on the productivity of a company.

The European Network of Workplace Health Promotion publishes results, concepts, and projects already implemented in all European regions, making them accessible to all interested parties by putting them in a database and ensuring their dissemination.

The existing quality criteria were developed in the 1990s, closely following the European Union's Luxembourg Declaration for Workplace Health Promotion, drawn up in 1997 and continuously developed (Luxembourg Declaration, 2007). The criteria were divided into six areas that provide a comprehensive picture of the quality of company health promotion measures, which are often insufficiently integrated into organizational structures and routines. This is often the case with individual, temporary measures. The European Network of Workplace Health Promotion criteria are therefore intended to form the strategic framework based on which an integrated health management system can be established.

6.3.4 United Kingdom—Scotland

The "Healthy Working Lives" award program (National Health Service, Health Scotland, 2017) supports employers and employees in implementing operational health management in a practical manner. After registering, companies can receive three different qualification levels (Bronze, Silver, and Gold).

The "Healthy Working Lives Award Program" is an agency of the National Health Service (NHS) and is thus under state aegis. The program is oriented towards results and applications.

First, a state profile is calculated through an online analysis. With this benchmark, action plans tailored to the company are developed. Appropriate progress is continuously measured and documented. In addition, a consultant of the agency navigates the company through the qualification program.

The distinction between the Bronze, Silver, and Gold levels of qualification is intended to encourage companies to continuously invest in the health of their employees. At the "Bronze" level, it is sufficient if the company is aware of the potential of Corporate Health Management. In addition, work safety programs must be implemented, which are always mandatory for industrial operators. Finally, a smoking ban must be established within the company.

At the Silver level, the company must already have established an integrated health policy. Guiding principles, processes, and case management are optimized according to Corporate Health Management measures. There are also preventive and intervention measures for the care of employees with stress symptoms. In addition to suitable care facilities for alcohol and drug abuse, behavioral programs must also be established to address nutrition, exercise, and relaxation issues.

The final Gold status is based on a company policy that is systematically oriented towards a healthy corporate culture. Participating companies must meet three obligatory, goal-oriented key criteria. A three-year action plan must be submitted to the agency. In addition, progress attributed to Corporate Health Management initiatives must be systematically documented and evaluated. Finally, problems for accessing Corporate Health Management services must be documented for all hierarchy levels. The company must also launch a focus program comprising a variety of measures.

6.3.5 The Netherlands

The Netherlands are known for a long tradition of programs that promote work safety, health protection, and health promotion. Two different Corporate Health Management labels are currently being awarded in the Netherlands. Since November 2016, a company can apply for the label "Gezond Bedrijf" ("Healthy enterprise"). The label is awarded by the "Healthy Netherlands Foundation" and can be purchased on an annual basis. To keep the label, each company has to re-apply. The focus for the label is on areas of health management, Corporate Health Management training, and medical check-ups (Keurmerk Gezond Bedrijf, 2017).

The "Nederlandse Organisatie voor toegepast" (TNO) is a national public body of the Netherlands. TNO annually awards projects that promote sustainable, healthy employability. The award "Kroon op het werk" ("Crown on your work") is a non-financially rewarded performance recognition assigned by an expert jury (Duurzame inzetbaarheid, 2017).

6.3.6 Germany

In Germany, there is a large number of organizations that award prizes and labels to healthy companies. What is striking about the German programs is that they have often been co-initiated by the government, but then implemented in cooperation with associations and company networks. This strategic orientation of public-private partnership seems ideal to us. In Switzerland, for example, such initiatives are much more difficult because they are seldom supported by public bodies.

The AOK-Leonardo, the Federal Association of the Health Insurer AOK awards digital programs and applications with prize money up to 25,000 Euros. The Federal Minister of Health sponsors the program. Their focus is on projects that combine health education with digital technologies. This will also open up prevention and health promotion-specific channels that have not been adequately covered so far, and will now also address the digitally-inclined Generation Y. In addition, projects are being awarded that promote health competences in general, and not only in company contexts (AOK Bundesverband, 2017).

The "employment and family-index" (berufundfamilie-Index) is an instrument with which companies can independently check the strengths and development potentials of their own personnel policy with regard to family awareness. This shows a German peculiarity because an active employment policy has been in force in Germany since the 1990s in favor of women who want to work part-time or full-time. In Germany, the establishment of family-friendly businesses is seen as an integral part of a health-promoting company. The profession and family index is a new management tool developed by FFP (Forschungszentrum Familienbewusste Personalpolitik), a research center focusing on family friendly HR policies. Here, too, government agencies and private non-profit foundations cooperated in the set-up of this organization. The project was commissioned by the berufundfamilie GmbH, an initiative of the Hertie Foundation, and is supported by the Federal Ministry for Family Affairs, Senior Citizens, Women, and Youth and financed through the European Social Fund.

The index value is determined by means of an online questionnaire and represents all three essential aspects of family awareness: dialogue between company management and employees, the implementation of company-specific family-friendly measures, and a family-conscious corporate culture. Company-specific factors are determined through a questionnaire that is relevant for the different dimensions of the family awareness (Berufundfamilie, 2017).

The "Corporate Health Award" ("Deutscher Unternehmenspreis Gesundheit") sees itself as "the leading quality initiative for sustainable Corporate Health Management". This is a program initiated by the private sector, which assigns the so-called Corporate Health Award by means of a multi-stage evaluation system. Audits have to be purchased.

The evaluation is based on validated quality criteria, which are supplemented by an expert opinion from an expert advisory board. The best participating companies have a chance to win the Corporate Health Award after completing the Corporate Health Audit. The audit results of the finalists are screened by an expert committee and a total of 15 winners are determined. In addition to funding the company's measures, the award is also used for employer branding. The application process consists of four stages, with the first three steps—application, benchmarking, and feedback—being free of charge. The fourth step, the expert assessment with recommendations for action, has to be paid (Corporate Health Award, 2017).

The German Association for Companies' Health Insurances (BKK-Dachverband, 2018) offers the so called "German Companies' Health Award" (Deutscher Unternehmenspreis Gesundheit). The Award is given to those companies that fully integrated Corporate Health Management into their strategy. The whole application and evaluation process is conducted online. Companies take an online survey of best practices. The award is given by a jury (BKK-Dachverband, 2018).

"Great Place to Work" is a for-profit private consulting firm focused on services providing Corporate Health Management programs. The company is active in 50 countries and measures employability, which can be estimated using employee surveys. The company's portfolio includes audits of measures and concepts of employee-oriented personnel and management work, as well as the development of health-promoting corporate cultures. Through international dissemination platforms, representatives from each country can access international Corporate Health Management databases and best practice pools. The best companies participating in the program will be recognized in an Awards Ceremony and through announced placements (Great Place to Work, 2017).

6.3.7 Austria

In Austria, a corporate management seal of approval exists. It is supported by a so-called Corporate Health Management network that, in good Austrian tradition, consists of public corporations and does not participate in any specific private enterprise networks. It is a federation of the State health insurance companies, the State accident insurance company, the main Austrian social insurance association, a number of social partners, and the "Austria Health Fund", which is taxpayer-funded. The network awards successfully completed Corporate Health Management projects, which applicants must submit. Participants' ranking and the decision to award the seal of approval are then considered by a jury. In case of a positive result, the company receives a seal of quality for three years. At the end of the three-year period, it may be requested again, with a re-examination being carried out. Here, too, the project is supported by the relevant ministry (Netzwerk BGF, 2018).

6.3.8 Switzerland

The Friendly Work Space label, issued by Health Promotion Switzerland (Gesundheitsförderung Schweiz, 2018), honors companies that have integrated Corporate Health Management into their corporate strategy and actively live it. Health Promotion Switzerland is a private foundation, which is mandated by the Swiss Confederation to foster health promotion and prevention programs.

Friendly Work Space comprises a criteria system for Corporate Health Management with six main criteria and a total of 26 sub-criteria. The concept can be explained upon the basis of this system of criteria. At the same time, it provides good support and guidelines for the introduction of Corporate Health Management in a company.

Renowned Swiss companies developed the criteria for the label in cooperation with Health Promotion Switzerland.

The six main criteria of the Friendly Work Space label are based on the six "Quality Criteria for Workplace Health Promotion" developed the European Network for

Workplace Health Promotion (European Network of Workplace Health Promotion, 1996), already described in a prior section.

- The first criterion, "Corporate Health Management and corporate policy", describes the prerequisites for Corporate Health Management on an organizational and strategic level: awareness of and attention to health must be anchored in corporate policy so that the planning and implementation of Corporate Health Management can be successful in the long term. Sufficient financial resources have to be guaranteed to set up a sustainable program.
- The second criterion, "Aspects of human resources management and work organization", describes the health-promoting design of the organization with a special focus on the processes and structures that characterize the relationship between the organization and its employees. For health promotion and maintenance to take place systematically, suitable structures must be established and maintained in the company. Accordingly, corresponding processes are also defined and implemented. Subjects include burnout prevention, leadership skills, absence management, reintegration, rehabilitation, and life-domain balance aspects.
- The third criterion encompasses the systematic planning of Corporate Health Management. It is recommended to employ a special Health Promotion Officer and create a Corporate Health Management steering committee.
- The fourth criterion deals with the social responsibility of the organization (Corporate Social Responsibility), which is understood here as part of Corporate Health Management, because only a company with a sustainable culture can substantially promote its employees' health.
- The fifth criterion describes the systematic implementation of specific Corporate Health Management measures. This is based on a survey of the current situation and the definition of targets and target groups.
- The sixth criterion comprises a systematic and regular evaluation of the whole Corporate Health Management System.

The combination of these six criteria forms the basis for systematic health promotion and prevention within the company. Only if all six levels are maintained simultaneously can a long-term and sustainable effect be achieved.

6.4 From Workplace Health Promotion to Systematic Corporate Health Management

Businesses that recognize the value of their employees' health for long-term company success address the issue systematically and have an institutional health policy.

The company health policy defines the fundamental values, standards, and principles of company health management. It structures and legitimizes the definition and implementation of measures to promote and maintain health. Company health policy makes the health of employees a matter of course.

The view that the improvement of employees' resources (in the above example, appreciation) has a positive influence on performance and willingness to perform, and thus on the reduction of absences and the improvement of productivity, can be tested at a higher level. Surveys of the Health Promotion Switzerland Job Stress Index appear to confirm these observations.

6.5 Concluding Remarks

Schools that want to succeed in the area of Corporate Health Management do not only ask themselves what can be done to prevent illness. They also ask themselves what can be done to improve health (according to the salutogenetic approach of Aaron Antonovsky; cf. Antonovsky, 1987). The answer often lies in the social relations between employees and concerns issues of appreciation and participation in important company decisions.

However, the behavior of each individual employee is decisive for his or her health. Responsibility for one's own health cannot be shifted to the company. Nevertheless, it is worthwhile for the organization to implement health-promoting measures, because employee health problems always have a negative impact on the company. It is crucial for companies to create the conditions for health-promoting behavior. In this way, the organization encourages employees' autonomy regarding health-related decisions in their daily work and often also in their private lives. At the same time, the company improves its own health in terms of competitiveness.

References

Antonovsky, A. (1987). *Unraveling the mystery of health. How people manage stress and stay well.* San Francisco: Jossey-Bass.

AOK Bundesverband. (2017). *AOK Leonardo.* http://www.aok-leonardo.de/. Accessed January 12, 2019.

Berufundfamilie. (2017). *Berufundfamilie-Index.* http://www.berufundfamilie-index.de. Accessed January 12, 2019.

BKK-Dachverband. (2018). *Deutscher Unternehmerpreis Gesundheit.* http://www.deutscher-unternehmenspreis-gesundheit.de. Accessed January 12, 2019.

Corporate Health Award. (2017). *Corporate Health Award.* http://www.corporate-health-award.de. Accessed January 12, 2019.

Duurzame Inzetbaarheid. (2017). *Duurzame.* http://www.duurzaaminjewerk.nl/343_kroon-op-het-werk. Accessed January 12, 2019.

Eichel, V., Dloughy, K., Schmitz, D., & Braun, O. (2013). Kleines Siegel, grosse Wirkung. Fachbeiträge der Personalarbeit. *MW online.* https://www.dgfp.de/wissen/personalwissen-direkt/dokument/91038. Accessed January 12, 2019.

European Network of Workplace Health Promotion. (1996). *Work. In tune with life.* http://www.enwhp.org/about-enwhp.html. Accessed January 19, 2019.

Gesundheitsförderung Schweiz. (2018). *Friendly Workspace.* https://friendlyworkspace.ch/. Accessed January 12, 2019.

Great Place to Work. (2017). *Better for Business. Better for People. Better for the World*, San Francisco. https://www.greatplacetowork.com. Accessed January 12, 2019.

Jennings, P., Brown, J., Frank, J., Doyle, S., Oh, Y., Davis, R., et al. (2017). Impacts of the CARE for teachers program on teachers' social and emotional competence and classroom interactions. *Journal of Educational Psychology, 109*(7), 1010–1028.

Keurmerk Gezond Bedrijf. (2017). *Keurmerk Gezond Bedrijf.* http://keurmerkgezondbedrijf.nl/. Accessed January 12, 2019.

Landstad, B., Hedlund, M., & Vinberg, S. (2017). How managers of small-scale enterprises can create a health promoting corporate culture. *International Journal of Workplace Health Management, 10*(3), 228–248.

Luxembourg Declaration on Workplace Health Promotion in the European Union. (2007). http://www.mentalhealthpromotion.net/resources/luxembourg-declaration.pdf. Accessed July 6, 2019.

Mattig, T., & Weber, L. (2016a). Betriebliches Gesundheitsmanagement heute. In V. Schulte & A. H. Verkuil (Eds.), *Management für Health Professionals* (pp. 153–162). Bern: Hogrefe.

Mattig, T., & Weber, L. (2016b). Betriebliches Gesundheitsmanagement im Krankenhaus. In W. Hellmann (Ed.), *Herausforderung Krankenhausmanagement* (pp. 181–192). Bern: Hogrefe.

National Health Service, Health Scotland. (2017). *Healthy Working Lives.* http://www.healthyworkinglives.com/. Accessed January 12, 2019.

Netzwerk BGF Austria. (2018). *Netzwerk Betriebliche Gesundheitsförderung.* https://www.netzwerk-bgf.at/cdscontent/?contentid=10007.701055&viewmode=content. Accessed January 12, 2019.

Radix. (2018). *RADIX Gesunde Schulen.* https://www.radix.ch/Gesunde-Schulen/PIlJV/. Accessed January 12, 2019.

Scheil-Adlung, X., & Kuhl, C. (2011). *Social security for all. Addressing inequities in access to health care for vulnerable groups in countries of Europe and Central Asia.* Geneva: ILO.

Schulte, V., & Verkuil, A. (Eds.). (2016). *Management für Health Professionals.* Bern: Hogrefe.

Chapter 7
Mindfulness as a Path Towards Sustainable Lifestyle Change, Resilience, and Well-Being: Community, Social, and Environmental Factors

Giuseppe Carrus and Angelo Panno

Abstract Recent developments in psychological theory and research offer arguments that help to promote a transition towards sustainable lifestyles. Based on these insights, we outline how the concept of mindfulness could be a key psychological mechanism to understand this process and provide arguments supporting this assumption. To illustrate this line of reasoning, we introduce the dual-process accounts of human decision making, as this theory provides support for a conceptual model linking mindfulness to more sustainable lifestyles, increased well-being, and resilience in daily life settings. Specifically, we argue that the mindfulness-based model of pro-environmental behavior and sustainable lifestyle presented in this article could be particularly well suited to contemporary adolescents and younger generations in general, as they might represent the ideal target of large-scale environmental awareness raising and education programs in today's digital society. In our theoretical proposal, mindfulness could thus be key to promoting adolescents' shift towards more sustainable, less consumption-based, and more nature-connected lifestyles that are also less carbon-intensive. Both the community and the physical settings could offer positive support in this transition.

Keywords Ecosystem · Sustainability · Sustainable lifestyle · Well-being · Values

7.1 Introduction

Ecosystems are under considerable pressure, as most of humanity is enjoying greater prosperity in more areas than ever before. The Millennium Ecosystem Assessment (https://www.millenniumassessment.org/en/index.html), examining the state of global ecosystems and the consequences of ecosystem change for human well-being from 2001 to 2005, found that 60% of these were degraded or being used in an unsustainable way. "Over the past 50 years, humans have changed ecosystems more rapidly and extensively than in any comparable period of time in human history, largely to meet rapidly growing demands for food, fresh water, timber, fiber

G. Carrus (✉) · A. Panno
Department of Education, Roma Tre University, Rome, Italy
e-mail: giuseppe.carrus@uniroma3.it

C. Steinebach and Á. I. Langer (eds.), *Enhancing Resilience in Youth*,
https://doi.org/10.1007/978-3-030-25513-8_7

and fuel. This resulted in a substantial and largely irreversible loss in the diversity of life on Earth" (Secretariat of the Convention on Biological Diversity, 2010, p. 94). The impact of climate change is now rapidly increasing in all ecosystems, changing human habitats. Apart from some minority positions of scepticism and denial (e.g. Carrus, Panno, & Leone, 2018), there currently is a wide scientific, political, and public opinion consensus that ecosystems, and human beings therein, must adapt to a global warming on top of their already weakened resilience. The implementation of solutions to address this issue is thus urgently needed. We would have to reduce the impact of our activities on the earth as the overconsumption of resources underlies all human activities, and this consumption will become more intense as middle-class consumers across the developing world now become increasingly numerous. Although the IPCC (2000) claimed that technological changes can significantly help reduce pollution, greater efforts to change human behaviour are needed, which should be aimed at using resources sustainably and reducing overconsumption, among other environmental goals.

Some authors argue that a transition to sustainability requires a "shift from materialist to post-materialist values, from anthropocentric to ecological world-views" (Leiserowitz, Kates, & Parris, 2005, p. 30); i.e. the problem is linked to "how we ought to live, and how humans should relate to each other and to the rest of nature" (Jamieson, 1992, p. 149). Unfortunately, a tradeoff between well-being and the environment has always been shown as a potential conflict, because of a shared common sense notion that the means to achieve well-being are exclusively materialistic rewards; therefore, to date, many assume that huge sacrifices have to be made to encourage change toward less material consumption and to foster a more sustainable way of life.

In this chapter, we argue how recent developments in psychological theory and research could offer arguments that challenge this straightforward assumption, while also helping promote a transition towards sustainable lifestyles. More specifically, we outline how the concept of mindfulness could be a key psychological mechanism to understand this process and provide arguments supporting this assumption. To illustrate this line of reasoning, the dual-process accounts of human decision making will also be shortly introduced, as this theory provides support for our conceptual model linking mindfulness to more sustainable lifestyles, increased well-being and resilience in daily life settings. We argue, in particular, that our mindfulness-based model of pro-environmental behaviour and sustainable lifestyle could be particularly well suited to contemporary adolescents and younger generations in general, as they might represent the ideal target of large-scale environmental awareness raising and education programs in today's digital society. In our theoretical proposal, mindfulness could thus be key to promoting adolescents' shift towards more sustainable, less consumption-based, and more nature-connected lifestyles that are also less carbon-intensive. Both the community and the physical settings could offer positive support in this transition.

In this chapter, we review an overarching theoretical framework developed in social cognitive psychology, namely the dual-process accounts of human decision making, which sees people's behaviour as an interplay between an automatic, impulsive, or "hot" mental system and another that is reasoned, reflexive, or "cold". Then, we discuss how a mindfulness-based psychological model can be useful to improve our understanding of the mechanisms governing the transition towards a sustainable way of life at the level of individuals, groups, and communities. Applied implications for future studies and interventions to promote sustainable lifestyle changes among young people and adolescents will be also envisaged.

7.2 Dual-Process Accounts: A Theoretical Framework to Understand Human Behaviour and Foster Environmentally-Relevant Behaviour

Sigmund Freud and other 20th century psychoanalysts introduced the notion of an unconscious mind motivating our behavior with a combination of innate drives and repressed emotions alongside a conscious mind prone to rationalization and "self-deception" (Freud, 1912). About two decades earlier, James (1890) had already put forward the idea of the automaticity of certain human cognitive processes. Within psychology, these could be regarded as the first explicit attempts to understand human behaviour through the lens of a dual-processes account. In present-day psychological science, dual-processing accounts explaining human behavior have risen sharply in the literature over the last 30 years, especially in cognitive and social psychology (e.g. Bargh & Chartrand, 1999; Fazio & Towles-Schwen, 1999; Kahneman, 2002; Strack & Deutsch, 2004). Given the aims of our study, we will try to explain what a dual-processes account is and what dual-process theories have in common, while also outlining how these accounts can be related to the link between mindfulness and sustainable lifestyles. The idea behind dual-process theories is that there are two different modes of mental processing, for which we use the terms "*hot*" and "*cold*" (Keren & Schul, 2009). According to these and other authors, mental characteristics like unconscious (or preconscious), implicit, automatic, effortless, rapid, holistic perceptual, associative, and parallel thinking can be associated with hot processes, while characteristics like conscious, explicit, controlled, effortful, slow, analytic reflective, rule based, and sequential thinking can be associated with cold processes.

Authors in this field agree on a distinction between processes that are unconscious, rapid, automatic, and high capacity (i.e. hot), and those that are conscious, slow, and deliberative (i.e. cold). Some authors ignore emotion altogether, but it should be clear that emotional and motivational factors belong to the hot rather than the cold system (Evans, 2003). Studies linking dual process accounts to decision making, such as Kahneman and Tversky's (1982) seminal research, are particularly useful for improving our understanding of sustainable lifestyles, since pro-environmental behavior is an outcome of human decision-making capacity.

To understand how dual-processes accounts can influence sustainable lifestyles and their relation to mindfulness, we need to point out some individual differences linked to the hot and cold system, as individual differences related to dual process accounts may be also linked to environmentally friendly behaviour. There are some person-based factors that could make the hot system prevail over the cold system and vice versa, such as general intelligence and working memory resources. In general, a strong basis for dual-systems theories is the evidence that "controlled" cognitive processing correlates with individual differences in general intelligence and working memory capacity, whereas "automatic" processing does not. Since human behaviour is an outcome of the interaction between cold and hot processes, it then seems that individuals' behaviour may be controlled both with and without the use of executive working memory resources. This aspect is particularly relevant to our discussion, since later we will see in more detail how present-centred attention and mindfulness could represent a driver of more environmentally aware behaviour, while automaticity, impulsive, and immediate materialistic reward-seeking action could undermine pro-environmental behavior and be less environmentally friendly.

There are also specific situational factors which can make the hot system prevail over the cold system. One of them is time pressure. For example, several circumstances where time pressure occurs (e.g. an impending deadline) might trigger automatic impulses, overriding the cold system. Time pressure has also been found to be a factor capable of triggering specific cognitive motivational states known as "need for cognitive closure" (see Webster & Kruglanski, 1994, for more details). Recent empirical evidence indeed shows that higher levels of need for cognitive closure can be linked to less pro-environmental behavior (Panno, Carrus, et al., 2018). People in their everyday lives strongly show the capacity to self-regulate to overcome the impulses resulting from the hot system, which induce us in well known temptations such as overeating, overconsumption, using illicit drugs and alcohol, and engaging in unprotected sex (e.g. Steel, 2007; Tice & Bratslavsky, 2000). This human capacity to exert control over the hot system through the predominance of the cold system is needed to delay gratification of immediate desires (Metcalfe & Mischel, 1999; Mischel, Shoda, & Rodriguez, 1989) and enables people to engage in goal-directed behaviour to bring about long-term desirable outcomes (Baumeister, 2005; Logue, 1988). The mechanism behind this relationship is that the time pressure rapidly uses up cognitive resources, making people less likely to act in an environmentally friendly way. Thus, we suggest that time pressure can be regarded as a factor that drains cognitive resources needed to behave in an environmentally friendly way. We argue that self-regulation mechanisms are crucial in this processes, and we will discuss how mindfulness could represent a positive psychological factor driving more sustainable and environmentally-aware choices in everyday life. For example, we can consider the fact that people often do not use recycled paper to print documents if an impending deadline is coming. Also, an array of activities carried out under time pressure conditions could make people more likely to engage in environmentally damaging behaviors, because some of these behaviors are thought to be restorative (e.g. compulsive shopping, overeating). On the other hand, one may delay immediate gratification by using public transport instead of driving one's car in order to get less pollution in the future. Indeed, recent studies suggest that both mindfulness and emotion regulation strategies, such as cognitive reappraisal, could help buffer this negative tendency (e.g. Panno, Carrus, Maricchiolo, & Mannetti, 2015; Panno,

Giacomantonio, et al., 2018). We will discuss these arguments in more detail in the next section, where we outline a conceptual model for sustainable mindfulness-based lifestyles.

7.3 Mindfulness to Foster Sustainable Lifestyle Change

In the following paragraph, we review empirical research that has shown how the psychological construct of mindfulness can help enhance adolescents' strength in the pursuit of sustainable lifestyles and well-being.

The concept of mindfulness has roots in Buddhist religion and other spiritual and contemplative traditions, where conscious attention and awareness are actively cultivated. It is most commonly defined as the state of being attentive to and aware of what is taking place in the present. For instance, Nyanaponika Thera (1972) called mindfulness "the clear and single-minded awareness of what actually happens to us and in us at the successive moments of perception" (p. 5). Empirical research has shown that the enhancement of mindfulness by training facilitates a number of well-being outcomes such as overcoming health-related problems (Kabat-Zinn, 1990). Because mindfulness bears some relation to other constructs that have received empirical attention, such as emotional intelligence, which includes perceptual clarity about one's emotional states (Salovey, Mayer, Goldman, Turvey, & Palfai, 1995), one should expect that mindfulness to be related to such clarity as it involves receptive attention to human psychological states and environmental stimuli.

Conversely, in less mindful states, emotions may partly occur outside of individual awareness or drive our behaviour before we clearly acknowledge them (Brown & Ryan, 2003). This process typically occurs when the hot system overrides the cold system. Mindfulness captures a quality of consciousness that is characterized by the clarity and vividness of the current experience and functioning. By contrast, the mindless state represents a less "awake" level of habitual or automatic functioning that can be chronic for many people. By adding clarity and vividness to common human experience, mindfulness may also contribute to well-being and happiness in a direct way. Relevant to environmentally responsible activities, mindfulness may play an important role in disengaging individuals from strong unsustainable habits and unhealthy behavioural patterns, thus fostering people's self-regulation, which has long been associated with well-being enhancement (Ryan & Deci, 2000). In other words, mindfulness might serve an important self-regulatory function which can at the same time foster people's sustainable lifestyles (e.g. Brown & Kasser, 2005) and be associated with children positive social adjustment and resilience (Eisenberg et al., 2003).

Mindfulness-based studies on pro-environmental behaviors and sustainable lifestyles outnumber those that follow other theoretical accounts that we have briefly described in previous sections (e.g. Brown & Kasser, 2005; Ericson, Kjønstad, & Barstad, 2014; Fischer, Stanszus, Geiger, Grossman, & Schrader, 2017; Geiger, Otto, & Schrader, 2018; Geiger, Grossman, & Schrader, 2019; Howell, Dopko, Passmore,

& Buro, 2011; Panno, Giacomantonio, et al., 2018). Recently, Ericson and colleagues showed that encouraging mindfulness practice in schools, workplaces, and elsewhere could contribute to more sustainable ways of life and promote well-being (Ericson et al., 2014). The proposed mechanism behind this link rests on the notion that mindfulness is strongly related to psychological well-being (PWB), which in turn is linked to sustainability through seeking gratification by means other than material rewards. As we have already mentioned, health resources are also under pressure because of our excessive levels of material consumption. Thus, seeking PWB through means different from material consumption could greatly contribute to global sustainability, and mindfulness can play a key role in this relationship. To corroborate these relationships among mindfulness, PWB, and environmentally friendly behaviours, we can also refer to studies showing strong associations among connectedness to nature, well-being, and mindfulness (Howell et al., 2011). Empirical evidence suggests that human health and well-being are associated with the possibility of repeated and systematic experiences of nature (e.g. Mitchell & Popham, 2008; Van den Berg, Hartig, & Staats, 2007; see also Carrus, Passiatore, Pirchio, & Scopelliti, 2015; Carrus et al., 2017). Thus, one could also claim that strong connectedness to nature can foster PWB through mindfulness by enhancing the positive emotions and perceptions that humans feel when experiencing contact with the natural world. In present-day human societies, a more generalized mindful consideration of one's inner states and behaviour should then be likely to bring simultaneous benefits to both individuals and ecosystems.

Regarding the idea of mindfulness as a tool to promote more sustainable lifestyles in adolescence, it is important to come back to the issue that we briefly discussed in the beginning of this chapter: the shared common sense assumption that sustainable behaviors do necessarily entail negative outcomes for the individual, such as self-sacrifice, discomfort, fatigue, or economic costs. Recently, several authors have started to question this straightforward assumption, suggesting that sustainable conducts might also represent a form of intrinsic reward for the individual (e.g. Bechtel & Corral, 2010; De Young, 2000; Veenhoven, 2006). For example, Brown and Kasser (2005) found that PWB and pro-environmental behaviours are complementary, as happier people live in more ecologically sustainable ways. The authors identified mindfulness as the core factor that promoted both happiness and ERB: "These results weigh against the oft-stated belief that personal well-being and ecologically supportive behaviour are necessarily in conflict, and instead suggest that a trade-off between the two is not a *fait accompli*" (Brown & Kasser, 2005, pp. 360–361). Thus, even though human happiness and ecological well-being are often portrayed as conflictual pursuits by consumption economics, they may be viewed as complementary by sustainable economics. We argue that promoting a stronger awareness of the compatibility between well-being and pro-environmental behaviours, through mindfulness, could be a crucial message to encourage sustainable lifestyles among adolescents.

The link between income, well-being, and sustainable lifestyles is also a relevant issue to discuss here. A problem associated with increases in material goods and income is that their effects on PWB seem to be rather short-lived, since people soon become accustomed to a given level of material welfare. This phenomenon of habituation and adaptation to the circumstances of life is called the "*hedonic treadmill effect*" (see Seligman, 2002, for more details). Thus, an interesting aspect of mindfulness is that mindfulness-based training techniques could be useful to undo the hedonic treadmill effect (Fredrickson, Cohn, Coffey, Pek, & Finkel, 2008). Mental training techniques aimed at improving mindfulness could have important applied implications, as many people could enhance their awareness of global ecosystems' resources and pursue PWB without falling prey to the hedonic treadmill effect. This suggests that policy makers should incentive collective programs aimed at fostering mindfulness-based interventions and practice.

To summarize, in our view mindfulness can make people's lifestyle more sustainable through two paths, as depicted in Fig. 7.1. First, mindfulness dampens the hedonic treadmill effect, which allows people to enhance PWB without focusing on material rewards and adopting a more sustainable lifestyle, in line with their outlook. Second, mindfulness leads to PWB through greater empathy and connectedness with nature, which are known to be relevant predictors of environmentally relevant behaviours (ERB). Indeed, there is empirical evidence showing a link between empathy for natural beings, positive attitudes towards nature, and pro-environmental behaviour (e.g. Berenguer, 2007). In both cases, a more habitual use of more environmentally aware and mindful strategies in daily life decisions can be expected to lead to a more sustainable lifestyle.

With respect to the relationship between mindfulness and sustainability, it is also worth pointing out that a mindfulness-based lifestyle may counteract unsustainable habits triggered by situational factors, such as time pressure. Specifically, the usual daily life experience shared by many citizens in western societies, characterized by increasing feelings of time scarcity (e.g. Wajcman, 2008) and the desire to quickly obtain material rewards, can be regarded as supporting a view of life that has no space or time for environmentally friendly habits. Accordingly, a mindfulness-based lifestyle might slacken impulses and block out the urges related to time pressure. This, in turn, should be reflected in the development of more sustainable habits in the long run. Indeed, recent studies on adolescents suggest that time affluence could

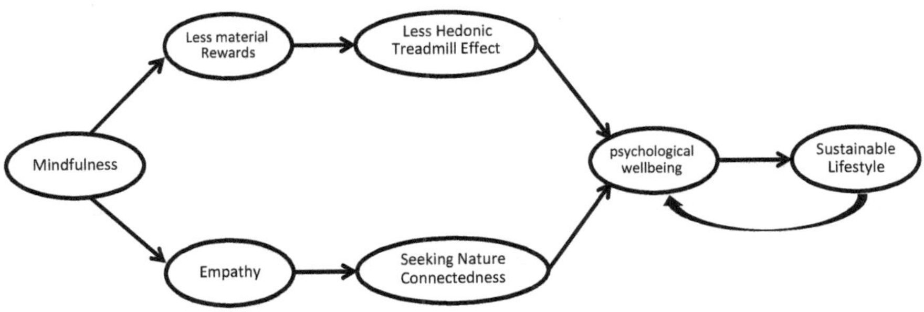

Fig. 7.1 Conceptual two-path model of the relationship between mindfulness, psychological well-being (PWB), and sustainable lifestyle

help in buffering the negative link between materialistic and compulsive consumption and well-being (e.g. Manolis & Roberts, 2012).

Abramovitz (2003) also pointed out that material consumption levels are rising worldwide and that, consequently, human quality of life may be at risk. Consistent with this idea, previous studies (e.g. Brown & Kasser, 2005; Ericson et al., 2014) show that achieving sustainable societies will mean scaling back on our material lives. Yet, convincing people to live in more ecologically sustainable ways will be challenging if they believe that their PWB will suffer. Taken together, the results of these studies are hopeful in pointing to a mutually beneficial relation between personal and planetary well-being, especially given that such supportive factors as mindfulness and intrinsic values can be cultivated among younger generations. In sum, one might claim that, in today's consumerism-prone culture, mindfulness may be necessary to develop more sustainable habits among young people and adolescents. Three billion more middle-class consumers will enter the market during the next 20 years, which will further increase the global consumption of the earth's resources. If billions of people across the world hold materialistic values, making perceived well-being heavily dependent on material consumption, it will be hard to achieve sustainable development goals. Global sustainability will be more easily achieved if well-being is pursued through means that are less dependent on material consumption. Preliminary environmental psychological research indicates that mindfulness is a fruitful path that may help enhance environmentally friendly activities as well as sustainable lifestyles.

There are, however, many things we do not know in this field of inquiry, especially as regards the effects that this change in attitude can have on sustainability. Long-term consequences in terms of environmental behaviour, political activism (or alienation), and lifestyle have seldom been explored in systematic experimental settings. Another question is how easy it is to sustain mindfulness meditation over time, and what role training plays in developing and sustaining the practice, especially among adolescents. To address these issues, longitudinal studies, both quantitative and qualitative, are needed. Last but not least, the practical feasibility of direct mindfulness training programs on large sectors of present-day adolescents should also be explored, as this can represent a barrier to concrete and cost-effective large–scale policy implementations.

References

Abramovitz, J. (2003). *Vital signs 2003: The trends that are shaping our future*. New York: W. W. Norton.

Bargh, J. A., & Chartrand, T. L. (1999). The unbearable automaticity of being. *American Psychologist, 54*(7), 462.

Baumeister, R. F. (2005). *The cultural animal: Human nature, meaning, and social life*. New York: Oxford University Press.

Bechtel, R. B., & Corral, V. (2010). Happiness and sustainable behavior. In V. Corral, C. García, & M. Frías (Eds.), *Psychological approaches to sustainability*. New York: Nova Science Publishers.

Berenguer, J. (2007). The effect of empathy in proenvironmental attitudes and behaviors. *Environment and Behavior, 39*(2), 269–283.
Brown, K. W., & Kasser, T. (2005). Are psychological and ecological well-being compatible? The role of values, mindfulness, and lifestyle. *Social Indicators Research, 74*(2), 349–368.
Brown, K. W., & Ryan, R. M. (2003). The benefits of being present: Mindfulness and its role in psychological well-being. *Journal of Personality and Social Psychology, 84*(4), 822.
Carrus, G., Panno, A., & Leone, L. (2018). The moderating role of interest in politics on the relations between conservative political orientation and denial of climate change. *Society & Natural Resources, 31*(10), 1103–1117. https://doi.org/10.1080/08941920.2018.1463422.
Carrus, G., Passiatore, Y., Pirchio, S., & Scopelliti, M. (2015). Contact with nature in educational settings might help cognitive functioning and promote positive social behavior. *Psyecology, 6*(2), 191–212.
Carrus, G., Scopelliti, M., Panno, A., Lafortezza, R., Colangelo, G., Pirchio, S., et al. (2017). A different way to stay in touch with 'urban nature': The perceived restorative qualities of botanical gardens. *Frontiers in Psychology, 8*, 914.
De Young, R. (2000). Expanding and evaluating motives for environmentally responsible behavior. *Journal of Social Issues, 56*, 509–526.
Eisenberg, N., Valiente, C., Fabes, R. A., Smith, C. L., Reiser, M., Shepard, S. A., et al. (2003). The relations of effortful control and ego control to children's resiliency and social functioning. *Developmental Psychology, 39*, 761–776.
Ericson, T., Kjønstad, B. G., & Barstad, A. (2014). Mindfulness and sustainability. *Ecological Economics, 104*, 73–79.
Evans, J. S. B. (2003). In two minds: dual-process accounts of reasoning. *Trends in cognitive sciences, 7*(10), 454–459.
Fazio, R. H., & Towles-Schwen, T. (1999). The MODE model of attitude-behavior processes. In S. Chaiken & Y. Trope (Eds.), *Dual process theories in social psychology* (pp. 97–116). New York: Guilford Press.
Fischer, D., Stanszus, L., Geiger, S., Grossman, P., & Schrader, U. (2017). Mindfulness and sustainable consumption: A systematic literature review of research approaches and findings. *Journal of Cleaner Production, 162*, 544–558.
Fredrickson, B. L., Cohn, M. A., Coffey, K. A., Pek, J., & Finkel, S. M. (2008). Open hearts build lives: Positive emotions, induced through loving-kindness meditation, build consequential personal resources. *Journal of Personality and Social Psychology, 95*(5), 1045.
Freud, S. (1963). Recommendations for physicians on the psycho-analytic method of treatment. In P. Reiff (Ed.), *Freud: Therapy and technique* (pp. 117–126). New York: Collier. (Original work published 1912).
Geiger, S. M., Grossman, P., & Schrader, U. (2019). Mindfulness and sustainability: Correlation or causation? *Current Opinion in Psychology, 28*, 23–27.
Geiger, S. M., Otto, S., & Schrader, U. (2018). Mindfully green and healthy: An indirect path from mindfulness to ecological behavior. *Frontiers in Psychology – Environmental Psychology, 8*, 2306. https://doi.org/10.3389/fpsyg.2017.02306.
Howell, A. J., Dopko, R. L., Passmore, H. A., & Buro, K. (2011). Nature connectedness: Associations with well-being and mindfulness. *Personality and Individual Differences, 51*(2), 166–171.
IPCC. (2000). *IPCC Special Report on Emissions Scenarios*. SRES, Technical Summary.
James, W. (1890/1950). *The principles of psychology* (Vol. 1, Authorized ed.). New York: Dover.
Jamieson, D. (1992). Ethics, public policy, and global warming. *Science Technology Human Values, 17*, 139–153.
Kabat-Zinn, J. (1990). *Full catastrophe living: Using the wisdom of your body and mind to face stress, pain, and illness*. New York: Delacourt.
Kahneman, D. (2002). Maps of bounded rationality: A perspective on intuitive judgment and choice. *Nobel Prize Lecture, 8*, 351–401.
Kahneman, D., & Tversky, A. (1982). The psychology of preferences. *Scientific American, 246*, 160–173.

Keren, G., & Schul, Y. (2009). Two is not always better than one. A critical evaluation of Two-System Theories. *Perspectives on psychological science*, *4*(6), 533–550.
Leiserowitz, A. A., Kates, R. W., & Parris, T. M. (2005). Do global attitudes and behaviors support sustainable development? *Environment, 47*(9), 28–38.
Logue, A. W. (1988). Research on self-control: An integrating framework. *Behavioral and Brain Sciences, 11,* 665–709.
Manolis, C., & Roberts, J. A. (2012). Subjective well-being among adolescent consumers: The effects of materialism, compulsive buying, and time affluence. *Applied Research in Quality of Life, 7*(2), 117–135.
Metcalfe, J., & Mischel, W. (1999). A hot/cool-system analysis of delay of gratification: Dynamics of willpower. *Psychological Review, 106*(1), 3.
Mischel, W., Shoda, Y., & Rodriguez, M. I. (1989). Delay of gratification in children. *Science, 244*(4907), 933–938.
Mitchell, R., & Popham, F. (2008). Effect of exposure to natural environment on health inequalities: An observational population study. *The Lancet, 372*, 1655–1660.
Nyanaponika Thera. (1972). *The power of mindfulness*. San Francisco, CA: Unity Press.
Panno, A., Carrus, G., Brizi, A., Maricchiolo, F., Giacomantonio, M., & Mannetti, L. (2018). Need for cognitive closure and political ideology: Predicting pro-environmental preferences and behavior. *Social Psychology, 49,* 103–112. https://doi.org/10.1027/1864-9335/a000333.
Panno, A., Carrus, G., Maricchiolo, F., & Mannetti, L. (2015). Cognitive reappraisal and pro-environmental behavior: The role of global climate change perception. *European Journal of Social Psychology, 45*(7), 858–867.
Panno, A., Giacomantonio, M., Carrus, G., Maricchiolo, F., Pirchio, S., & Mannetti, L. (2018). Mindfulness, pro-environmental behavior, and belief in climate change: The mediating role of social dominance. *Environment and Behavior, 50*(8), 864–888. https://doi.org/10.1177/0013916517718887.
Ryan, R. M., & Deci, E. L. (2000). Self-determination theory and the facilitation of intrinsic motivation, social development, and well-being. *American Psychologist, 55,* 68–78.
Salovey, P., Mayer, J. D., Goldman, S. L., Turvey, C., & Palfai, T. F. (1995). Emotional attention, clarity, and repair: Exploring emotional intelligence using the Trait Meta-Mood Scale. In J. W. Pennebaker (Ed.), *Emotion, disclosure, and health* (pp. 125–154). Washington, DC: American Psychological Association.
Secretariat of the Convention on Biological Diversity. (2010). *Global Biodiversity Outlook 3*. Montréal: Secretariat of the Convention on Biological Diversity. https://www.cbd.int/doc/publications/gbo/gbo3-final-en.pdf. Accessed January 18, 2019.
Seligman, M. E. P. (2002). *Authentic happiness*. New York: Free Press.
Steel, P. (2007). The nature of procrastination: A meta-analytic and theoretical review of quintessential self-regulatory failure. *Psychological Bulletin, 133*(1), 65–83.
Strack, F., & Deutsch, R. (2004). Reflective and impulsive determinants of social behavior. *Personality and Social Psychology Review, 8*(3), 220–247.
Tice, D. M., & Bratslavsky, E. (2000). Giving into feel good: The place of emotion regulation in the context of general self-control. *Psychological Inquiry, 11*(3), 149–159.
Van den Berg, A. E., Hartig, T., & Staats, H. (2007). Preference for nature in urbanized societies: Stress, restoration, and the pursuit of sustainability. *Journal of Social Issues, 63,* 79–96.
Veenhoven, R. (2006). Is life getting better? How long and happy people live in modern society. *European Psychologist, 10,* 330–343.
Wajcman, J. (2008). Life in the fast lane? Towards a sociology of technology and time. *The British Journal of Sociology, 59*(1), 59–77.
Webster, D. M., & Kruglanski, A. W. (1994). Individual differences in need for cognitive closure. *Journal of Personality and Social Psychology, 67*(6), 1049–1062.

Part III
Interventions for Enhancing Resilience: Mindfulness and Peer Relations

Chapter 8
Recommendations for Mindfulness Interventions in the Educational Context

Matías Irarrázaval

Abstract Significant clinical problems in children are affecting academic achievement. One of the most important and influential factors is sustained stress in and outside of school. Excessive or sustained stress without the mechanisms to manage it properly impacts the brain structures involved in cognition and emotion regulation in a developing brain. As a consequence, academic performance can be diminished and mental disorders are more likely to occur, especially in children and adolescents who have risk factors and socio-environmental determinants for illness. The application of mindfulness-based interventions (MBIs) with children and adolescents is a newly evolving field, and has become increasingly popular in recent years, both in research and practice. In this chapter, several reviews and meta-analyses are included, which show that mindfulness-based interventions are effective in healthy individuals and for a wide range of stress related and clinical problems. A key feature of contemplative practices is that they represent forms of mental training that cultivate more positive habits of mind by incorporating repetition and practice exercises. Thus, mindfulness is well aligned with the neuroscientific understanding of how new connections are formed in the brain and how regular mental practice influences brain circuits and complex cognitive function. Research exploring the determinants of meditation practice for adolescents can provide school health programs with critical knowledge when developing and implementing future initiatives that promote at-home practice, thus optimizing their effects.

Keywords Brain structures · Attentional problems · Mindfulness programs · Standards · Implementation

---

M. Irarrázaval (✉)
Department of Mental Health, Ministry of Health, Santiago, Chile
e-mail: mirarrazavald@uchile.cl

Millennium Institute for Research in Depression and Personality, Santiago, Chile

Department of Psychiatry, University of Chile, Santiago, Chile

C. Steinebach and Á. I. Langer (eds.), *Enhancing Resilience in Youth*,
https://doi.org/10.1007/978-3-030-25513-8_8

8.1 Introduction

Nowadays, teachers and schools are faced with the task of not only delivering a formal education, but also considering the mental health and well-being of children. Academic achievement, social and emotional competence and physical and mental health are inter-related and must be addressed together. Significant clinical problems in children are worrying and affecting academic achievement (Card & Hodges, 2008; Currie et al., 2004). One of the most important and influential factors is sustained stress in and outside of school (Lupien, McEwen, Gunnar, & Heim, 2009). Excessive or sustained stress without the mechanism to manage it properly impacts the brain structures involved in cognition and emotion regulation in a developing brain. As a consequence, academic performance can be diminished and mental disorders are more likely to occur, especially in children and adolescents who have risk factors and socio-environmental determinants for illness (Chen & Baram, 2016; Evans & Schamberg, 2009). It has been reported that 21% of young people aged 13–18 in the United States are currently suffering, or have at some point during their life, suffered from a mental disorder, with ADHD, conduct disorder, anxiety and depression as the most prevalent diagnoses (Merikangas et al., 2010; Perou et al., 2013).

Since many children and youth exhibit learning, behavioral and attentional problems that are stress-sensitive or stress-induced, the school setting offers an ideal environment for using interventions that promote healthy brain development and function. It is for this reason, and because of the convenience of conducting low-cost interventions in a setting where young people spend much of their time, that schools have become one of the most important settings for health promotion and preventive interventions among children and adolescents (Weare & Nind, 2011). These needs have driven educators, teachers, and psychologists to seek novel ways to improve academic outcomes, but also well-being and healthy development at schools.

The application of mindfulness-based interventions (MBIs) with children and adolescents is a newly evolving field, and has become increasingly popular in recent years, both in research and practice. Research in mindfulness is still in early stages and stems largely from clinical studies with adults. However, initial reviews suggest that mindfulness-based interventions are feasible with children and adolescents, and some of them have demonstrated beneficial in both clinical and non-clinical samples (Black, Milam, & Sussman, 2009; Burke, 2010). In this chapter, several reviews and meta-analyses are included, which show that mindfulness-based interventions are effective in healthy individuals (Chiesa & Serretti, 2009; Khoury, Sharma, Rush, & Fournier, 2015) and for a wide range of stress related and clinical problems (Fjorback, Arendt, Ornbøl, Fink, & Walach, 2011; Grossman, Niemann, Schmidt, & Walach, 2004; Piet & Hougaard, 2011; Piet, Würtzen, & Zachariae, 2012; Zenner, Herrnleben-Kurz, & Walach, 2014). They have been successfully applied to adolescents with a variety of externalizing disorders (Bögels, Hoogstad, van Dun, de Schutter, & Restifo, 2008), symptoms of depression (Liehr & Diaz, 2010), attention deficit hyperactivity disorder symptoms (Cassone, 2015; van de Weijer-Bergsma, Formsma, de Bruin, & Bögels, 2012; van der Oord, Bögels & Peijnenburg, 2012) and

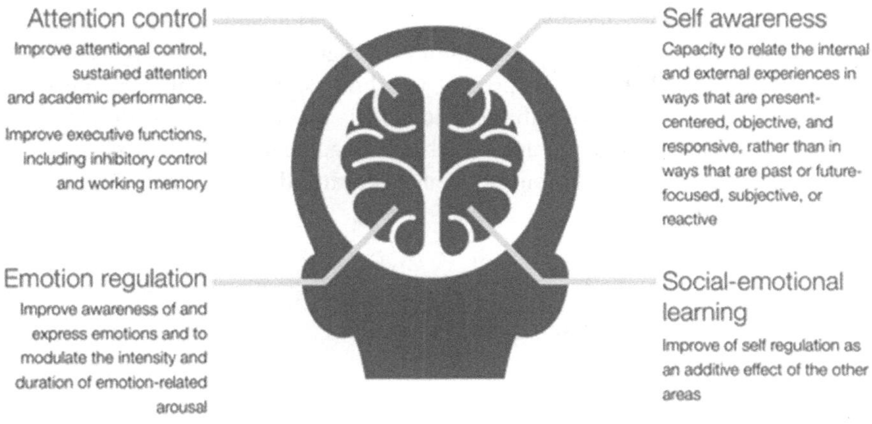

Fig. 8.1 Mindfulness meditation components: the interaction of the components constitutes a process of enhanced self-regulation

anxiety (Beauchemin, Hutchins, & Patterson, 2008). A qualitative study indicated improvements in academic performance, interpersonal relations, stress-reduction, and physical health (Kerrigan et al., 2011; Sibinga et al., 2011). An additional and interesting aspect of mindfulness is its preventive and health-promoting potential in non-clinical populations: reducing the subjective sense of stress; enhancing the subjective sense of well-being; improving immune function (Chiesa & Serretti, 2009; Davidson et al., 2003; Sedlmeier et al., 2012); promoting personal development such as self-compassion, empathy and perspective taking (Birnie, Speca, & Carlson, 2010; Jain et al., 2007; Shapiro, Schwartz, & Bonner, 1998); and increasing attentional capacity (Haukaas, Gjerde, Varting, Hallan, & Solem, 2018; Jha, Krompinger, & Baime, 2007; Tang et al., 2007) (Fig. 8.1).

8.2 Evidence and Recommendations for School-Based Mindfulness Programs

The following section will review evidence and recommendations from different studies, which have investigated the evidence of school-based mindfulness programs (for example: Carsley, Khoury, & Heath, 2018; Dunning et al., 2018; Zenner, 2014). The programs included in this section were implemented with students at school, as opposed to programs run in other settings, and describe outcomes using quantitative and qualitative data. The inclusion of qualitative studies adds an important perspective on the effects of mindfulness because they help researchers and educators to more deeply understand student experiences of mindfulness (Maxwell, 2012).

It should be also noted that the current evidence base for mindfulness-based interventions for children and adolescents is limited due to problems of sample size, design, and measurement methods. In general, research methodologies are still evolving and lack sufficient precision, which limits the validity of the findings. However, the studies described below shows positive feasibility and acceptability results in the implementation process of mindfulness at schools and changes in different areas, such as: (1) emotion regulation and social–emotional learning; (2) social competition; (3) self-care and compassion; (4) mental health and welfare; and (5) executive functions (Table 8.1).

8.3 Program Recommendations

Implementing a mindfulness program in any environment, but particularly in schools, is a challenge. Unlike most educational activities that seek to be applied to all students regularly, mindfulness is intended to deliver a personal experience that does not fit entirely into a conceptualization of learning based on 'right answers'. Adding one more program to a school curriculum that may already be overloaded can be difficult, especially if that curriculum already offers similar content in relation to stress or well-being (Broderick & Metz, 2009; Semple, Droutman, & Reid, 2017).

In the context of implementation, there are elements that are important for determining the feasibility and acceptability of using mindfulness in a particular school (Table 8.2).

8.3.1 Type of Program

A solid understanding of the theoretical foundations of existing programs can inform teachers about the objectives, content, techniques and evaluation of a mindfulness-based program. The underlying assumptions about the mechanisms of change that serve as the basis of the program should be as clear as possible. In most cases, the theory is linked to previously existing mindfulness programs such as Mindfulness Based Stress Reduction (MBSR), Mindfulness-Based Cognitive Therapy (MBCT), Dialectical Behavior Therapy (DBT) and Acceptance and Commitment Therapy (ACT). Some interventions also refer to theories and findings of positive psychology or combine mindfulness with special group-based intervention programs at school, such as social-emotional learning.

Most programs contain more than one component to facilitate mindfulness, with observation of breathing as the traditional essential exercise, as well as psychoeducation and group discussions. The interventions most commonly used in school studies are based on mindfulness-based stress reduction (MBSR) and mindfulness-based cognitive therapy (MBCT) programs. Current efforts to clarify the components of mindfulness interventions provide a useful approach for researchers and users of mindfulness programs (Baer, 2015; Broderick & Metz, 2016).

Table 8.1 Sample of mindfulness-based programs for children and adolescents in schools

Program	Age group targeted	Theoretical framework/methods	Duration; characteristics	Resources
Inner Explorer	Pre-K to K Grades 1–5 Grades 6–8	Mindfulness education, breath meditation, body scan, progressive muscle relaxation, personal journaling	5–10 min, daily for 10 to 18 weeks Pre-K to K has 50 × 5-min segments Strengthen self–awareness; promote self–management of emotions	www.innerexplorer.org (Bakosh, Snow, Tobias, Houlihan, & Barbosa-Leiker, 2015)
Inner Kids Program	Pre-K-8	It is based on the New ABCs—Attention, balance and compassion—framework.	A general formula is used of play, followed by introspection, and then sharing to help children to: better understand their introspective experience; relate it to their daily lives; and understand the importance of helping within both their families and their communities	www.susankaisergreenland.com (Flook et al., 2010)
Inner Resilience Program (IRP)	K-8 Students, teachers, parents, and administrators	It uses a mindfulness-based approach for contemplative practice, integrating social and emotional learning	In general, young children meet twice a week for 30-min sessions for 8 weeks. Older children meet once a week for approx. 45 min for 10–12 weeks It includes regular classroom instruction to develop students' social, emotional and inner life skills; a more mindful approach to behavior and classroom management aligned with Inner Resilience methods; a safe, orderly and peaceful classroom climate which values reflection; mindfulness-based practices integrated throughout the curriculum; Inner Resilience workshops that inform and engage parents; professional development for staff on their personal learning of these skills as well as support for implementing this work in the classroom	www.innerresiliencetidescenter.org (Lantieri & Malkmus, 2011)

(continued)

Table 8.1 (continued)

Program	Age group targeted	Theoretical framework/methods	Duration; characteristics	Resources
Learning to BREATHE	Adolescents	MBSR	The program includes six structured of class sessions of 30–45 min, which may be adapted for different groups and ages Six lessons are built around the BREATHE acronym, and each lesson has a core theme. The six themes include body awareness, understanding and working with thoughts, understanding and working with feelings, integrating awareness of thoughts feelings and bodily sensations, reducing harmful judgments, and integrating mindful awareness into daily life	http://learning2BREATHE.org (Broderick & Metz, 2009; Broderick, 2013; Campion & Rocco, 2009; Metz et al., 2013)
Master Mind	Grades 4–5	Mindful breathing; "mindful journeys" (e.g., body scan and mindful eating); mindful movement; everyday mindfulness; daily home practice	15 min, daily for 4 weeks Teacher-led curriculum Mindfulness education; substance abuse prevention	www.irtinc.us (Parker et al., 2014)
Mindfulness and Mind-Body Skills for Children (MMBS)	Ages 3–13	Awareness of breath and body sensations, sounds, movement, thoughts, and emotions. Yoga, "loving kindness" practice, guided imagery; and "mindful circles"	45 min, once weekly for a minimum of 2 years MMBS trained instructor-led classes, which teachers then integrate into a "whole school" curriculum Enhance self–awareness; improve self–efficacy and resilience; develop social–emotional skills; prevent risky behaviors; improve learning potential	http://mindbody-il.com (Limone, 2011)

(continued)

Table 8.1 (continued)

Program	Age group targeted	Theoretical framework/methods	Duration; characteristics	Resources
Mindful Schools	Grades K-5 Grades 6–12	Breath and body exercises; mindfulness in sensory modes; mindfulness of thoughts and emotions	15 min, 2–3 times weekly for 10–15 weeks K-5 program has 30 modules 6–12 program has 25 modules Teacher-led classes, facilitated by teachers who have attended an MS training program	www.mindfulschools.org (Black & Fernando, 2014; Fernando, 2013)
Mindfulness in Schools Project (MiSP)	14–18 years	MBSR/MBCT	9-week course Teachings include: mindfulness of breath, body scan, mindful eating, mindful movement, mindfulness of thought and sound, several variations on the 3 min silence, and mindful texting. The program is offered during normal school lessons	www.mindfulnessinschools.org (Huppert & Johnson, 2010)
Mindful Schools	K-12 Students and parents	Integrate of mindfulness into education approach	The program involves direct teaching to students in 15-sessions delivered over 8 weeks The program engages children through lessons including mindfulness of sound, breath, body, emotions, test taking, generosity, appreciation, kindness and caring, and others	www.mindfulschools.org (Liehr & Diaz, 2010)
MindUP	Pre-K-8	Classroom-tested, evidence-based curriculum which pursues objectives roughly parallel to those of the five-point framework of competencies laid out in the work of the Collaborative for Academic, Social and Emotional Learning (CASEL)	15 lessons that foster social and emotional awareness, enhance psychological well-being, and promote academic success The core practice of MindUP is mindful breathing which is ideally done three times a day (for a few minutes each time) at intervals reflective of classroom culture and needs	www.thehawnfoundation.org (Schonert-Reichl & Lawlor, 2010)

(continued)

Table 8.1 (continued)

Program	Age group targeted	Theoretical framework/methods	Duration; characteristics	Resources
Sfat Hakeshev (The Mindfulness Language)	6–13 years Students, parents and teachers	Mindfulness of: breath, body boundaries, body sensations	Goals include mindful learning (experiential awareness and mind–body practices) as a way to: develop cognitive and emotional skills; guide students to "stop", "tune in", "pay attention to what's inside"; and teach constructive rest as a useful catalyst in cognitive learning	
Still Quiet Place	Pre-K-12 Ages 5–18	Mindfulness practices taught include awareness of: breath, body, thoughts, feelings, loving kindness, and walking, as well as yoga, mindfulness in daily life, and responding versus reacting	Sessions are 45–90 min once weekly for 8 weeks Trained instructor-led classes It focuses on developing mindful awareness to support participants in responding rather than reacting to difficult situations, and in cultivating peace and happiness	www.stillquietplace.com (Saltzman & Goldin, 2008)
Stress Reduction and Mindfulness Curriculum	Elementary and middle school	Yoga, meditation, breathing, tai-chi, centering, and other mindfulness techniques	45 min, 4 times weekly for 12 weeks or 2 times weekly for 24 weeks Trained instructor-led classes Improve affective self–regulation; social–emotional wellness; anger management; problem resolution; and interpersonal relationships	http://hlfinc.org (Mendelson et al., 2010, 2013)
Stressed Teens	13–18 years	MBSR	This is an 8-week program for 1.5–2 h per week The primary focus is on formal and informal mindfulness practices Specific mindfulness practices taught include: Body scan, Walking meditation, Sitting meditation, Sitting meditation with heartfulness, Yoga, Mindful stopping, Mindful homework/test taking	www.stressedteens.com (Biegel, Brown, Shapiro, & Schubert, 2009)

MBSR mindfulness-based stress reduction; *MBCT* mindfulness-based cognitive therapy

Table 8.2 Elements to consider in the mindfulness school-based program implementation

1. Type of program
2. Characteristics of the program
3. Program and lessons duration
4. Developmental adaptation of activities
5. Participants
6. Level of implementation
7. Sustainability

Mindfulness-based stress reduction (MBSR) is a program that incorporates mindfulness to assist people with pain and a range of conditions or life issues that were initially difficult to treat in a hospital setting. Developed at the University of Massachusetts Medical Center in the 1970s by Professor Jon Kabat-Zinn, MBSR uses a combination of mindfulness meditation, body awareness, and yoga to help people become more mindful. The MBSR program consists of 8 weekly sessions of 2.5 h, and a day of mindfulness practice. Mindfulness is practiced through sitting meditation, simple yoga movements, and body-scan, which is a progressive sweep of attention through the body. Mindfulness is also cultivated in everyday activities, such as eating, and as a resource in emotionally challenging situations or in the treatment of physical pain. Daily practice in the home for approximately 45 min is recommended. Additionally, the program includes psychoeducation and attitudinal foundations, such as non-judging, trust, non-striving, acceptance, letting go, patience, and beginner's mind (Kabat-Zinn, 1982, 1990, 2003).

Mindfulness-based cognitive therapy (MBCT) incorporates elements of cognitive-behavioral therapy with mindfulness-based stress reduction. Initially conceived as an intervention for relapse prevention in people with recurrent depression, it has been applied to various psychiatric conditions (Bishop et al., 2004; Segal, Williams, & Teasdale, 2018).

In other therapies, such as acceptance and commitment therapy (ACT, Hayes, 2004) and dialectical behavior therapy (DBT, Linehan, 1993), the emphasis of treatment resides both in acceptance and change.

8.3.2 *Characteristics of the Program*

In addition to considering factors such as the duration and costs of implementing the program, in educational settings it is important to clearly define the objectives of the mindfulness program and link them with the established objectives of schools, school districts and national standards. Most schools have to meet certain curriculum objectives for each grade level. If teachers create instructional objectives that do not meet their grade level standards, then they have less time available for their main and mandatory objectives. The school's mindfulness programs should guarantee that teaching skills are consistent with grade level standards and are aligned with the appropriate common core standards. It is recommended that teachers be provided with additional instructional materials and tools to supplement their existing curriculum so that they can also teach and practice mindfulness with their students. On the side of decision makers, aligning each program activity with academic standards creates greater acceptance in the school system, including among administrators, principals, and teachers.

Mindfulness programs may have a better chance of sustainability in educational settings if they can be clearly linked in some way to the objectives of the institution. One way to address this standard is through a activity completion checklist (process evaluation) and a questionnaire involving an evaluation of results, in order to assess whether the proposed objectives were met.

To achieve the objectives, manualized programs have an advantage. A manualized program implies that the goals, objectives, theory of change, and instructions of a program are available, and students are trained in the program. A professional graphic design artist can design age-appropriate and easy-to-interpret materials, with input from psychologists, teachers, and instructional designers, for the layout and content of the instructional materials used in the program. The use of these support instruction materials can improve the effectiveness of program implementation, decreasing training time and facilitating the teaching of mindfulness. As a result, program implementation can gain ease of use and fidelity (Parker & Kupersmidt, 2016). More than half of the programs described in this chapter, such as 'Mindful Schools' and 'Learning to BREATHE' are examples of manual programs.

8.3.3 Program and Lessons Duration

Program and lesson duration are important factors that facilitate the delivery of the program. Teachers have many competing demands during a typical school day. Therefore, despite the multiple benefits of a mindfulness program, teachers may not have the time to add an additional activity to their already demanding and full school day.

In relation to duration characteristics, it has been observed that interventions with shorter duration (<6 weeks) have shown a lower percentage of significant findings compared to longer interventions. Daily meditation sessions have a higher percentage of significant findings compared with weekly practice.

A small number of studies have considered time devoted to the intervention. For example, Warner (2005) found a positive correlation between the time devoted to practice and performance in working memory, flexibility, reflectivity and conservation tasks (e.g. detecting the conservation attributes of number, substance, weight and volume displacement) (Warner, 2005). Huppert and Johnson (2010) also found a relationship between the length of meditation time and well-being (Huppert & Johnson, 2010). In some studies, meditation for 27 min a day produces changes in 8 weeks (Hölzel et al., 2011). However, sessions of this length are not feasible for school programs. Programs with short, daily lessons that can be easily integrated into the curriculum can improve the fidelity and effectiveness of the implementation of the program (Semple et al., 2005). There are many mindfulness programs that are designed to fit a typical class period of 45–50 min, however, lessons as short as 15 min have been tested with good results (Parker, Kupersmidt, Mathis, Scull, & Sims, 2014). Furthermore, it can be recommended that the program is integrated into natural transition points in the school day, for example, when students first arrive at school in the morning, or when they return to class after lunch, recess, or physical education. This can help students to pay more attention and adapt their behavior appropriately, and teachers can continue the rest of the activities after the mindfulness lessons (Parker & Kupersmidt, 2016).

In a systematic review and meta-analysis of mindfulness-based interventions in schools, in some studies, 81% of students rated the school mindfulness program sessions as extremely useful, 83% as satisfying (Anand & Sharma, 2014) and 89% would recommend the training to others (Broderick & Metz, 2009; Metz et al., 2013). Three quarters of students said that they would like to continue and thought that it should have lasted longer (Beauchemin et al., 2008; Huppert & Johnson, 2010), or that it was the right length (Anand & Sharma, 2014). Only 5% thought that it was too long (Huppert & Johnson, 2010). Some programs also contain an individual home practice. When this component is added, one third of students practiced at least three times a week and two thirds once a week or less (Huppert & Johnson, 2010). In Broderick and Metz's study (2009), two thirds of the participants practiced mindfulness techniques outside the classroom. However, not all students practiced the lessons at home. In fact, Frenkel et al. found that no student practiced the full amount of weekly exercises, and two thirds failed to do their homework at least once (Zenner et al., 2014).

Trying to summarize the available information on psychological outcomes of school-based mindfulness programs, Zenner et al. (2014) conducted a meta-analysis which included a total of eight studies with 1348 elementary, middle and high school students (Zenner et al., 2014). The effect sizes were in the same range as in other school-based prevention programs such as social–emotional programs. Time analysis showed a substantial effect between effect size and minutes in mindfulness. The authors found that dedication to practice represented more than half of the variance and was a critical factor in the effect of the programs. Likewise, they recommended training teachers in mindfulness so that they can deliver the intervention and model the behavior. This also may help prevent teacher burnout while promoting resilience (Zenner et al., 2014).

8.3.4 Developmental Adaptation of Activities

Some activities of mindfulness programs are beyond the capabilities of most children, and even many adolescents. Therefore, it is recommended that educators adapt the basic elements of mindfulness training so that they are more appropriate for children and adolescents in schools. These adaptations generally include a reduction in the duration of the practice, the use of less abstract exercises with the introduction of physical materials, and the use of more activities based on movement (Zelazo & Lyons, 2012). For example, to help children understand the notion of a body scan, a teacher can tell children to use a hula-hoop as a scanner, like the scanner of the supermarket (Zelazo & Lyons, 2012). To improve children's concentration on their breathing, a teacher can place a stuffed animal on the abdomen of a child and give them instructions to put the bear to sleep with soft breaths (Kaiser-Greenland, 2010). Additionally, to encourage conscious awareness, children can be asked to manipulate a common object without seeing it and describe how the object feels (Saltzman & Goldin, 2008). Asking children to focus their attention on their feelings can lay the foundation for conscious awareness of more complex aspects of their subjective experience, such as emotions or thoughts. For example, children can be told that thoughts pass through the mind like floats in a parade; some of the floats (thoughts) may catch their attention more than others, but just as they do not jump into a parade, they can simply watch their thoughts as they occur (Saltzman & Goldin, 2008).

With older children and adolescents, the training activities may be gradually more abstract, including metacognitive reflections. For example, adolescents may practice full awareness of the thoughts by imagining that they are standing on the top of a hill, looking down on a train, with each train car carrying one of their thoughts. The task is to observe each thought as it passes without adding emotional responses or cognitive judgments (Broderick, 2013). Older teenagers can practice mindfulness by being told to ride on the waves of their emotions like a surfer riding a wave (Broderick, 2013).

These examples show that students of all grades and ability levels can practice mindfulness if educators implement it appropriately by the level of cognitive and emotional maturity of their students.

In substance use prevention programs, the inclusion of interactive activities and teaching methods in mindfulness school programs has been associated with better participation, and improvement in the fidelity of the implementation (Ennett et al., 2003). Interaction between students in the classroom can include the exchange of ideas, role-plays or feedback on newly acquired skills, or the discussion of possible ways of handling challenging situations inside or outside the classroom (Tobler et al., 2000). One method used to integrate interactivity into mindfulness programs is to make students participate in group discussions addressing mindfulness concepts and the implementation of new practices to cope with everyday stressful experiences (Vidmar & Kerman, 2016).

8.3.5 Participants

An important feature of effective school-based preventive and promotion programs is the inclusion of peer-led activities (Botvin, Griffin, & Nichols, 2006; Cuijpers, 2002). In the case of fellow facilitators, they already know the topics and are usually very motivated to collaborate. It is likely that this familiarity and motivation may allow adolescents to relax and learn more quickly and easily during attention exercises as well as benefit more from the experience (Galla, Kaiser-Greenland, & Black, 2016). A limitation of using peer facilitators is their level of competence. The best effort should be made for the peer facilitator to have experience in mindfulness and the protocols that will be used with the peer group (Jennings & Jennings, 2013).

While it is beyond the scope of this chapter to review and analyze the research on mindfulness for teachers and school personnel, this work has been reviewed elsewhere (see the chapter 'Attention, compassion and resilience for teachers' in this book). However, it should be emphasized that mindfulness can help to foster teacher resilience and prevent teacher burnout, promote self-control and emotional regulation, and improve empathy and the student-teacher relationship (Meiklejohn et al., 2012; Zenner et al., 2014). Despite the positive effect of mindfulness on teachers, there are a series of challenges related to teacher training in the implementation of mindfulness programs in educational settings. Many educators have not been adequately prepared to create the necessary comprehensive and supportive classroom environments nor received the support and training to effectively teach mindfulness to their students.

The involvement of parents in the training of mindfulness programs for school children has proven to be viable, acceptable and effective (Bögels et al., 2008; van der Oord et al., 2012). The involvement of parents has the potential to increase the practice of the techniques at home, leading to greater benefits in reducing parental stress and promoting a positive effect on the family environment (Biegel et al., 2009; Goyal et al., 2014; Huppert & Johnson, 2010; Kuyken et al., 2013; Zenner et al., 2014).

8.3.6 Level of Implementation

A mindfulness program can be delivered as part of a school-based curriculum or after-school program, and to the entire school population or some more targeted group. The adjustment of program delivery (universal, selective, indicated) often determines the level of impact (Haggerty & Mrazek, 1994). Selective intervention, on the one hand, is aimed at young people at risk of behavioral, social or emotional problems, while indicated interventions are aimed at adolescents who present early symptoms such as school absenteeism, aggressive behavior or symptoms of depression or anxiety.

Universal interventions—aimed at the entire school population—have broad coverage and are more effective if administered in a school setting. Universal programs also increase the likelihood of sustainability and consistent positive results over time (Hawkins, Kosterman, Catalano, Hill, & Abbott, 2005). The specific level of intervention is an important consideration for selecting a program, its implementation and sustainability.

Schools can promote school-wide mindfulness interventions through the use of signs and posters to promote mindful behaviors, and the provision of physical spaces for students to meditate in during lunch or free periods. One of the advantages of using this approach is that it can create a healthy school environment, and reduce stress and other negative psychological outcomes, while improving a series of positive health-related outcomes. As students develop these skills within the school environment, it is likely to lead to a healthier school climate that positively affects the socio-emotional climate (Lawlor, 2014). Despite the benefits of universal implementation, in some studies, teachers suggested that intervention was more feasible when performed in a classroom with voluntary participation (Beauchemin et al., 2008).

Mindfulness interventions can easily be incorporated into physical education programs through physical activity related practices, such as yoga. Physical educators can develop flexibility lessons, incorporate mindfulness into lessons focusing on yoga or include brief mindfulness sessions in lessons on other fitness components at the beginning or end of physical education classes (Mendelson et al., 2010). The integration of mindfulness movements into activities to promote flexibility, strength and balance can provide children with the opportunity to not only know their bodies and their breathing, but also to increase their daily physical activity.

Mental health and psychological services could benefit greatly from incorporating mindfulness into their practice and work with students struggling with stress and other related issues. Care and consideration on a case-by-case basis is essential when determining if mindfulness is an appropriate intervention for such students. School mental health professionals could help their students develop mindfulness skills and equip them with resources. Specific recommendations for school social workers and other mental health related professionals can be found elsewhere (Wisner, Jones, & Gwin, 2010).

8.3.7 *Sustainability*

The development of plans for sustainability, including the participation and training of the entire school and the community, is essential. Sharing program materials and making them more accessible, cost–effective and culturally sensitive is also of paramount importance. Programs that provide principles or frameworks for practice and that encourage the participation of educators in their design, development and implementation can empower communities and foster sustainability. To ensure the sustainability of the program, it is also crucial to improve the acceptance and support of teachers and administrative personnel before starting the implementation of new programs in the classroom (Reyes, Brackett, Rivers, White, & Salovey, 2012).

8.4 Difficulties in Implementation

Some studies have provided information about the feasibility of different program elements, though very few have reported complete information on the implementation process (detailed protocols, scripts, feedback formulas or fidelity logs). Joyce,

Etty-Leal, Zazryn, and Hamilton (2010) mention specific factors that facilitated successful implementation, such as teaching along with colleagues, administrative and parental support and child enthusiasm. What hindered implementation were the lack of time and students who could not participate in the program. Desmond and Hanich (2010) cite problems related to scheduling, completion of administrative tasks, school holidays and difficulties with participants who arrived late (Desmond, Hanich, & Millersville, 2010).

8.5 Conclusions

This chapter reviewed the evidence regarding the effects of mindfulness on student welfare, social competence, and academic performance, and offers some broad conclusions. First, school-based mindfulness is beneficial in most cases. Second, most effects of mindfulness on student outcomes are small, yet at least one third of studies show medium or strong effect sizes. This finding is not unexpected given the multitude of factors that contribute to student welfare, social competence and academic performance. And finally, mindfulness programs can be more effective by increasing the acceptability and implementation components of the program. Mindfulness programs will be more effective when they are designed considering: (1) Type and characteristics of the program; (2) Program and lessons duration; (3) Developmental adaptation of activities; (4) Participants; (5) Level of implementation; and (6) Sustainability.

The results of the different studies presented appear promising for mindfulness programs in schools. Mindfulness seems to have positive effects on the psychological health of students, including the reduction of depression, anxiety and stress; greater general well-being; the regulation of self and emotions; positive affect; and resilience. Mindfulness training can also enhance students' capacities in self-regulation of attention and emotions and buffer the developing brain from the deleterious effects of excessive stress. Related academic outcomes described in the studies include increased attention, cognitive and academic performance. As expected, the more time spent in mindfulness practice, the greater the benefits experienced.

A key feature of contemplative practices is that they represent forms of mental training that cultivate more positive habits of mind by incorporating repetition and practice exercises. The idea of regularity of practice and repetition is well aligned with the neuroscientific understanding of how new connections are formed in the brain and the impact of regular practice on brain circuits and complex cognitive function.

Although initial studies are limited by small sample sizes and the lack of RCTs, some more recent studies have included larger sample sizes and a randomized control design. The promise of mindfulness training in schools is appealing, and much could be gained by improving research and best implementation practices in this area. Research exploring the determinants of meditation practice for adolescents can provide school health programs with critical knowledge when developing and implementing future programs that promote at-home practice, thus optimizing the effects of the programs.

We hope this review chapter offers a solid platform for future researchers to design high quality mindfulness-based programs for schools.

References

Anand, U., & Sharma, M. P. (2014). Effectiveness of a mindfulness-based stress reduction program on stress and well-being in adolescents in a school setting. *Indian Journal of Positive Psychology, 5*(1), 17.

Baer, R. (2015). Ethics, values, virtues, and character strengths in mindfulness-based interventions: A psychological science perspective. *Mindfulness, 6*(4), 956–969.

Bakosh, L. S., Snow, R. M., Tobias, J. M., Houlihan, J. L., & Barbosa-Leiker, C. (2015). Maximizing mindful learning: An innovative mindful awareness intervention improves elementary school students' quarterly grades. *Mindfulness, 7*(1), 59–67.

Beauchemin, J., Hutchins, T. L., & Patterson, F. (2008). Mindfulness meditation may lessen anxiety, promote social skills, and improve academic performance among adolescents with learning disabilities. *Complementary Health Practice Review, 13*(1), 34–45.

Biegel, G. M., Brown, K. W., Shapiro, S. L., & Schubert, C. M. (2009). Mindfulness-based stress reduction for the treatment of adolescent psychiatric outpatients: A randomized clinical trial. *Journal of Consulting and Clinical Psychology, 77*(5), 855–866. https://doi.org/10.1037/a0016241.

Birnie, K., Speca, M., & Carlson, L. E. (2010). Exploring self-compassion and empathy in the context of mindfulness-based stress reduction (MBSR). *Stress and Health, 26*(5), 359–371.

Bishop, S. R., Lau, M., Shapiro, S., Carlson, L., Anderson, N. D., Carmody, J., et al. (2004). Mindfulness: A proposed operational definition. *Clinical Psychology: Science and Practice, 11*(3), 230–241.

Black, D. S., & Fernando, R. (2014). Mindfulness training and classroom behavior among lower-income and ethnic minority elementary school children. *Journal of Child and Family Studies, 23*(7), 1242–1246.

Black, D. S., Milam, J., & Sussman, S. (2009). Sitting-meditation interventions among youth: A review of treatment efficacy. *Pediatrics, 124*(3), e532–e541. https://doi.org/10.1542/peds.2008-3434.

Bögels, S., Hoogstad, B., van Dun, L., de Schutter, S., & Restifo, K. (2008). Mindfulness training for adolescents with externalizing disorders and their parents. *Behavioural and Cognitive Psychotherapy, 36*(2), 193–209.

Botvin, G. J., Griffin, K. W., & Nichols, T. D. (2006). Preventing youth violence and delinquency through a universal school-based prevention approach. *Prevention Science, 7*(4), 403–408.

Broderick, P. C. (2013). *Learning to breathe: A mindfulness curriculum for adolescents to cultivate emotion regulation, attention, and performance*. New Harbinger Publications.

Broderick, P. C., & Metz, S. (2009). Learning to BREATHE: A pilot trial of a mindfulness curriculum for adolescents. *Advances in School Mental Health Promotion, 2*(1), 35–46.

Broderick, P. C., & Metz, S. M. (2016). Working on the inside: Mindfulness for adolescents. In *Handbook of mindfulness in education* (pp. 355–382). Springer.

Burke, C. A. (2010). Mindfulness-based approaches with children and adolescents: A preliminary review of current research in an emergent field. *Journal of Child and Family Studies, 19*(2), 133–144.

Campion, J., & Rocco, S. (2009). Minding the mind: the effects and potential of a school-based meditation programme for mental health promotion. *Advances in School Mental Health Promotion, 2*(1), 47–55.

Card, N. A., & Hodges, E. V. E. (2008). Peer victimization among schoolchildren: Correlations, causes, consequences, and considerations in assessment and intervention. *School Psychology Quarterly, 23*(4), 451.

Carsley, D., Khoury, B., & Heath, N. L. (2018). Effectiveness of mindfulness interventions for mental health in schools: A comprehensive meta-analysis. *Mindfulness, 9*(3), 693–707.

Cassone, A. R. (2015). Mindfulness training as an adjunct to evidence-based treatment for ADHD within families. *Journal of Attention Disorders, 19*(2), 147–157. https://doi.org/10.1177/1087054713488438.

Chen, Y., & Baram, T. Z. (2016). Toward understanding how early-life stress reprograms cognitive and emotional brain networks. *Neuropsychopharmacology: Official Publication of the American College of Neuropsychopharmacology, 41*(1), 197–206. https://doi.org/10.1038/npp.2015.181.

Chiesa, A., & Serretti, A. (2009). Mindfulness-based stress reduction for stress management in healthy people: A review and meta-analysis. *Journal of Alternative and Complementary Medicine (New York, N.Y.), 15*(5), 593–600. https://doi.org/10.1089/acm.2008.0495.

Cuijpers, P. (2002). Effective ingredients of school-based drug prevention programs: A systematic review. *Addictive Behaviors, 27*(6), 1009–1023.

Currie, C., Roberts, C., Morgan, A., Smith, R., Settertobulte, W., Samdal, O., & Rasmussen, V. B. (2004). *Young people's health in context.* World Health Organization Regional Office for Europe.

Davidson, R. J., Kabat-Zinn, J., Schumacher, J., Rosenkranz, M., Muller, D., Santorelli, S. F. … Sheridan, J. F. (2003). Alterations in brain and immune function produced by mindfulness meditation. *Psychosomatic Medicine, 65* (4), 564–570. Retrieved from http://www.ncbi.nlm.nih.gov/pubmed/12883106.

Desmond, C. T., Hanich, L., & Millersville, P. A. (2010). *The effects of mindful awareness teaching practices on the executive functions of students in an urban, low income middle school.* PA: Millersville.

Dunning, D. L., Griffiths, K., Kuyken, W., Crane, C., Foulkes, L., Parker, J., et al. (2018). The effects of mindfulness-based interventions on cognition and mental health in children and adolescents: A meta-analysis of randomised controlled trials.

Ennett, S. T., Ringwalt, C. L., Thorne, J., Rohrbach, L. A., Vincus, A., Simons-Rudolph, A., et al. (2003). A comparison of current practice in school-based substance use prevention programs with meta-analysis findings. *Prevention Science, 4*(1), 1–14.

Evans, G. W., & Schamberg, M. A. (2009). Childhood poverty, chronic stress, and adult working memory. *Proceedings of the National Academy of Sciences, 106*(16), 6545–6549.

Fernando, R. (2013). Measuring the efficacy and sustainability of a mindfulness-based in-class intervention. In *Bridging the Hearts and Minds of Youth: Mindfulness in Clinical Practice, Education, and Research conference, San Diego, CA.*

Fjorback, L. O., Arendt, M., Ornbøl, E., Fink, P., & Walach, H. (2011). Mindfulness-based stress reduction and mindfulness-based cognitive therapy: A systematic review of randomized controlled trials. *Acta Psychiatrica Scandinavica, 124*(2), 102–119. https://doi.org/10.1111/j.1600-0447.2011.01704.x.

Flook, L., Smalley, S. L., Kitil, M. J., Galla, B. M., Kaiser-Greenland, S., Locke, J., et al. (2010). Effects of mindful awareness practices on executive functions in elementary school children. *Journal of Applied School Psychology, 26*(1), 70–95.

Galla, B. M., Kaiser-Greenland, S., & Black, D. S. (2016). Mindfulness training to promote self-regulation in youth: Effects of the inner kids program. In *Handbook of mindfulness in education* (pp. 295–311). Springer.

Goyal, M., Singh, S., Sibinga, E. M. S., Gould, N. F., Rowland-Seymour, A., Sharma, R. … Shihab, H. M. (2014). Meditation programs for psychological stress and well-being: A systematic review and meta-analysis. *JAMA Internal Medicine, 174*(3), 357–368.

Graziano, P. A., Reavis, R. D., Keane, S. P., & Calkins, S. D. (2007). The role of emotion regulation and children's early academic success. *Journal of School Psychology, 45*(1), 3–19. https://doi.org/10.1016/j.jsp.2006.09.002.

Grossman, P., Niemann, L., Schmidt, S., & Walach, H. (2004). Mindfulness-based stress reduction and health benefits. A meta-analysis. *Journal of Psychosomatic Research, 57*(1), 35–43. https://doi.org/10.1016/S0022-3999(03)00573-7.

Haggerty, R. J., & Mrazek, P. J. (1994). *Reducing risks for mental disorders: Frontiers for preventive intervention research*. National Academies Press.

Haukaas, R. B., Gjerde, I. B., Varting, G., Hallan, H. E., & Solem, S. (2018). A randomized controlled trial comparing the attention training technique and mindful self-compassion for students with symptoms of depression and anxiety. *Frontiers in Psychology, 9*. https://doi.org/10.3389/fpsyg.2018.00827.

Hawkins, J. D., Kosterman, R., Catalano, R. F., Hill, K. G., & Abbott, R. D. (2005). Promoting positive adult functioning through social development intervention in childhood: Long-term effects from the Seattle Social Development Project. *Archives of Pediatrics and Adolescent Medicine, 159*(1), 25–31.

Hayes, S. C. (2004). Acceptance and commitment therapy, relational frame theory, and the third wave of behavioral and cognitive therapies. *Behavior Therapy, 35*(4), 639–665.

Hölzel, B. K., Lazar, S. W., Gard, T., Schuman-Olivier, Z., Vago, D. R., & Ott, U. (2011). How does mindfulness meditation work? Proposing mechanisms of action from a conceptual and neural perspective. *Perspectives on Psychological Science, 6*(6), 537–559. https://doi.org/10.1177/1745691611419671.

Huppert, F. A., & Johnson, D. M. (2010). A controlled trial of mindfulness training in schools: The importance of practice for an impact on well-being. *The Journal of Positive Psychology, 5*(4), 264–274.

Jain, S., Shapiro, S. L., Swanick, S., Roesch, S. C., Mills, P. J., Bell, I., et al. (2007). A randomized controlled trial of mindfulness meditation versus relaxation training: Effects on distress, positive states of mind, rumination, and distraction. *Annals of Behavioral Medicine, 33*(1), 11–21. https://doi.org/10.1207/s15324796abm3301_2.

Jennings, S. J., & Jennings, J. L. (2013). Peer-directed, brief mindfulness training with adolescents: A pilot study. *International Journal of Behavioral Consultation and Therapy, 8*(2), 23.

Jha, A. P., Krompinger, J., & Baime, M. J. (2007). Mindfulness training modifies subsystems of attention. *Cognitive, Affective & Behavioral Neuroscience, 7*(2), 109–119. Retrieved from http://www.ncbi.nlm.nih.gov/pubmed/17672382.

Joyce, A., Etty-Leal, J., Zazryn, T., & Hamilton, A. (2010). Exploring a mindfulness meditation program on the mental health of upper primary children: A pilot study. *Advances in School Mental Health Promotion, 3*(2), 17–25.

Kabat-Zinn, J. (1982). An outpatient program in behavioral medicine for chronic pain patients based on the practice of mindfulness meditation: Theoretical considerations and preliminary results. *General Hospital Psychiatry, 4*(1), 33–47.

Kabat-Zinn, J. (1990). *Full catastrophe living: The program of the stress reduction clinic at the University of Massachusetts Medical Center*. New York: Delta.

Kabat-Zinn, J. (2003). Mindfulness-based interventions in context: Past, present, and future. *Clinical Psychology: Science and Practice, 10*(2), 144–156.

Kaiser-Greenland, S. (2010). The mindful child. *How to Help Your Kid Manage Stress*.

Kerrigan, D., Johnson, K., Stewart, M., Magyari, T., Hutton, N., Ellen, J. M., et al. (2011). Perceptions, experiences, and shifts in perspective occurring among urban youth participating in a mindfulness-based stress reduction program. *Complementary Therapies in Clinical Practice, 17*(2), 96–101. https://doi.org/10.1016/j.ctcp.2010.08.003.

Khoury, B., Lecomte, T., Fortin, G., Masse, M., Therien, P., Bouchard, V., et al. (2013). Mindfulness-based therapy: A comprehensive meta-analysis. *Clinical Psychology Review, 33*(6), 763–771. https://doi.org/10.1016/j.cpr.2013.05.005.

Khoury, B., Sharma, M., Rush, S. E., & Fournier, C. (2015). Mindfulness-based stress reduction for healthy individuals: A meta-analysis. *Journal of Psychosomatic Research, 78*(6), 519–528. https://doi.org/10.1016/j.jpsychores.2015.03.009.

Kuyken, W., Weare, K., Ukoumunne, O. C., Vicary, R., Motton, N., Burnett, R., et al. (2013). Effectiveness of the Mindfulness in Schools Programme: Non-randomised controlled feasibility study. *The British Journal of Psychiatry: The Journal of Mental Science, 203*(2), 126–131. https://doi.org/10.1192/bjp.bp.113.126649.

Lantieri, L., & Malkmus, C. D. (2011). *Building inner resilience in teachers and their students*. New York: Metis Associates Evaluation. http://www.innerresiliencetidescenter.org/documents/IRP_Pilot_Program_Results_AERA2011_updated_6.

Lawlor, M. S. (2014). Mindfulness in practice: Considerations for implementation of mindfulness-based programming for adolescents in school contexts. *New Directions for Youth Development, 2014*(142), 83–95.

Liehr, P., & Diaz, N. (2010). A pilot study examining the effect of mindfulness on depression and anxiety for minority children. *Archives of Psychiatric Nursing, 24*(1), 69–71. https://doi.org/10.1016/j.apnu.2009.10.001.

Limone, N. (2011). Opening the new school year with mindfulness.

Linehan, M. (1993). *Cognitive-behavioral treatment of borderline personality disorder*. Guilford Press.

Lupien, S. J., McEwen, B. S., Gunnar, M. R., & Heim, C. (2009). Effects of stress throughout the lifespan on the brain, behaviour and cognition. *Nature Reviews Neuroscience, 10*(6), 434–445. https://doi.org/10.1038/nrn2639.

Maxwell, J. A. (2012). *Qualitative research design: An interactive approach* (Vol. 41). Sage Publications.

Meiklejohn, J., Phillips, C., Freedman, M. L., Griffin, M. L., Biegel, G., Roach, A., et al. (2012). Integrating mindfulness training into K-12 education: Fostering the resilience of teachers and students. *Mindfulness, 3*(4), 291–307.

Mendelson, T., Dariotis, J. K., Feagans Gould, L., Smith, A. S. R., Smith, A. A., Gonzalez, A. A., et al. (2013). Implementing mindfulness and yoga in urban schools: A community-academic partnership. *Journal of Children's Services, 8*(4), 276–291.

Mendelson, T., Greenberg, M. T., Dariotis, J. K., Gould, L. F., Rhoades, B. L., & Leaf, P. J. (2010). Feasibility and preliminary outcomes of a school-based mindfulness intervention for urban youth. *Journal of Abnormal Child Psychology, 38*(7), 985–994. https://doi.org/10.1007/s10802-010-9418-x.

Merikangas, K. R., He, J.-P., Burstein, M., Swanson, S. A., Avenevoli, S., Cui, L., et al. (2010). Lifetime prevalence of mental disorders in U.S. adolescents: Results from the National Comorbidity Survey Replication–Adolescent Supplement (NCS-A). *Journal of the American Academy of Child and Adolescent Psychiatry, 49*(10), 980–989. https://doi.org/10.1016/j.jaac.2010.05.017.

Metz, S. M., Frank, J. L., Reibel, D., Cantrell, T., Sanders, R., & Broderick, P. C. (2013). The effectiveness of the learning to BREATHE program on adolescent emotion regulation. *Research in Human Development, 10*(3), 252–272.

Mind and Life Education Research Network (MLERN):, Davidson, R. J., Dunne, J., Eccles, J. S., Engle, A., Greenberg, M., Jennings, P. … Vago, D. (2012). Contemplative practices and mental training: Prospects for American Education. *Child Development Perspectives, 6*(2), 146–153. https://doi.org/10.1111/j.1750-8606.2012.00240.x.

Parker, A. E., & Kupersmidt, J. B. (2016). Two universal mindfulness education programs for elementary and middle-school students: Master Mind and Moment. In *Handbook of mindfulness in education* (pp. 335–354). Springer.

Parker, A. E., Kupersmidt, J. B., Mathis, E. T., Scull, T. M., & Sims, C. (2014). The impact of mindfulness education on elementary school students: Evaluation of the Master Mind program. *Advances in School Mental Health Promotion, 7*(3), 184–204.

Perou, R., Bitsko, R. H., Blumberg, S. J., Pastor, P., Ghandour, R. M., Gfroerer, J. C. … Huang, L. N. (2013). Mental health surveillance among children–United States, 2005–2011. *MMWR Supplements, 62*(2), 1–35.

Piet, J., & Hougaard, E. (2011). The effect of mindfulness-based cognitive therapy for prevention of relapse in recurrent major depressive disorder: A systematic review and meta-analysis. *Clinical Psychology Review, 31*(6), 1032–1040.
Piet, J., Würtzen, H., & Zachariae, R. (2012). The effect of mindfulness-based therapy on symptoms of anxiety and depression in adult cancer patients and survivors: A systematic review and meta-analysis. *Journal of Consulting and Clinical Psychology, 80*(6), 1007.
Reyes, M. R., Brackett, M. A., Rivers, S. E., White, M., & Salovey, P. (2012). Classroom emotional climate, student engagement, and academic achievement. *Journal of Educational Psychology, 104*(3), 700.
Saltzman, A., & Goldin, P. (2008). Mindfulness-based stress reduction for school-age children.
Schonert-Reichl, K. A., & Lawlor, M. S. (2010). The effects of a mindfulness-based education program on pre-and early adolescents' well-being and social and emotional competence. *Mindfulness, 1*(3), 137–151.
Sedlmeier, P., Eberth, J., Schwarz, M., Zimmermann, D., Haarig, F., Jaeger, S., et al. (2012). The psychological effects of meditation: A meta-analysis. *Psychological Bulletin, 138*(6), 1139–1171. https://doi.org/10.1037/a0028168.
Segal, Z. V., Williams, J. M. G., & Teasdale, J. D. (2018). *Mindfulness-based cognitive therapy for depression*. Guilford Publications.
Semple, R. J., Droutman, V., & Reid, B. A. (2017). Mindfulness goes to school: Things learned (so far) from research and real-world experiences. *Psychology in the Schools, 54*(1), 29–52. https://doi.org/10.1002/pits.21981.
Semple, R. J., Reid, E. F. G., & Miller, L. (2005). Treating anxiety with mindfulness: An open trial of mindfulness training for anxious children. *Journal of Cognitive Psychotherapy, 19*(4), 379–392. https://doi.org/10.1891/jcop.2005.19.4.379.
Shapiro, S. L., Carlson, L. E., Astin, J. A., & Freedman, B. (2006). Mechanisms of mindfulness. *Journal of Clinical Psychology, 62*(3), 373–386. https://doi.org/10.1002/jclp.20237.
Shapiro, S. L., Schwartz, G. E., & Bonner, G. (1998). Effects of mindfulness-based stress reduction on medical and premedical students. *Journal of Behavioral Medicine, 21*(6), 581–599. Retrieved from http://www.ncbi.nlm.nih.gov/pubmed/9891256.
Sibinga, E. M. S., Kerrigan, D., Stewart, M., Johnson, K., Magyari, T., & Ellen, J. M. (2011). Mindfulness-based stress reduction for urban youth. *The Journal of Alternative and Complementary Medicine, 17*(3), 213–218. https://doi.org/10.1089/acm.2009.0605.
Tang, Y.-Y., Holzel, B. K., & Posner, M. I. (2015). The neuroscience of mindfulness meditation. *Nature Reviews Neuroscience, 16*(4), 213–225. https://doi.org/10.1038/nrn3916.
Tang, Y.-Y., Ma, Y., Wang, J., Fan, Y., Feng, S., Lu, Q., et al. (2007). Short-term meditation training improves attention and self-regulation. *Proceedings of the National Academy of Sciences, 104*(43), 17152–17156. https://doi.org/10.1073/pnas.0707678104.
Tobler, N. S., Roona, M. R., Ochshorn, P., Marshall, D. G., Streke, A. V., & Stackpole, K. M. (2000). School-based adolescent drug prevention programs: 1998 meta-analysis. *Journal of Primary Prevention, 20*(4), 275–336.
van de Weijer-Bergsma, E., Formsma, A. R., de Bruin, E. I., & Bögels, S. M. (2012). The effectiveness of mindfulness training on behavioral problems and attentional functioning in adolescents with ADHD. *Journal of Child and Family Studies, 21*(5), 775–787. https://doi.org/10.1007/s10826-011-9531-7.
van der Oord, S., Bögels, S. M., & Peijnenburg, D. (2012). The effectiveness of mindfulness training for children with ADHD and mindful parenting for their parents. *Journal of Child and Family Studies, 21*(1), 139–147. https://doi.org/10.1007/s10826-011-9457-0.
Vidmar, M., & Kerman, K. (2016). The development of Teacher's Relational Competence scale: Structural validity and reliability. *Solsko Polje, 27.*
Warner, T. Q. (2005). Awareness and cognition: The role of awareness training in child development. *Journal of Social Behavior and Personality, 17*(1), 47.

Weare, K., & Nind, M. (2011). Mental health promotion and problem prevention in schools: What does the evidence say? *Health Promotion International, 26*(suppl_1), i29–i69. https://doi.org/10.1093/heapro/dar075.

Wisner, B. L., Jones, B., & Gwin, D. (2010). School-based meditation practices for adolescents: A resource for strengthening self-regulation, emotional coping, and self-esteem. *Children & Schools, 32*(3), 150–159.

Zelazo, P. D., & Lyons, K. E. (2012). The potential benefits of mindfulness training in early childhood: A developmental social cognitive neuroscience perspective. *Child Development Perspectives, 6*(2), 154–160.

Zenner, C., Herrnleben-Kurz, S., & Walach, H. (2014). Mindfulness-based interventions in schools: A systematic review and meta-analysis. *Frontiers in Psychology, 5,* 603. https://doi.org/10.3389/fpsyg.2014.00603.

Chapter 9
How Does Mindfulness Work in Schools? An Integrative Model of the Outcomes and the Mechanisms of Change of Mindfulness-Based Interventions in the Classroom

Catherine I. Andreu and Carlos García-Rubio

Abstract There is a need for theoretical models explaining the functioning of Mindfulness-Based Interventions (MBIs) in the school context to guide the research on the mechanisms of action and the effects that mindfulness practice may have on children and adolescents. In response, we develop and present here an integrative model of mindfulness in the school context. Concretely, we try to clarify and simplify the complexity of the MBIs outcomes and mechanisms in the classroom. In the model, the main outcomes of MBIs in the classrooms are presented, including mental health, well-being, peer relationships, classroom behavior, and academic performance. Besides, we suggest that different skills and processes developed during an MBI in the classroom, such as mindfulness, multiple cognitive and emotional processes (i.e., attention and self-regulation), and prosocial behavior may contribute indirectly, as mechanisms of action, to promoting these outcomes. Also, we propose that boosting these outcomes can lead to the improvement of mindfulness skills, multiple cognitive and emotional processes (i.e., attention and self-regulation), and social competence through an upward spiral process or positive feedback loops. Finally, some conditions that could moderate the effectiveness of the MBIs in the classroom are proposed. Nowadays, many mindfulness programs are implemented in educational settings, all of which display significant differences in term of structure, methodology, and mindfulness practices used. Therefore, this model can inform the design of the future studies in the field of mindfulness in schools to determine which program is particularly useful for obtaining specific results, through which specific mechanism, and under which specific conditions. Implications and limitations of

Note of interest about authors: Both authors contribute equally as first authors.

C. I. Andreu
Millennium Institute for Research in Depression and Personality (MIDAP), Santiago, Chile

School of Psychology, Pontificia Universidad Católica de Chile, Santiago, Chile

C. García-Rubio (✉)
Department of Biological and Health Psychology, Faculty of Psychology, Universidad Autónoma de Madrid, Madrid, Spain
e-mail: garciarubio.carlos@gmail.com

C. Steinebach and Á. I. Langer (eds.), *Enhancing Resilience in Youth*,
https://doi.org/10.1007/978-3-030-25513-8_9

the model in the framework of mindfulness-based interventions in the school are discussed.

Keywords Mindfulness · Mindfulness-based intervention (MBI) · School · Mechanisms of change · Children and adolescents

9.1 Mindfulness in Schools

During childhood and adolescence, the school is an active agent of development (Vygotsky, 1978). Schools are a critical context where children must be educated to foster positive development, including the promotion of both cognitive and non-cognitive skills and eventually the implementation of mental health prevention initiatives (Greenberg et al., 2003). 21st century schools not only provide a broad set of academic skills (e.g. math, reading, writing, math, and science), but they also promote the healthy development and mental health of children and adolescents through strengths-based education and the cultivation of socio-emotional and behavioral skills (Mind & Life Education Research, 2012).

Recently, mindfulness-based initiatives have been incorporated in schools aligned with the goals of the Social-Emotional Learning (SEL), with both initiatives being focused on the education of the "whole child" and positive development (Lawlor, 2016). A widely accepted definition of mindfulness is "*the awareness that emerges through paying attention on purpose, in the present moment, and nonjudgmentally to the unfolding of experience moment by moment*" (Kabat-Zinn, 2003, p. 145). Mindfulness-based interventions (MBIs) in the school context provide a set of practices that help children and adolescents to be more aware and be able to recognize their mental and behavioral habits to learn new ways to transcend their habitual patterns of behavior and develop healthy habits of the mind (Jennings, 2008).

In the last decade, interest in mindfulness applied in public and educational settings had a rapid expansion, accompanied by the exponential growth of empirical research documenting the benefits of mindfulness practices in educational contexts (Mind & Life Education Research, 2012; Schonert-Reichl & Roeser, 2016). Several meta-analyses have been conducted to study the effects of MBIs in youth. In the latest published meta-analysis (Dunning et al., 2018), to our knowledge, only studies employing randomized controlled trials (RCTs) were included, with significant effects on mindfulness, executive functioning, attention, depression, anxiety/stress, and negative behaviors being found, with small effect sizes. Interestingly, when only RCTs with active control groups were included, significant effects were restricted to mindfulness, depression, and anxiety/stress. In school contexts, significant effects were found on cognitive performance and resilience to stress (Zenner, Herrnleben-Kurz, & Walach, 2014), and small to moderate effects on mental health (Carsley, Khoury, & Heath, 2018). Importantly, the considerable heterogeneity of the studies, high diversity of samples, variety in implementation methods, and the wide range of measures made it difficult to compare between studies, so specific recommendations for future studies have been made (Felver, Celis-de Hoyos, Tezanos, & Singh, 2016). In the research field of mindfulness with adults, several models are available that try to explain how mindfulness works and what the mechanisms underlying mindfulness effects are. However, there are very few models explaining possible mechanisms about how MBIs with children and adolescents work in school contexts. Given this deficit, we propose a model on the mechanisms of change and outcomes of MBIs in the classroom at the individual and classroom level.

9.2 An Integrative Model of Mindfulness in the Classroom

After observing the systematic benefits shown by the practice of mindfulness with adults in a healthy and clinical population (De Vibe et al., 2017; Goldberg et al., 2017), research on the impact of MBIs with adults has yielded several theoretical models trying to describe the psychological and neurobiological mechanisms that explain their effectiveness (Hölzel et al., 2011; Vago & Silbersweig, 2012). Although empirical studies on these mechanisms are still scarce, there is increasing empirical evidence that the impact of mindfulness practice on improving mental health and well-being may be due to an enhancement in attentional regulation skills, cognitive and emotional self-regulation skills, and mindfulness skills (Gu, Strauss, Bond, & Cavanagh, 2015). Likewise, some studies have pointed to the importance of increases in self-compassion skills and psychological flexibility (Gu et al., 2015). Also, MBIs have also shown their effectiveness in the development of prosocial behaviors (Kemeny et al., 2012).

Although evidence about the efficacy of mindfulness-based training in adults is increasing, research on the effects of MBIs in children and adolescents is in its infancy, and it is especially significant in the school context (Felver et al., 2016). Even though during the last decade there has been an exponential increase in the number of studies on the effectiveness of MBIs in the school context, very few have explored the psychological and neurobiological mechanisms that underlie their effectiveness (Van der Gucht, Takano, Raes, & Kuppens, 2018). In addition, very few theoretical models have been proposed to explain how MBIs with children and adolescents work in school contexts (e.g., Roeser, Skinner, Beers, & Jennings, 2012). From our perspective, in order to continue gaining a deeper understanding of mindfulness in the school context, theoretical models are needed to guide applied research.

Drawing on the science of mindfulness with adults, children, and adolescents, and taking into consideration research in developmental and school psychology, cognitive neuroscience, clinical psychology, and prevention science, we propose a model that aims to present the main outcomes of MBIs in the school context and the mechanisms that underlie their impact (Fig. 9.1). The model emphasizes that MBIs in the school context have an impact on (*outcomes in* Fig. 9.1): (1) the improvement of mental health, well-being, and self-concept, (2) the improvement of peer-relationships, peer-acceptance, and peer-support and the decrease in bullying behaviors, (3) the improvement of emotional and behavioral engagement with classroom activities,

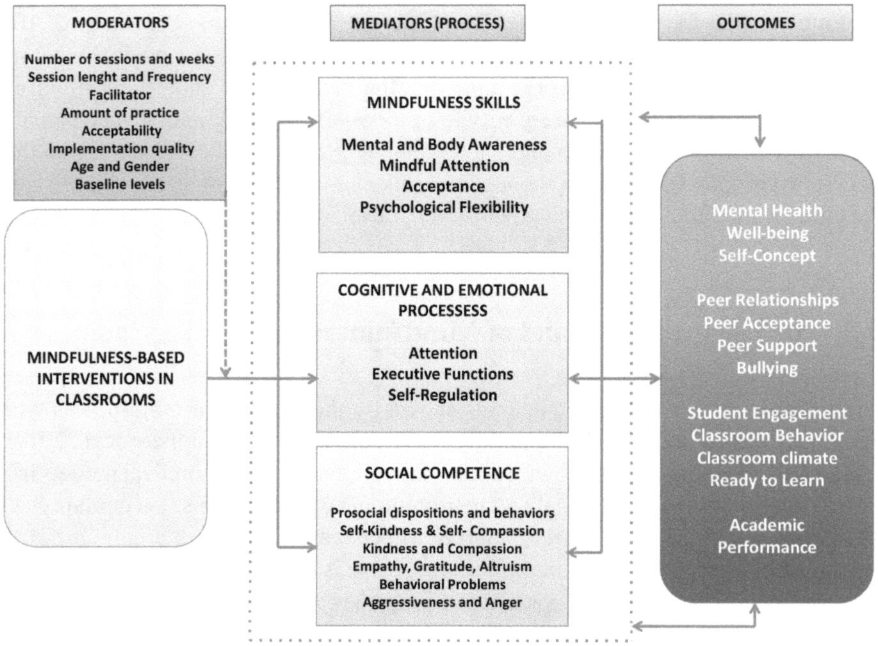

Fig. 9.1 Integrative Model of the Outcomes and the Mechanisms of Change of MBIs in the Classroom

classroom behavior, and the increase of ready-to-learn skills, and (4) the increase in academic performance. The effects of MBIs on outcomes could be produced through a set of skills and processes (*mediators in* Fig. 9.1): (1) the increase in mindfulness skills, (2) the improvement in cognitive and emotional processes such as attention, executive function, and self-regulation, and (3) the development of prosocial dispositions and behaviors towards oneself and towards others (e.g. kindness, compassion, and empathy), as well as through the reduction of behavioral problems and an improvement in the management of anger and aggression.

The model emphasizes that the impact of MBIs on outcomes can occur through the parallel increase of various skills and processes (e.g. improvement in mental health occurs through the simultaneous improvement of mindfulness skills and self-regulation) or sequential increase (e.g. the MBI has an effect on inhibitory control, which in turn increases peer acceptance, and the cumulative indirect effect improves academic performance). Besides, taking into consideration the broaden-and-build theory (Fredrickson, 2001), it is stated that the improvement of student outcomes also influences the development of skills and processes, generating new personal resources in children and adolescents through an upward spiral process or positive feedback loops.

Finally, it is stated that the effects of mindfulness based-interventions on processes and outcomes could be influenced by a group of characteristics of the intervention (*moderators in* Fig. 9.1), such as age and gender, the number of sessions and weeks, session length and frequency, type of facilitator, amount of practice, acceptability and implementation quality of the intervention, and baseline levels of the participants in the processes and outcomes before the intervention.

9.2.1 *Mindfulness Skills*

Mindfulness has been conceptualized in many different ways (Grossman & Van Dam, 2011). Mindfulness is used as an umbrella term that can refer to a set of practices, processes, and characteristics, and it is usually related to attention skills, memory, acceptance, and awareness (Van Dam et al., 2018). Historically, the practice of meditation has been regarded as a skillful way to develop mindfulness skills (Bodhi, 2011; Kabat-Zinn, 2003). Different types of meditation practices (e.g. sitting meditation and yoga) have been used to increase skills such as mindful attention, body and mind awareness (thoughts, feelings, emotions), acceptance, or psychological flexibility. MBIs with adults, whose central practices are a set of meditation practices (e.g. sitting meditation, mindful movement, body scan, informal practice), have been shown to be effective in developing mindfulness skills (Khoury et al., 2013). Several studies with adults have shown how increases in mindfulness skills are the fundamental mechanism that underlies the effect of MBIs on mental health and well-being (Gu et al., 2015; Nyklíček & Kuijpers, 2008).

In children and adolescents, *mindfulness skills* have been associated with fewer behavioral problems and better mental health, quality of life, social skills, and academic competence (Greco, Baer, & Smith, 2011). Specifically, mindfulness skills in children are related to less negative affect, anxiety, depression, and rumination, and greater optimism, school self-concept, self-efficacy, and school competence (Lawlor, Schonert-Reichl, Gadermann, & Zumbo, 2014). In adolescents, mindfulness has been associated with lower levels of stress and negative affect, depression, and anxiety, as well as greater life satisfaction, school self-concept, and self-efficacy (Pallozzi, Wertheim, Paxton, & Ong, 2017). Recently, a longitudinal study with adolescents showed that mindful attention reduces the association between maladaptive schemas and depressive symptoms, suggesting that MBIs can diminish depressive symptoms in adolescents by reducing the maladaptive schemas' impact (Calvete, Morea, & Orue, 2018). Likewise, a diary study with adolescents showed that less mindful individuals were particularly vulnerable to the negative effects of stress (Ciesla, Reilly, Dickson, Emanuel, & Updegraff, 2012). The empirical evidence supports the notion that mindfulness skills play a protective role during child and adolescent development (*arrows from mindfulness skills to outcomes in* Fig. 9.1).

Regarding the evidence on whether MBIs with children and adolescents are effective in promoting mindfulness skills (*arrows from MBIs to mindfulness skills in* Fig. 9.1), several studies have shown that practicing mindfulness is an effective way of developing mindfulness skills in school contexts (Schonert-Reichl et al., 2015; Viafora, Mathiesen, & Unsworth, 2015). However, results are contradictory, since recent studies have found no improvements (Johnson, Burke, Brinkman, & Wade,

2017). A recent meta-analysis revealed that MBIs in the school context only increased mindfulness skills when the facilitator of the intervention (moderator) was an outside mindfulness expert (Carsley et al., 2018). This result reveals the importance of studying under what specific conditions the practice of mindfulness in the school context is beneficial. More specifically, this finding suggests that a program characteristic, the type of facilitator during the MBI, can change the effectiveness of the intervention for the promotion of mindfulness skills. More research is needed on which moderating variables influence the development of mindfulness skills in MBIs at school.

Little is known about the role of mindfulness skills as a mechanism of the efficacy of MBIs in the school context (*mediators in* Fig. 9.1). Although theory suggests that the impact of MBIs on different outcomes is due to the development of mindfulness skills, very few empirical studies have addressed this question. Only a few studies suggest that changes in mindfulness skills after an MBI are related to changes in reactivity to anger (Sibinga et al., 2013) and well-being (Vickery & Dorjee, 2016). It is too early to assert that mindfulness skills are one of the specific mechanisms that explain the effectiveness of MBIs in the school context. Although preliminary research is promising, more studies are needed.

Theoretically, another critical skill that MBIs in school contexts seek to develop is *psychological flexibility*. In the scientific framework, psychological flexibility has been defined as "*the ability to contact the present moment more fully as a human being and to change or persist in behavior when doing so serves valued ends*" (Hayes, Luoma, Bond, Masuda, & Lillis, 2006, p. 7). Psychological flexibility is considered a fundamental aspect of health (Kashdan & Rottenberg, 2010). The opposite of psychological flexibility is psychological inflexibility. Psychological inflexibility occurs through two processes: cognitive fusion and experiential avoidance. Cognitive fusion refers to the connection with mental phenomena (thoughts, sensations, emotions), while experiential avoidance refers to the strategies put into practice to avoid mental phenomena or situations instead of living them with openness and acceptance, without struggle or defense (Hayes, Luoma, Bond, Masuda, & Lillis, 1999). According to this approach, the greater the cognitive fusion and experiential avoidance, the greater the psychological inflexibility. In children and adolescents, psychological inflexibility has been related to greater somatization, perceived stress, internalizing problems, externalizing problems, attention problems, rumination, and suppression of thoughts (*arrows from mindfulness skills to outcomes in* Fig. 9.1). It is also related to less self-compassion, self-worth, quality of life, social skills, and academic competence (Greco, Lambert, & Baer, 2008; Fung et al., 2018; Muris et al., 2017; Simon & Verboon, 2016); also, a strong inverse correlation has been reported between dispositional mindfulness and psychological inflexibility (Greco et al., 2011). Overall, the empirical evidence supports the protective nature during the development of a lower psychological inflexibility.

The impact of MBIs on children's and adolescents' psychological inflexibility is scarce, but promising results have been reported (Tan & Martin, 2015); (*arrows from mindfulness-based intervention to mindfulness skills in* Fig. 9.1). In the school context, a randomized controlled trial evaluated the impact of an MBI on young people from ethnic minority backgrounds (Fung et al., 2018). Results showed a tendency for psychological inflexibility to decrease after the intervention. However, the mediating effect of psychological inflexibility on mental health was not significant. The authors argued that the sample might have been too small to have sufficient statistical power to detect any effects. Therefore, more rigorous studies are needed to determine the impact of MBIs on psychological inflexibility and their role as a mediating mechanism.

9.2.2 Cognitive and Emotional Processes

Both MBIs and mindfulness skills in adults and also in children and adolescents have been consistently related with important cognitive and emotional processes, including attention, executive functions (EFs), and self-regulation abilities (Diamond & Ling, 2016; Hölzel et al., 2011; Schonert-Reichl & Roeser, 2016).

Attentional skills are essential not only for academic performance in school and behavior in the classroom but also for mental health and peer relationships (Schulte-Körne, 2016; DuPaul, McGoey, Eckert, & VanBrakle, 2001; Northup et al., 1995; DeHaas, 1986; Mrug, Hoza, & Gerdes, 2001); (*arrows from attention to outcomes in* Fig. 9.1). In a recent study, poor social and school functioning was found to be associated with symptoms of ADHD and poor EFs (Diamantopoulou, Rydell, Thorell, & Bohlin, 2007). As mindfulness practices require individuals to exercise volitional control to sustain the focus of attention on particular objects, it is widely hypothesized that attentional skills increase by MBIs (Mind & Life Education Research, 2012; Lutz, Slagter, Dunne, & Davidson, 2008; Slagter, Davidson, & Lutz, 2011). Growing evidence had shown that mindfulness training improves adults' ability to regulate attention (including orienting attention and monitoring conflict), showing improved performance in different attentional tasks and modified underlying neural attentional networks (Jha, Krompinger, & Baime, 2007; Tang, Hölzel, & Posner, 2015; Slagter et al., 2007). Several studies have shown that different MBIs applied in schools can also train and modify attention in children and adolescents, showing improvements in concentration (Ricarte, Ros, Latorre, & Beltrán, 2015), attentional measures (Napoli, Krech, & Holley, 2005), and attentional focus (Poehlmann-Tynan et al., 2016), together with a reduction in attentional problems (Crescentini, Capurso, Furlan, & Fabbro, 2016; Semple, Lee, Rosa, & Miller, 2010); (*arrows from MBIs to attention in* Fig. 9.1). With a different design, one recent randomized study assessed behavioral measures of attention using the Attention Network Test (ANT) in children who participated in a MBI for parents and children (Mindful Family Stress Reduction) and found decreased conflict monitoring and increased orienting subsystems in children in the intervention group compared with controls (Felver, Tipsord, Morris, Racer, & Dishion, 2017). Additionally, a recent systematic review found statistically significant MBI effects on attentional outcomes in children and adolescents, with medium to large effect sizes (Mak, Whittingham, Cunnington, & Boyd, 2018). Despite the promising results, more research is needed to establish the possible mediating role of attention in mental health, emotional, social, and behavioral outcomes after an MBI in schools.

Closely related to attention, *EFs* are a group of essential skills for our development from childhood onward. EFs refer to a family of cognitive control abilities that organize, sequence, and regulate behavior, mainly relying on prefrontal cortex areas (Diamond, 2013). There are different models, but a general agreement divides EFs into three core groups: inhibitory control, working memory, and cognitive flexibility; from these, higher order EFs (reasoning, planning, problem-solving) are built (Diamond, 2013). Inhibitory control involves being able to control one's attention, behavior, thoughts, and/or emotions; working memory refers to holding information in mind and mentally working with it; and cognitive flexibility relates to changing perspectives or approaches to a problem, flexibly adjusting to new demands or priorities (Diamond, 2013). Children with poor executive functioning have been shown to have poorer outcomes in adulthood such as worse health, worse self-regulation, and inferior prosocial behavior, being less happy, committing more crimes, and developing several EF-related disorders (Diamond & Ling, 2016; Diamond & Lee, 2011). Also, EFs are strongly related to children's social-emotional development and may affect SEL interventions as a mediator, moderator, or as an outcome of intervention effects (Riggs, Jahromi, Razza, Dillworth-Bart, & Mueller, 2006). EFs predict academic achievement, learning-related classroom behaviors, and observed engagement in preschoolers (Brock, Rimm-Kaufman, Nathanson, & Grimm, 2009; Blair & Razza, 2007), as well as school success, school readiness (Blair & Diamond, 2008; St Clair-Thompson & Gathercole, 2006; Blair & Raver, 2015), social functioning, peer problems, and aggressive and prosocial behavior (O'Toole, Monks, & Tsermentseli, 2017; Diamantopoulou et al., 2007; Holmes, Kim-Spoon, & Deater-Deckard, 2016). Thus, in general, EFs are critical for success in school, for the development of academic abilities, in friendships, for mental/physical health, and quality of life (*arrows from EFs to outcomes in* Fig. 9.1).

Given the importance of EFs for the whole child development, several authors have linked mindfulness dispositional skills and the importance of MBIs in schools for EF improvement in a theoretical way (Mind & Life Education Research, 2012; Sanger & Dorjee, 2015). Together with the theoretical approach, growing evidence has shown that MBIs applied in schools can improve or train EFs in children and/or adolescents, with the support of several systematic reviews that found significant results of interventions on EFs (Mak et al., 2018; Maynard, Solis, Miller, & Brendel, 2017); (*arrows from MBIs to EFs in* Fig. 9.1). The improvement in self-regulation and other EFs (such as inhibitory control, working memory, and cognitive flexibility) related to dispositional mindfulness skills or MBIs have been described in preschoolers (Flook, Goldberg, Pinger, & Davidson, 2015; Zelazo, Forston, Masten, & Carlson, 2018; Poehlmann-Tynan et al., 2016), children (Ricarte et al., 2015; Flook et al., 2010), and adolescents (Oberle, Schonert-Reichl, Lawlor, & Thomson, 2012; Riggs, Black, & Ritt-Olson, 2015; Schonert-Reichl & Lawlor, 2010). Thus, more consistent and promising results have been found regarding the effects of MBIs on EFs. However, more research is still needed, particularly with children and adolescents, including the use of diverse methodologies to assess these results (e.g. neuroscientific methods as electroencephalography or neuroimaging techniques) and establish the mediating role of the EFs on the effectiveness of MBIs.

Together with cognitive abilities like attention and EFs, *emotional processes* (e.g. emotional self-regulation strategies) have been related with several health outcomes, psychological well-being, and psychopathology (Aldao, Nolen-Hoeksema, & Schweizer, 2010; Carl, Soskin, Kerns, & Barlow, 2013). Emotional processes are strongly related to critical outcomes like mental health (e.g. anxiety and depression), peer relationships, academic performance, classroom behavior, and classroom climate (Graziano, Reavis, Keane, & Calkins, 2007; Kim & Cicchetti, 2010; Wyman et al., 2010). Socio-emotional competences are associated with academic and behavioral results significant for adult life (Domitrovich, Durlak, Staley, & Weissberg, 2017); likewise, interventions designed to promote emotional self-regulation have also been proven to reduce behavioral problems and increase prosocial abilities (Wyman et al., 2010). From a neuroscientific perspective, emotional regulation processes are essential for maximizing cognitive control (executive functions, based on prefrontal cortex areas) and diminishing emotional reactivity (based on limbic system areas). Through the integration of both systems, it is possible to promote self-regulation, academic achievement, and overall school success, while also preventing school failure (Blair & Diamond, 2008; Ursache, Blair, & Raver, 2012); (*arrows from self-regulation to outcomes in* Fig. 9.1).

Several studies have reported changes in emotional processes in children or adolescents after an MBI in school, including less rumination (Sibinga, Perry-Parrish, et al., 2013; Sibinga, Webb, Ghazarian, & Ellen, 2016; Mendelson et al., 2010), decreased negative coping (Deplus, Billieux, Scharff, & Philippot, 2016; Sibinga, Perry-Parrish, et al., 2013; Sibinga, Webb, et al., 2016), decreased impulsivity (Deplus et al., 2016), lower stress, and decreased intrusive thoughts (Mendelson et al., 2010). In a recent longitudinal randomized trial of an MBI with children with high depressive symptoms, effects were found on internalizing and externalizing symptoms, perceived stress, emotional regulation, cognitive reappraisal, expressive suppression, rumination, and avoidance fusion (Fung et al., 2018); (*arrows from MBIs to emotional processes in* Fig. 9.1). Interestingly, expressive suppression and rumination mediated the effects of the MBI on internalizing symptoms and perceived stress. Also, a moderation effect was found: the children with higher baseline levels of perceived stress and internalizing and externalizing problems benefited the most from the intervention (Fung et al., 2018). Likewise, a recent study with adolescents described lower depression symptoms, anxiety, and stress after a school-based mindfulness intervention. It was found that cognitive reactivity and self-coldness (an aspect of self-compassion) were the mediators that explained the decrease in depressive symptoms after the intervention (Van der Gucht et al., 2018). Therefore, both studies suggested that mindfulness training was associated with reduced mental health symptoms via improvements in emotion regulation.

9.2.3 Social Competence and Prosociality

Prosocial dispositions and behaviors are a result of our evolution (De Waal, 2009). Prosocial dispositions are natural and innate (Warneken & Tomasello, 2006). Prosociality can be expressed in many different ways, such as through caring, protecting, cooperating, helping, or sharing. Prosociality is part of social competence, which it is an early predictor of relevant outcomes during adolescence and early adulthood at the individual and public health levels (Jones, Greenberg, & Crowley, 2015). A child's greater social competence predicts better educational outcomes (graduating in time from school and university), better employment status (having a stable job and employment), minor problems with the law (less contact with the police and fewer arrests), less substance abuse, and less medication consumption. Social competence, therefore, is a determinant factor in healthy development.

In the school setting, early prosocial behaviors predict academic performance and peer acceptance in later years (Caprara, Barbaranelli, Pastorelli, Bandura, & Zimbardo, 2000). Children who behave more kindly increase their well-being and acceptance by their peers (Layous, Nelson, Oberle, Schonert-Reichl, & Lyubomirsky, 2012), and empathy predicts peer acceptance in adolescence (Sahdra, Ciarrochi, Parker, Marshall, & Heaven, 2015). The social connection during childhood and adolescence is crucial for healthy development since it is associated with better mental health outcomes and less substance abuse, as well as a higher probability of finishing secondary school (Bond et al., 2007). On the contrary, experiencing problems with peers has been associated with greater mental health problems, greater adjustment problems at school, greater social isolation, worse academic performance, less well-being, and less trust in others (Esbensen & Carson, 2009; Hawker & Boulton, 2000; You et al., 2008; Løhre, Lydersen, Paulsen, Mæhle, & Vatten, 2011; Flaspohler, Elfstrom, Vanderzee, Sink, & Birchmeier, 2009; Velderman et al., 2008). A broad and diverse set of social skills based on prosocial behaviors instead of aggressive behaviors predict greater success in peer interactions, improving peer acceptance and emotional regulation and generating higher quality relationships (Blair et al., 2015) (*arrows from social competence to outcomes in* Fig. 9.1). Thus, peer relationships are central to development in both childhood and adolescence. Effective evidence-based interventions are needed to promote the cultivation of a set of social skills-based on prosocial behaviors and dispositions.

In the school context, MBIs are effective to improve prosocial dispositions and behaviors, reducing behavioral problems, and improving school climate (Black & Fernando, 2014). A recent study showed that children who participated in an MBI, versus a control group, increased their empathy and perspective taking (Schonert-Reichl et al., 2015). In addition, peer-nomination measurements showed that children in the mindfulness group increased their prosocial behaviors and acceptance among their peers. Likewise, a study with preschoolers, which evaluated the impact of a Mindfulness-Based Kindness Curriculum relative to a control group, found improvements in the social competence and academic performance of those children who participated in the mindfulness group (Flook et al., 2015). Interestingly, children in the mindfulness group who had lower baseline levels (moderator) of social competence and inhibitory control showed a greater improvement in social competence. Also, several studies have shown increases in respect for others (Black & Fernando, 2014), a greater feeling of gratitude (Bluth & Eisenlohr-Moul, 2017), better regulation of anger (Viafora et al., 2015), and a decrease in aggressive behaviors (Franco, Amutio, López-González, Oriol, & Martínez-Taboada, 2016) after the completion of an MBI at school (*arrows from MBIs to social competence in* Fig. 9.1).

In addition to interpersonal benefits, numerous studies have shown the effectiveness of MBIs in promoting a better relationship with oneself (Marsh, Chan, & MacBeth, 2017). In particular, the practice of mindfulness in school has shown positive impact on self-compassion skills (de Carvalho, Pinto, & Marôco, 2017). Self-compassion refers to an individual's ability to show compassion towards oneself in the face of suffering (Neff, 2003). In children, self-compassion has been positively associated with self-concept, well-being, positive affect, empathy, and prosocial orientation. Conversely, lower levels of self-compassion in children have been associated with greater negative affect and stronger symptoms of depression and anxiety (Sutton, Schonert-Reichl, Wu, & Lawlor, 2018). In adolescents, self-compassion has been considered a protective factor for mental health, as it is inversely related to anxiety, depression, and psychological distress (Marsh et al., 2017).

Finally, few studies have investigated if changes in social competence processes help to explain how MBIs conducted at school influence several outcomes (*social competence as a mediator process in* Fig. 9.1). However, recent results support this notion. One study with adolescents found that changes in self-compassion were related to changes in perceived stress and depressive symptoms after an MBI (Bluth & Eisenlohr-Moul, 2017). Another study showed how the co-development of mindfulness and self-compassion skills could lead to the strengthening of emotional well-being (Bluth & Blanton, 2014). Thus, preliminary empirical evidence supports the importance of the prosocial dispositions as a mechanism that underlies the impact of the MBIs in school, but more rigorous mediation studies are necessary.

9.3 Conclusions, Limitations and Future Directions

Over the last years, research on the effects of MBIs in the school context has grown exponentially, but it is still in its infancy. There is a need for theoretical models explaining the functioning of MBIs in the school context in order to guide research on the mechanisms of action and the effects that mindfulness practice may have on children and adolescents. We have developed an integrative model of mindfulness in the school context, trying to clarify and simplify the complexity of MBI outcomes and mechanisms in schools. In the model, the main outcomes of MBIs in schools are presented, including mental health, well-being, peer relationships, classroom behavior, and academic performance. We have suggested that different skills and processes developed during an MBI in schools, such as mindfulness skills, multiple cognitive and emotional processes, and prosocial behaviors may contribute indirectly, as mechanisms of action, to promoting these outcomes. Also, we propose that boosting these outcomes can lead to the improvement of mindfulness skills, cognitive and emotional processes, and social competence through an upward spiral process or positive feedback loops.

The proposed model has several limitations. At the individual level, it focuses primarily on the impact that MBIs have on the processes and results of children and adolescents, as well as on the impact of these interventions on students' social relationships, classroom climate, and engagement. However, the model does not explicitly include the effects of MBIs on the teacher-student relationship. Roeser et al. (2012) previously proposed a model that included the impact of MBIs on teachers and particularly on teacher-student interaction. Thus, we consider that both models can complement each other to offer a broad view of the functioning of MBIs in the school context and may be useful to guide future research on mindfulness in education. Also, it is necessary to mention that our model does not consider the impact of MBIs on the organizational climate of the school and parent-child and parent-school interaction. Future models could focus on the impact of the MBIs at the organizational level.

Another limitation of the model is the possible overlap among the different processes proposed (e.g. EFs and self-regulation). Although we made an effort to clarify and specify the constructs included in the model, we must acknowledge that some of them may overlap to some extent. However, because it is challenging but necessary to clearly explain the different mechanisms involved in MBIs in the school context, we have tried to detail the specific contribution of the different processes, constructs, and perspectives included in the model.

In conclusion, in future years, it will be a challenge to continue researching the unique effects of MBIs in schools. It is necessary to understand in greater depth the mechanisms that underlie the effectiveness of MBIs in the school context, while also determining under what conditions they are most effective and for whom. The model proposed can help clarify how mindfulness works in schools and can also inform the design of future studies. Nowadays, many mindfulness programs are implemented in educational settings (e.g. b, MindUp, Growing Up Breathing [Crecer Respirando in Spanish], Mindful Schools), all of which display significant differences in terms of structure, methodology, and the mindfulness practices used. Our model can help determine which program is particularly useful for obtaining specific results, through which specific mechanisms, and under which specific conditions.

Funding Information This manuscript was supported by a grant from the Spanish Ministry of Education, Culture, and Sport (FPU13/01677) to García-Rubio, Carlos. In addition, this work was supported by the Fund for Innovation and Competitiveness (FIC) of the Chilean Ministry of Economy, Development, and Tourism, through the Millennium Scientific Initiative, Grant [IS 130005-MIDAP to C.I.A.].

References

Aldao, A., Nolen-Hoeksema, S., & Schweizer, S. (2010). Emotion-regulation strategies across psychopathology: A meta-analytic review. *Clinical Psychology Review, 30*(2), 217–237. https://doi.org/10.1016/j.cpr.2009.11.004.

Black, D. S., & Fernando, R. (2014). Mindfulness training and classroom behavior among lower-income and ethnic minority elementary school children. *Journal of Child and Family Studies, 23*(7), 1242–1246. https://doi.org/10.1007/s10826-013-9784-4.

Blair, C., & Diamond, A. (2008). Biological processes in prevention and intervention: The promotion of self-regulation as a means of preventing school failure. *Development and Psychopathology, 20*(3), 899–911. https://doi.org/10.1017/S0954579408000436.

Blair, B. L., Perry, N. B., O'Brien, M., Calkins, S. D., Keane, S. P., & Shanahan, L. (2015). Identifying developmental cascades among differentiated dimensions of social competence and emotion regulation. *Developmental Psychology, 51*(8), 1062. https://doi.org/10.1037/a0039472.

Blair, C., & Raver, C. (2015). School readiness and self-regulation: A developmental psychobiological approach. *Annual Review of Psychology, 66,* 711–731. https://doi.org/10.1146/annurev-psych-010814-015221.

Blair, C., & Razza, R. P. (2007). Relating effortful control, executive function, and false belief understanding to emerging math and literacy ability in kindergarten. *Child Development, 78*(2), 647–663. https://doi.org/10.1111/j.1467-8624.2007.01019.x.

Bluth, K., & Blanton, P. W. (2014). Mindfulness and self-compassion: Exploring pathways to adolescent emotional well-being. *Journal of Child and Family Studies, 23*(7), 1298–1309. https://doi.org/10.1007/s10826-013-9830-2.

Bluth, K., & Eisenlohr-Moul, T. A. (2017). Response to a mindful self-compassion intervention in teens: A within-person association of mindfulness, self-compassion, and emotional well-being outcomes. *Journal of Adolescence, 57,* 108–118. https://doi.org/10.1016/j.adolescence.2017.04.001.

Bodhi, B. (2011). What does mindfulness really mean? A canonical perspective. *Contemporary Buddhism, 12*(1), 19–39. https://doi.org/10.1080/14639947.2011.564813.

Bond, L., Butler, H., Thomas, L., Carlin, J., Glover, S., Bowes, G., et al. (2007). Social and school connectedness in early secondary school as predictors of late teenage substance use, mental health, and academic outcomes. *Journal of Adolescent Health, 40*(4), 357. https://doi.org/10.1016/j.jadohealth.2006.10.013.

Brock, L. L., Rimm-Kaufman, S. E., Nathanson, L., & Grimm, K. J. (2009). The contributions of 'hot' and 'cool' executive function to children's academic achievement, learning-related behaviors, and engagement in kindergarten. *Early Childhood Research Quarterly, 24*(3), 337–349. https://doi.org/10.1016/j.ecresq.2009.06.001.

Calvete, E., Morea, A., & Orue, I. (2018). The role of dispositional mindfulness in the longitudinal associations between stressors, maladaptive schemas, and depressive symptoms in adolescents. *Mindfulness,* 1–12. https://doi.org/10.1007/s12671-018-1000-6.

Caprara, G. V., Barbaranelli, C., Pastorelli, C., Bandura, A., & Zimbardo, P. G. (2000). Prosocial foundations of children's academic achievement. *Psychological Science, 11*(4), 302–306. https://doi.org/10.1111/1467-9280.00260.

Carl, J. R., Soskin, D. P., Kerns, C., & Barlow, D. H. (2013). Positive emotion regulation in emotional disorders: A theoretical review. *Clinical Psychology Review, 33*(3), 343–360. https://doi.org/10.1016/j.cpr.2013.01.003.

Carsley, D., Khoury, B., & Heath, N. L. (2018). Effectiveness of mindfulness interventions for mental health in schools: A comprehensive meta-analysis. *Mindfulness, 9*(3), 693–707. https://doi.org/10.1007/s12671-017-0839-2.

Ciesla, J. A., Reilly, L. C., Dickson, K. S., Emanuel, A. S., & Updegraff, J. A. (2012). Dispositional mindfulness moderates the effects of stress among adolescents: Rumination as a mediator. *Journal of Clinical Child & Adolescent Psychology, 41*(6), 760–770. https://doi.org/10.1080/15374416.2012.698724.

Crescentini, C., Capurso, V., Furlan, S., & Fabbro, F. (2016). Mindfulness-oriented meditation for primary school children: Effects on attention and psychological well-being. *Frontiers in Psychology, 7,* 805. https://doi.org/10.3389/fpsyg.2016.00805.

de Carvalho, J. S., Pinto, A. M., & Marôco, J. (2017). Results of a mindfulness-based social-emotional learning program on portuguese elementary students and teachers: A quasi-experimental study. *Mindfulness, 8*(2), 337–350. https://doi.org/10.1007/s12671-016-0603-z.

De Vibe, M. F., Bjørndal, A., Fattah, S., Dyrdal, G. M., Halland, E., & Tanner-Smith, E. E. (2017). Mindfulness-based stress reduction (MBSR) for improving health, quality of life and social functioning in adults: A systematic review and meta-analysis. *Campbell Systematic Reviews, 2017,* 11. https://doi.org/10.4073/csr.2017.11.

De Waal, F. (2009). *The age of empathy*. New York: Harmony.

DeHaas, P. A. (1986). Attention styles and peer relationships of hyperactive and normal boys and girls. *Journal of Abnormal Child Psychology, 14,* 457–467.

Deplus, S., Billieux, J., Scharff, C., & Philippot, P. (2016). A mindfulness-based group intervention for enhancing self-regulation of emotion in late childhood and adolescence: A pilot study. *International Journal of Mental Health and Addiction, 14*(5), 775–790. https://doi.org/10.1007/s11469-015-9627-1.

Diamantopoulou, S., Rydell, A.-M., Thorell, L. B., & Bohlin, G. (2007). Impact of executive functioning and symptoms of attention deficit hyperactivity disorder on children's peer relations and school performance. *Developmental Neuropsychology, 32*(1), 521–542. https://doi.org/10.1080/87565640701360981.

Diamond, A. (2013). Executive functions. *Annual Review of Psychology, 64,* 135–168. https://doi.org/10.1146/annurev-psych-113011-143750.

Diamond, A., & Lee, K. (2011). Interventions shown to aid executive function development in children 4 to 12 years old. *Science, 333*(6045), 959–964. https://doi.org/10.1126/science.1204529.

Diamond, A., & Ling, D. S. (2016). Conclusions about interventions, programs, and approaches for improving executive functions that appear justified and those that, despite much hype, do not. *Developmental Cognitive Neuroscience, 18,* 34–48. https://doi.org/10.1016/j.dcn.2015.11.005.

Domitrovich, C. E., Durlak, J. A., Staley, K. C., & Weissberg, R. P. (2017). Social-emotional competence: An essential factor for promoting positive adjustment and reducing risk in school children. *Child Development, 88*(2), 408–416. https://doi.org/10.1111/cdev.12739.

Dunning, D. L., Griffiths, K., Kuyken, W., Crane, C., Foulkes, L., Parker, J., et al. (2018). Research review: The effects of mindfulness-based interventions on cognition and mental health in children and adolescents–a meta-analysis of randomized controlled trials. *Journal of Child Psychology and Psychiatry.* https://doi.org/10.1111/jcpp.12980.

DuPaul, G. J., McGoey, K. E., Eckert, T. L., & VanBrakle, J. (2001). Preschool children with attention-deficit/hyperactivity disorder: Impairments in behavioral, social, and school functioning. *Journal of the American Academy of Child and Adolescent Psychiatry, 40*(5), 508–515. https://doi.org/10.1097/00004583-200105000-00009.

Esbensen, F., & Carson, D. (2009). Consequences of being bullied: Results from a longitudinal assessment of bullying victimization in a multisite sample of American students. *Youth & Society, 41*(2), 209–233. https://doi.org/10.1177/0044118X09351067.

Felver, J. C., Celis-de Hoyos, C. E., Tezanos, K., & Singh, N. N. (2016). A systematic review of mindfulness-based interventions for youth in school settings. *Mindfulness, 7*(1), 34–45. https://doi.org/10.1007/s12671-015-0389-4.

Felver, J. C., Tipsord, J. M., Morris, M. J., Racer, K. H., & Dishion, T. J. (2017). The effects of mindfulness-based intervention on children's attention regulation. *Journal of Attention Disorders, 21*(10), 872–881. https://doi.org/10.1177/1087054714548032.

Flaspohler, P. D., Elfstrom, J. L., Vanderzee, K. L., Sink, H. E., & Birchmeier, Z. (2009). Stand by me: The effects of peer and teacher support in mitigating the impact of bullying on quality of life. *Psychology in the Schools, 46*(7), 636–649. https://doi.org/10.1002/pits.20404.

Flook, L., Goldberg, S. B., Pinger, L., & Davidson, R. J. (2015). Promoting prosocial behavior and self-regulatory skills in preschool children through a mindfulness-based kindness curriculum. *Developmental Psychology, 51*(1), 44. https://doi.org/10.1037/a0038256.

Flook, L., Smalley, S. L., Kitil, M. J., Galla, B. M., Kaiser-Greenland, S., Locke, J., et al. (2010). Effects of mindful awareness practices on executive functions in elementary school children. *Journal of Applied School Psychology, 26*(1), 70–95. https://doi.org/10.1080/15377900903379125.

Franco, C., Amutio, A., López-González, L., Oriol, X., & Martínez-Taboada, C. (2016). Effect of a mindfulness training program on the impulsivity and aggression levels of adolescents with behavioral problems in the classroom. *Frontiers in Psychology, 7,* 1385. https://doi.org/10.3389/fpsyg.2016.01385.

Fredrickson, B. (2001). The role of positive emotions in positive psychology: The broaden-and-build theory of positive emotions. *American Psychologist, 56*(3), 218. https://doi.org/10.1037/0003-066X.56.3.218.

Fung, J., Kim, J. J., Jin, J., Chen, G., Bear, L., & Lau, A. S. (2018). A randomized trial evaluating school-based mindfulness intervention for ethnic minority youth: exploring mediators and moderators of intervention effects. *Journal of Abnormal Child Psychology,* 1–19. https://doi.org/10.1007/s10802-018-0425-7.

Goldberg, S. B., Tucker, R. P., Greene, P. A., Davidson, R. J., Wampold, B. E., Kearney, D. J., et al. (2017). Mindfulness-based interventions for psychiatric disorders: A systematic review and meta-analysis. *Clinical Psychology Review, 59,* 52–60. https://doi.org/10.1016/j.cpr.2017.10.011.

Graziano, P. A., Reavis, R. D., Keane, S. P., & Calkins, S. D. (2007). The role of emotion regulation in children's early academic success. *Journal of School Psychology, 45*(1), 3–19. https://doi.org/10.1016/j.jsp.2006.09.002.

Greco, L. A., Baer, R. A., & Smith, G. T. (2011). Assessing mindfulness in children and adolescents: Development and validation of the child and adolescent mindfulness measure (CAMM). *Psychological Assessment, 23*(3), 606. https://doi.org/10.1037/a0022819.

Greco, L. A., Lambert, W., & Baer, R. A. (2008). Psychological inflexibility in childhood and adolescence: Development and evaluation of the Avoidance and Fusion Questionnaire for Youth. *Psychological Assessment, 20*(2), 93. https://doi.org/10.1037/1040-3590.20.2.93.

Greenberg, M. T., Weissberg, R. P., O'Brien, M. U., Zins, J. E., Fredericks, L., Resnik, H., et al. (2003). Enhancing school-based prevention and youth development through coordinated social, emotional, and academic learning. *American Psychologist, 58*(6–7), 466. https://doi.org/10.1037/0003-066X.58.6-7.466.

Grossman, P., & Van Dam, N. T. (2011). Mindfulness, by any other name…: Trials and tribulations of sati in western psychology and science. *Contemporary Buddhism, 12*(1), 219–239. https://doi.org/10.1080/14639947.2011.564841.

Gu, J., Strauss, C., Bond, R., & Cavanagh, K. (2015). How do mindfulness-based cognitive therapy and mindfulness-based stress reduction improve mental health and wellbeing? A systematic review and meta-analysis of mediation studies. *Clinical Psychology Review, 37,* 1–12. https://doi.org/10.1016/j.cpr.2015.01.006.

Hawker, D. S., & Boulton, M. J. (2000). Twenty years' research on peer victimization and psychosocial maladjustment: A meta-analytic review of cross-sectional studies. *The Journal of Child Psychology and Psychiatry and Allied Disciplines, 41*(4), 441–455. https://doi.org/10.1111/1469-7610.00629.

Hayes, S. C., Luoma, J. B., Bond, F. W., Masuda, A., & Lillis, J. (2006). Acceptance and commitment therapy: Model, processes and outcomes. *Behaviour Research and Therapy, 44*(1), 1–25. https://doi.org/10.1016/j.brat.2005.06.006.

Hayes, S. C., Strosahl, K. D., & Wilson, K. G. (1999). *Acceptance and commitment therapy.* New York: Guilford Press.

Holmes, C. J., Kim-Spoon, J., & Deater-Deckard, K. (2016). Linking executive function and peer problems from early childhood through middle adolescence. *Journal of Abnormal Child Psychology, 44*(1), 31–42. https://doi.org/10.1007/s10802-015-0044-5.

Hölzel, B. K., Lazar, S. W., Gard, T., Schuman-Olivier, Z., Vago, D. R., & Ott, U. (2011). How does mindfulness meditation work? Proposing mechanisms of action from a conceptual and neural perspective. *Perspectives on Psychological Science, 6*(6), 537–559. https://doi.org/10.1177/1745691611419671.

Jennings, P. A. (2008). Contemplative education and youth development. *New Directions for Youth Development, 2008*(118), 101–105. https://doi.org/10.1002/yd.262.

Jha, A. P., Krompinger, J., & Baime, M. J. (2007). Mindfulness training modifies subsystems of attention. *Cognitive, Affective & Behavioral Neuroscience, 7*(2), 109–119. https://doi.org/10.3758/CABN.7.2.109.

Johnson, C., Burke, C., Brinkman, S., & Wade, T. (2017). A randomized controlled evaluation of a secondary school mindfulness program for early adolescents: Do we have the recipe right yet? *Behaviour Research and Therapy, 99,* 37–46. https://doi.org/10.1016/j.brat.2017.09.001.

Jones, D. E., Greenberg, M., & Crowley, M. (2015). Early social-emotional functioning and public health: The relationship between kindergarten social competence and future wellness. *American Journal of Public Health, 105*(11), 2283–2290. https://doi.org/10.2105/AJPH.2015.302630.

Kabat-Zinn, J. (2003). Mindfulness-based interventions in context: Past, present, and future. *Clinical Psychology: Science and Practice, 10*(2), 144–156. https://doi.org/10.1093/clipsy.bpg016.

Kashdan, T., & Rottenberg, J. (2010). Psychological flexibility as a fundamental aspect of health. *Clinical Psychology Review, 30*(7), 865–878. https://doi.org/10.1016/j.cpr.2010.03.001.

Kemeny, M. E., Foltz, C., Cavanagh, J. F., Cullen, M., Giese-Davis, J., Jennings, P., et al. (2012). Contemplative/emotion training reduces negative emotional behavior and promotes prosocial responses. *Emotion, 12*(2), 338. https://doi.org/10.1037/a0026118.

Khoury, B., Lecomte, T., Fortin, G., Masse, M., Therien, P., Bouchard, V., et al. (2013). Mindfulness-based therapy: A comprehensive meta-analysis. *Clinical Psychology Review, 33*(6), 763–771. https://doi.org/10.1016/j.cpr.2013.05.005.

Kim, J., & Cicchetti, D. (2010). Longitudinal pathways linking child maltreatment, emotion regulation, peer relations, and psychopathology. *Journal of Child Psychology and Psychiatry, 51*(6), 706–716. https://doi.org/10.1111/j.1469-7610.2009.02202.x.

Lawlor, M. S. (2016). Mindfulness and social emotional learning (SEL): A conceptual framework. In K. A. Schonert-Reichl & R. W. Roeser (Eds.), *Handbook of mindfulness in education: Integrating theory and research into practice* (pp. 65–80). New York, NY: Springer.

Lawlor, M. S., Schonert-Reichl, K. A., Gadermann, A. M., & Zumbo, B. D. (2014). A validation study of the mindful attention awareness scale adapted for children. *Mindfulness, 5*(6), 730–741. https://doi.org/10.1007/s12671-013-0228-4.

Layous, K., Nelson, S. K., Oberle, E., Schonert-Reichl, K. A., & Lyubomirsky, S. (2012). Kindness counts: Prompting prosocial behavior in preadolescents boosts peer acceptance and well-being. *PloS One, 7*(12), https://doi.org/10.1371/journal.pone.0051380.

Løhre, A., Lydersen, S., Paulsen, B., Mæhle, M., & Vatten, L. J. (2011). Peer victimization as reported by children, teachers, and parents in relation to children's health symptoms. *BMC Public Health, 11*(1), 278. https://doi.org/10.1186/1471-2458-11-278.

Lutz, A., Slagter, H. A., Dunne, J. D., & Davidson, R. J. (2008). Attention regulation and monitoring in meditation. *Trends in Cognitive Sciences, 12*(4), 163–169. https://doi.org/10.1016/j.tics.2008.01.005.

Mak, C., Whittingham, K., Cunnington, R., & Boyd, R. N. (2018). Efficacy of mindfulness-based interventions for attention and executive function in children and adolescents—A systematic review. *Mindfulness, 9*(1), 59–78. https://doi.org/10.1007/s12671-017-0770-6.

Marsh, I. C., Chan, S. W., & MacBeth, A. (2017). Self-compassion and psychological distress in adolescents—A meta-analysis. *Mindfulness, 9*(4), 1–17. https://doi.org/10.1007/s12671-017-0850-7.

Maynard, B. R., Solis, M., Miller, V., & Brendel, K. E. (2017). Mindfulness-based interventions for improving cognition, academic achievement, behavior and socio-emotional functioning of primary and secondary students. *Campbell Systematic Reviews, 13*. https://doi.org/10.4073/csr.2017.5.

Mendelson, T., Greenberg, M. T., Dariotis, J. K., Gould, L. F., Rhoades, B. L., & Leaf, P. J. (2010). Feasibility and preliminary outcomes of a school-based mindfulness intervention for urban youth. *Journal of Abnormal Child Psychology, 38*(7), 985–994. https://doi.org/10.1007/s10802-010-9418-x.

Mind & Life Education Research Network. (2012). Contemplative practices and mental training: Prospects for American education. *Child Development Perspectives, 6*(2), 146–153. https://doi.org/10.1111/j.1750-8606.2012.00240.x.

Mrug, S., Hoza, B., & Gerdes, A. C. (2001). Children with attention-deficit/hyperactivity disorder: Peer relationships and peer-oriented interventions. *New Directions for Child and Adolescent Development, 2001*(91), 51–78. https://doi.org/10.1002/cd.5.

Muris, P., Meesters, C., Herings, A., Jansen, M., Vossen, C., & Kersten, P. (2017). Inflexible youngsters: Psychological and psychopathological correlates of the avoidance and fusion questionnaire for youths in nonclinical dutch adolescents. *Mindfulness, 8*(5), 1381–1392. https://doi.org/10.1007/s12671-017-0714-1.

Napoli, M., Krech, P. R., & Holley, L. C. (2005). Mindfulness training for elementary school students: The attention academy. *Journal of Applied School Psychology, 21*(1), 99–125. https://doi.org/10.1300/J370v21n01_05.

Neff, K. D. (2003). The development and validation of a scale to measure self-compassion. *Self and Identity, 2*(3), 223–250. https://doi.org/10.1080/15298860309027.

Northup, J., Broussard, C., Jones, K., George, T., Vollmer, T. R., & Herring, M. (1995). The differential effects of teacher and peer attention on the disruptive classroom behavior of three children with a diagnosis of attention deficit hyperactivity disorder. *Journal of Applied Behavior Analysis, 28*(2), 227–228. https://doi.org/10.1901/jaba.1995.28-227.

Nyklíček, I., & Kuijpers, K. (2008). Effects of mindfulness-based stress reduction intervention on psychological well-being and quality of life: is increased mindfulness indeed the mechanism? *Annals of Behavioral Medicine, 35*(3), 331–340. https://doi.org/10.1007/s12160-008-9030-2.

O'Toole, S. E., Monks, C. P., & Tsermentseli, S. (2017). Executive function and theory of mind as predictors of aggressive and prosocial behavior and peer acceptance in early childhood. *Social Development, 26*(4), 907–920. https://doi.org/10.1111/sode.12231.

Oberle, E., Schonert-Reichl, K. A., Lawlor, M. S., & Thomson, K. C. (2012). Mindfulness and inhibitory control in early adolescence. *The Journal of Early Adolescence, 32*(4), 565–588. https://doi.org/10.1177/0272431611403741.

Pallozzi, R., Wertheim, E., Paxton, S., & Ong, B. (2017). Trait mindfulness measures for use with adolescents: A systematic review. *Mindfulness, 8*(1), 110–125. https://doi.org/10.1007/s12671-016-0567-z.

Poehlmann-Tynan, J., Vigna, A. B., Weymouth, L. A., Gerstein, E. D., Burnson, C., Zabransky, M., et al. (2016). A pilot study of contemplative practices with economically disadvantaged preschoolers: Children's empathic and self-regulatory behaviors. *Mindfulness, 7*(1), 46–58. https://doi.org/10.1007/s12671-015-0426-3.

Ricarte, J., Ros, L., Latorre, J., & Beltrán, M. (2015). Mindfulness-based intervention in a rural primary school: Effects on attention, concentration and mood. *International Journal of Cognitive Therapy, 8*(3), 258–270. https://doi.org/10.1521/ijct_2015_8_03.

Riggs, N. R., Black, D. S., & Ritt-Olson, A. (2015). Associations between dispositional mindfulness and executive function in early adolescence. *Journal of Child and Family Studies, 24*(9), 2745–2751. https://doi.org/10.1007/s10826-014-0077-3.

Riggs, N. R., Jahromi, L. B., Razza, R. P., Dillworth-Bart, J. E., & Mueller, U. (2006). Executive function and the promotion of social–emotional competence. *Journal of Applied Developmental Psychology, 27*(4), 300–309. https://doi.org/10.1016/j.appdev.2006.04.002.

Roeser, R. W., Skinner, E., Beers, J., & Jennings, P. A. (2012). Mindfulness training and teachers' professional development: An emerging area of research and practice. *Child Development Perspectives, 6*(2), 167–173. https://doi.org/10.1111/j.1750-8606.2012.00238.x.

Sahdra, B. K., Ciarrochi, J., Parker, P. D., Marshall, S., & Heaven, P. (2015). Empathy and nonattachment independently predict peer nominations of prosocial behavior of adolescents. *Frontiers in Psychology, 6,* 263. https://doi.org/10.3389/fpsyg.2015.00263.

Sanger, K. L., & Dorjee, D. (2015). Mindfulness training for adolescents: A neurodevelopmental perspective on investigating modifications in attention and emotion regulation using event-related brain potentials. *Cognitive, Affective & Behavioral Neuroscience, 15*(3), 696–711. https://doi.org/10.3758/s13415-015-0354-7.

Schonert-Reichl, K. A., & Lawlor, M. S. (2010). The effects of a mindfulness-based education program on pre-and early adolescents' well-being and social and emotional competence. *Mindfulness, 1*(3), 137–151. https://doi.org/10.1007/s12671-010-0011-8.

Schonert-Reichl, K. A., Oberle, E., Lawlor, M. S., Abbott, D., Thomson, K., Oberlander, T. F., et al. (2015). Enhancing cognitive and social–emotional development through a simple-to-administer mindfulness-based school program for elementary school children: A randomized controlled trial. *Developmental Psychology, 51*(1), 52. https://doi.org/10.1037/a0038454.

Schonert-Reichl, K. A., & Roeser, R. W. (2016). *Handbook of mindfulness in education: Integrating theory and research into practice*. New York: Springer.

Schulte-Körne, G. (2016). Mental health problems in a school setting in children and adolescents. *Deutsches Ärzteblatt International, 113*(11), 183. https://doi.org/10.3238/arztebl.2016.0183.

Semple, R. J., Lee, J., Rosa, D., & Miller, L. F. (2010). A randomized trial of mindfulness-based cognitive therapy for children: Promoting mindful attention to enhance social-emotional resiliency in children. *Journal of Child and Family Studies, 19*(2), 218–229. https://doi.org/10.1007/s10826-009-9301-y.

Sibinga, E. M., Perry-Parrish, C., Chung, S.-E., Johnson, S. B., Smith, M., & Ellen, J. M. (2013). School-based mindfulness instruction for urban male youth: A small randomized controlled trial. *Preventive Medicine, 57*(6), 799–801. https://doi.org/10.1016/j.ypmed.2013.08.027.

Sibinga, E. M., Webb, L., Ghazarian, S. R., & Ellen, J. M. (2016). School-based mindfulness instruction: An RCT. *Pediatrics, 137*(1). https://doi.org/10.1542/peds.2015-2532.

Simon, E., & Verboon, P. (2016). Psychological inflexibility and child anxiety. *Journal of Child and Family Studies, 25*(12), 3565–3573. https://doi.org/10.1007/s10826-016-0522-6.

Slagter, H. A., Davidson, R. J., & Lutz, A. (2011). Mental training as a tool in the neuroscientific study of brain and cognitive plasticity. *Frontiers in Human Neuroscience, 5,* 17. https://doi.org/10.3389/fnhum.2011.00017.

Slagter, H. A., Lutz, A., Greischar, L. L., Francis, A. D., Nieuwenhuis, S., Davis, J. M., et al. (2007). Mental training affects distribution of limited brain resources. *PLoS Biology, 5*(6), e138. https://doi.org/10.1371/journal.pbio.0050138.

St Clair-Thompson, H. L., & Gathercole, S. E. (2006). Executive functions and achievements in school: Shifting, updating, inhibition, and working memory. *The Quarterly Journal of Experimental Psychology, 59*(4), 745–759. https://doi.org/10.1080/17470210500162854.

Sutton, E., Schonert-Reichl, K. A., Wu, A. D., & Lawlor, M. S. (2018). Evaluating the reliability and validity of the self-compassion scale short form adapted for children ages 8–12. *Child Indicators Research, 11*(4), 1217–1236. https://doi.org/10.1007/s12187-017-9470-y.

Tan, L., & Martin, G. (2015). Taming the adolescent mind: A randomised controlled trial examining clinical efficacy of an adolescent mindfulness-based group programme. *Child and Adolescent Mental Health, 20*(1), 49–55. https://doi.org/10.1111/camh.12057.

Tang, Y., Hölzel, B., & Posner, M. (2015). The neuroscience of mindfulness meditation. *Nature Reviews Neuroscience, 16*(4), 213. https://doi.org/10.1038/nrn3916.

Ursache, A., Blair, C., & Raver, C. C. (2012). The promotion of self-regulation as a means of enhancing school readiness and early achievement in children at risk for school failure. *Child Development Perspectives, 6*(2), 122–128. https://doi.org/10.1111/j.1750-8606.2011.00209.x.

Vago, D. R., & Silbersweig, D. A. (2012). Self-awareness, self-regulation, and self-transcendence (S-ART): A framework for understanding the neurobiological mechanisms of mindfulness. *Frontier Human Neuroscience, 6,* 296. https://doi.org/10.3389/fnhum.2012.00296.

Van Dam, N., van Vugt, M. K., Vago, D. R., Schmalzl, L., Saron, C. D., Olendzki, A., et al. (2018). Mind the hype: A critical evaluation and prescriptive agenda for research on mindfulness and meditation. *Perspectives on Psychological Science, 13*(1), 36–61. https://doi.org/10.1177/1745691617709589.

Van der Gucht, K., Takano, K., Raes, F., & Kuppens, P. (2018). Processes of change in a school-based mindfulness programme: Cognitive reactivity and self-coldness as mediators. *Cognition and Emotion, 32*(3), 658–665. https://doi.org/10.1080/02699931.2017.1310716.

Velderman, M. K., van Dorst, A. G., Wiefferink, C. H., Detmar, S. B., Paulussen, T. G., & The KIDSCREEN group. (2008). Quality of life of victims bullies, and bully/victims among school-aged children in the Netherlands. *Advances in School Mental Health Promotion, 1*(4), 42–52. https://doi.org/10.1080/1754730X.2008.9715738.

Viafora, D. P., Mathiesen, S. G., & Unsworth, S. J. (2015). Teaching mindfulness to middle school students and homeless youth in school classrooms. *Journal of Child and Family Studies, 24*(5), 1179–1191. https://doi.org/10.1007/s10826-014-9926-3.

Vickery, C. E., & Dorjee, D. (2016). Mindfulness training in primary schools decreases negative affect and increases meta-cognition in children. *Frontiers in Psychology, 6,* 2025. https://doi.org/10.3389/fpsyg.2015.02025.

Vygotsky, L. S. (1978). Interaction between learning and development. In M. Cole, V. John-Steiner, S. Scribner, & E. Souber-Man (Eds.), *Mind in society: The development of higher psychological processes* (pp. 79–91). Cambridge, MA: Harvard University Press.

Warneken, F., & Tomasello, M. (2006). Altruistic helping in human infants and young chimpanzees. *Science, 311*(5765), 1301–1303. https://doi.org/10.1126/science.1121448.

Wyman, P. A., Cross, W., Brown, C. H., Yu, Q., Tu, X., & Eberly, S. (2010). Intervention to strengthen emotional self-regulation in children with emerging mental health problems: Proximal impact on school behavior. *Journal of Abnormal Child Psychology, 38*(5), 707–720. https://doi.org/10.1007/s10802-010-9398-x.

You, S., Furlong, M. J., Felix, E., Sharkey, J. D., Tanigawa, D., & Green, J. G. (2008). Relations among school connectedness, hope, life satisfaction, and bully victimization. *Psychology in the Schools, 45*(5), 446–460. https://doi.org/10.1002/pits.20308.

Zelazo, P. D., Forston, J. L., Masten, A. S., & Carlson, S. M. (2018). Mindfulness plus reflection training: Effects on executive function in early childhood. *Frontiers in Psychology, 9,* 208. https://doi.org/10.3389/fpsyg.2018.00208.

Zenner, C., Herrnleben-Kurz, S., & Walach, H. (2014). Mindfulness-based interventions in schools—A systematic review and meta-analysis. *Frontiers in Psychology, 5,* 603. https://doi.org/10.3389/fpsyg.2014.00603.

Chapter 10
Basic Needs, Resilience, and General Principles in Counseling

Marcel Schaer and Imke Knafla

Abstract Even though basic needs are independent of cultures and development stages, there are clear inter-individual differences in how they can be fulfilled. Thus, while basic needs are universal, the ways in which people seek to satisfy them are highly personal. In the course of their development, people amass the most diverse experiences as to the strategies for fulfilling these basic needs (approach) and for avoiding harm (avoidance). When adolescents succeed in satisfying their basic needs, these positive experiences result in positive assumptions about themselves, their environment, and their future. However, these strategies are not always successful. The environment can change, for instance, confronting the adolescent with a new situation where the old strategies and patterns are no longer effective. It is important for the psychological health of adolescents how much they persevere in finding new ways to fulfill their basic needs and how they succeed in fulfilling them. Professional psychological support can encourage and support adolescents to achieve this goal in a better way and help them to grow towards greater resilience. In addition, we illustrate which factors are important for providing adolescents with effective support in counseling and psychotherapy.

Keywords Psychological needs · Approach patterns · Avoidance patterns · Common factors · Therapeutic relationship

10.1 Basic Needs, Psychological Well-Being, and Resilience

What does it take to enable young people to develop well? How can they stay—or become—psychologically healthy, in spite of various obstacles in life?

These are some of the big and crucial questions in psychotherapy and counseling with adolescents. And, as with the big questions in so many areas, Psychology has a wide variety of answers. One answer focuses on the satisfaction of fundamental

M. Schaer (✉) · I. Knafla
School of Applied Psychology, ZHAW Zürich University of Applied Sciences, Zürich, Switzerland
e-mail: shma@zhaw.ch

C. Steinebach and Á. I. Langer (eds.), *Enhancing Resilience in Youth*,
https://doi.org/10.1007/978-3-030-25513-8_10

psychological needs, called basic needs: the better the individual succeeds in fulfilling these needs, the more stable and resistant is his or her psyche.

These needs are basic for various reasons (e.g. Ryan & Deci, 2017; Grawe, 2004). First, they are universal, i.e. independent of development stages or cultural settings (Ryan & Deci, 2017). Second, our experiences with fulfillment or frustration of these basic needs during childhood and youth are formative for our later lives. Third, they cannot be compensated for or ignored without a disorder developing, i.e. without damage to psychological and social balance. Thus, fulfillment of these basic needs is essential for our mental health. In the long run, frustrations lead to psychological imbalance and corresponding disorders (Ryan & Deci, 2017; Grawe, 2004; Maslow, 1954).

When it comes to fulfilling such basic needs, adolescents in particular (and their parents) are faced with a great developmental challenge. One prime developmental goal for adolescents is to part from their parents and their household. In parallel, they need to build stable and reliable extrafamilial contacts, but without completely severing contact with their parents. In view of the fact that basic needs are fulfilled with and by the social environment, they are now faced with the task to no longer satisfy their basic needs via their parents, but to broaden and fashion their living environment themselves for that fulfillment. For this, adolescents need courage, personal initiative, and social support (among others, from their parents).

Below, we will introduce the various basic psychological needs and place them in a theoretical model of resilience development.

10.1.1 Basic Needs

What a human being needs for healthy development is a question that was already pondered by Epicurus. He held that for a good life, a person needs friendships, freedoms, and reflection (de Botton, 2001). But more recent thinkers, psychologists, and researchers have worked on the subject of basic needs as well, developing a wide range of models (e.g. Brazelton & Greenspan, 2002; Grawe, 2004; Maslow, 1954; Young, Klosko, & Weishaar, 2008). Even though these theories vary strongly in content, they all agree on one basic psychological need—the need for attachment and belonging. Concerning the other basic needs, two theories seem particularly comprehensive and fruitful: Epstein's "Cognitive-Experimental Self-Theory" (1990) and the "Self-Determination Theory" by Deci and Ryan (2000). Both of these are very well empirically examined and validated. To develop a provisional working model, we suggest combining these two theories, since they complement each other in an ideal way. Against this backdrop, we postulate four different clusters of basic needs (c.f. Schaer & Steinebach, 2015):

Attachment and belonging: The need for attachment, social integration, and love is, certainly, one of the most primal. This insight owes a great deal to the groundbreaking research by Spitz, Bowlby, and Ainsworth. This need is satisfied when other people are felt to be helpful, benevolent, trustworthy, and supportive. Thus, good attachment persons provide protection, closeness, consolation, and safety, serving as an important and accessible haven in difficult situations. This need is violated when parents' reactions to their children's signals are not empathic, but stalled, inconsistent, inadequate or nonexistent. When trying to make contact with these parents, children experience rejection and/or a lack of reliability. As a consequence, they develop a conviction that other people are not reliable.

In the beginning of a child's development, in particular, the need for attachment is very closely connected to the other basic needs (c.f. Grawe, 2004). A sensitive and responsive attachment person allows the infant to experience, for example, that his or her behavior (e.g. crying) can cause the mother to react in order to fulfill his or her needs (e.g. for nourishment). Fulfillment leads to positive, agreeable, and comforting conditions; frustration leads to aversive, disagreeable, and activating moods. Thus, positive attachment experiences are relevant experiences of control and self-worth as well ("I can make others take care of me"). Since a good attachment is a place of safety, it allows individuals to explore unknown things, too ("In case of danger, I can go to a safe place"), and start venturing towards autonomy. In the course of development, these basic needs become more separate and more independent.

Control and orientation: All of their lives, people strive to attain influence, effectuality, and control over their environment. For some authors like Heckhausen (Heckhausen & Heckhausen, 2010) and Epstein (1990), this is one of the most fundamental of all needs. The need for control has been the subject of countless theoretical and empirical studies as well. Connected concepts are, for instance, Rotter's "sense of control" (1966) or Bandura's "self-efficacy" (1977). This need is satisfied if the world is felt to be (sufficiently) influenceable, predictable, and controllable, and therefore just to some extent. And even if some events do not correspond to what we expect or what we would like, there is the conviction that we could influence and change them. Learning and understanding rules and boundaries are essential factors for experiencing events as controllable and predictable. These help children to orient themselves and find their bearings in a complex world.

The need for control, orientation, and effectuality is frustrated when the child or adolescent receives unjust punishments from attachment persons, and/or if boundaries and rules are lacking, intransparent, or diffuse. Neglect and abuse are among the most massive breaches of this need.

Self-worth and self-acceptance: Developing an accepting and positive self is seen by many psychologists as one of the most important tasks in life (e.g. Adler, 1920; Rogers, 2004). As already pointed out by Rogers, an appreciative, empathic, and supportive environment is central to developing a healthy self. In a child's development, self-worth forms over several years and becomes stable in mid-childhood. The cognitive basis for this is the ability to become aware of self and the capacity of self-reflective thinking. In cases of negative development, children and adolescents feel incompetent, not loveable, worthless, and weak. For young people, experiences in school as well as the transition to college and working life are extremely important, because in these environments they often receive direct feedback on themselves, their performance, and their capabilities more directly and immediately than before (Berk, 2011).

Freedom and autonomy: The need for freedom and autonomy can be understood as the need for one's thoughts and actions to be self-determined and self-chosen (Ryan & Deci, 2017). Although autonomy and social integration/attachment are sometimes in conflict, they also depend on each other: experiences towards autonomy are only possible if there is a safe haven and if orientation in the world is possible. If the basis of a safe attachment is not given, or if the need for autonomy is repeatedly frustrated, a feeling arises of not being allowed to be independent and to think independently. In other words, autonomy is the basis for creativity and experimentation.

A frequent constellation that impedes healthy autonomy development arises in emotionally very strained families. First, the accompanying parentification of children can lead to excessive demands and expectations that prevent them from developing their autonomy. In addition, the atmosphere in such families is often depressed and tense, making it hard for children to live out important aspects of childhood (e.g. spontaneity, liveliness, carelessness). This makes it impossible for them to experience the independence of their own feelings ("I can still laugh and be happy although my Mom is depressive") (c.f. Beardslee, 2009).

10.1.2 Approach and Avoidance Strategies

Even though these different basic needs are independent of cultures and development stages, there are clear inter-individual differences in *how* these basic needs can be fulfilled. Thus, while basic needs are universal, the ways in which people seek to satisfy them are highly personal. In the course of their development, people amass the most diverse experiences as to the strategies for fulfilling these basic needs (approach) and for avoiding harm (avoidance). These strategies are internalized in the form of patterns or "inner working models". This means we develop approach as well as avoidance patterns.

Thus, basic needs do not influence behavior directly, but via these patterns. The patterns represent the individual possibilities for basic need satisfaction (Grosse, Holtforth, & Grawe, 2004). That said, both approach and avoidance patterns can be functional or dysfunctional. Approach patterns are functional when sensible goals are chosen and sufficient means to attain them are available. The more friction these goals and means cause with other goals or needs (a person's own or other people's), the more dysfunctional they are. Avoidance patterns help to prevent anticipated harm. As long as the danger of harm actually exists, and the child or adolescent has no choice of alternative behaviors, these patterns are highly expedient. However, because harm concerning basic needs is experienced as very grievous, avoidance patterns tend to persist. This means they are applied, too, when they would no longer be necessary, which makes them dysfunctional (see next section). Moreover, it must be observed that avoidance "only" prevents harm, but the underlying basic needs remain unfulfilled.

10.1.3 The Pyramid of Basic Needs

These four basic needs can be visualized in the form of an upside-down pyramid. The underlying idea is threefold (Fig. 10.1):

First, in keeping with the attachment theories, we assume that the attachment experiences generated during development are decisive factors for experiences in other areas.
Second, this visualization expresses an unstable balance: consistent and balanced satisfaction of these needs is a complex endeavor. The balance needs constant readjustment because, on the one hand, the world around us changes constantly—and with it, the requirements we face; on the other hand, so do we. Therefore, we need to constantly change our strategies for *how* we fulfill these basic needs as well.
Third, needs and their related patterns can be interdependent and competing at the same time. For instance, positive and fulfilling experiences in attachment can lead to higher self-worth, a sense of autonomy, and orientation. Depending on the way basic needs are acted out, they may conflict more or less strongly with each other. If a person seeks to be close to another person, he or she risks rejection. If someone becomes attached to someone else, he or she always surrenders a certain measure of control and freedom. Or when adolescents venture to do something new, they risk failure. Thus, the attempt to fulfill one need can lead to frustration of another need, and the pyramid loses its balance.

Seen from this angle, it could be said that the art of living consists in keeping this pyramid of basic needs in balance. This entails permanently ensuring that one's basic needs can be fulfilled without excessive internal and external conflict. And the fewer conflicts one has, the better one's psychological health.

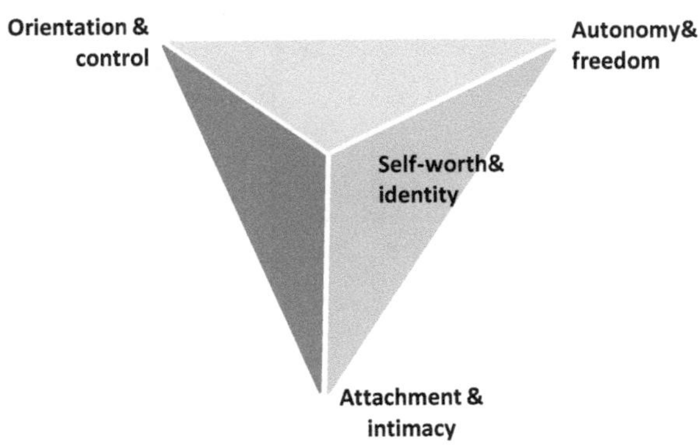

Fig. 10.1 The pyramid of basic needs (Schär, 2016)

10.1.4 Resilience and Basic Needs

The theory of basic needs lends itself well to a connection with the concept of resilience. For instance, several studies show that, for adolescents in highly conflictual environments, the fulfillment of basic needs has a positive effect on their resilience and psychological well-being (Abualkibash & Lera, 2017; Deci & Ryan, 2000; Kaydkhorde, 2014). Below, we show in a theoretical model how the fulfillment of basic needs, moderated by approach and avoidance strategies, can lead to higher resilience (Fig. 10.2).

When adolescents succeed in satisfying their basic needs, these positive experiences result in positive assumptions about themselves, their environment, and their future. This occurs because the fulfillment of basic needs and the way in which this goal is achieved result from a complex interaction between individual and environment. Also, this learning process is a major determinant of a person's future. If a person has built positive assumptions about himself/herself and the world, this favors, of course, the development of approach patterns. This means that adolescents develop approach goals and look for means and strategies to attain them. When these are successful, a range of positive emotions are experienced (e.g. joy, pride). This reinforces the behaviors practiced, internalizes the patterns, and heightens the probability that these successful behaviors will become more frequent in the future.

However, these strategies are not always successful. The environment can change, for instance, confronting the adolescent with a new situation where the old strategies and patterns are no longer effective: new requirements arise, the pressure to perform is heightened, certain behaviors are no longer tolerated, etc. As a consequence, negative emotions such as disappointment arise. Accordingly, the probability of these

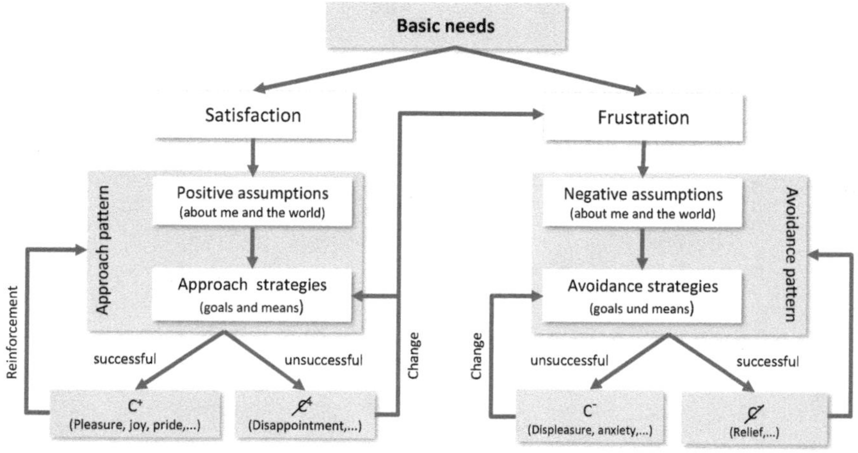

Fig. 10.2 Theoretical model of the influence of basic needs, approach and avoidance strategies, and resilience (Schär & Steinebach, 2015)

behaviors occurring is reduced, and the person needs to look for alternative approach goals and means in order to fulfill his or her basic needs in a new way.

Repeated disappointment becomes frustration: Sooner or later, however, repeated disappointments lead to growing frustration. In its wake, patterns also change step by step. Slowly, but continually, more negative assumptions build up about the individual himself or herself, the environment, or the future. And so, more and more avoidance goals and means take center stage. This is how the vicious circle sets in.

- Unsuccessful avoidance. If the attempted avoidance strategies are unsuccessful, i.e. if the breach of basic needs cannot be averted, this has two consequences: first, it reinforces negative assumptions about self, the environment, and the future. Second, while new strategies are tested, these are avoidance oriented again, because the individual's idea that the world is dangerous and protection is needed has been reinforced.
- Successful avoidance. If these new avoidance strategies are successful, negative emotions cease because the breach of basic needs has been averted. This is felt, for instance, as relief. Due to avoidance, though, there is no experience able to correct the negative assumptions; therefore, these persist. And due to reinforcement, the specific avoidance behavior is likely to be repeated more often in the future.

This means that, when basic needs are frustrated over a longer period, and when avoidance strategies and negative assumptions have become too deeply ingrained, there is (almost) no way out of avoidance any more. Now, avoidance patterns are internalized, and they take control: more and more energy is used for avoiding harm, leaving less and less energy free for practicing approach strategies and thus fulfilling basic needs.

10.2 Objectives of Psychotherapy and Counseling

From this perspective, resilience is the ability to not become inherently frustrated in spite of negative experiences and disappointments, instead continuing to seek and find new and more effective approach strategies to fulfill one's basic needs. *The better and the longer an adolescent is able to do this, the more resilient he or she will be*. Based on this, the fundamental objectives of psychotherapy and counseling with adolescents can be deduced:

On the one hand, a fundamental objective is to guide adolescents back from avoidance to approach—to encourage and support them in trying out new behaviors in order to gain new corrective experiences.

On the other hand, it is also necessary to bear with them when not all of the new behaviors work out. Counseling and psychotherapy does not mean to give them approach strategies that work for them, or to avoid disappointments. On the contrary, such resilience-oriented counseling is about learning to deal with disappointments in a good way. The aim is to integrate the resulting disappointments into one's self-concept in such a way that they can be acknowledged and accepted as a normal and important experiential reality, and do not have to result in deprecation of self and others. Adolescents become more resilient when they try out new approach strategies with more courage and persistence.

10.2.1 Fundamental Principles of Effective Counseling

As shown above, it is important for the psychological health of adolescents how much they persevere in finding new ways to fulfill their basic needs and how they succeed in fulfilling them. Professional psychological support can encourage and support adolescents to achieve this goal in a better way and help them to grow towards greater resilience.

In the second part of this chapter, we would like to illustrate which factors are important for providing adolescents with effective support. In our definition, counseling, particularly in non-directive client-centered approaches, overlaps with psychotherapy, so both words are used synonymously in this text.

A short history of common factors: As early as 1936, Saul Rosenzweig showed in his still-noted publication "Some implicit common factors in diverse methods of psychotherapy" that, in psychotherapy, changes are brought about by implicit processes common to all psychotherapies rather than by the techniques used. He ascribed therapeutic change to clients gaining a different, new, and adaptive understanding of their problems in a sustainable relationship with a safe and consistent psychotherapist. The changes that follow the formation of alternative perspectives, he wrote, have positive effects on other aspects of behavior and experience. Jerome Frank, an American psychotherapy researcher, ascribed the effectiveness of psychotherapy to common factors as well. He saw the transformation of meaning, from demoralization to moralization, as a key process in psychotherapy, postulating four sufficient and necessary conditions (Frank, 1997):

(1) a trusting and emotional relationship with the psychotherapist;
(2) a professional context;
(3) a plausible explanatory model (myth); and
(4) a therapeutic procedure (ritual) based on that myth.

This view—ascribing the effectiveness of psychotherapy and counseling to common factors, and focusing on the therapeutic relationship as well as on clients' and therapists' expectations and beliefs—runs counter to the "medical model". According to that model, disorders have specific causes calling for specific interventions, a view based on belief in the therapeutic importance of method- and disorder-specific techniques.

In a comprehensive, much-noted research undertaking, Wampold and Imel (2015) examined two paradigms and contrasted the medical model with their own context model based on common factors. The sum of psychotherapy research points towards the context model being preferable. First, proof of specificity has yet to be produced,

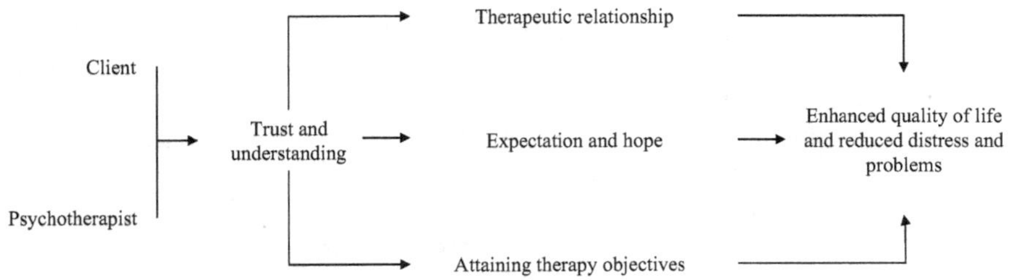

Fig. 10.3 Therapeutic components and processes from the perspective of a contextual understanding of psychotherapy, following Wampold and Budge (2011)

i.e. the differences between various lines of psychotherapy are minor. Second, non-specific factors explain success of psychotherapy to a great extent (for more detail, see Wampold & Imel, 2015).

According to the context model (Wampold & Budge, 2011), effective psychotherapy comprises three therapeutic components. These are (1) a real therapeutic relationship, a feeling of connectedness and belonging, (2) clients' expectation and hope in the therapy (and the consultants' expertise and trustworthiness) as well as the therapists' expectations, and (3) the attainment of therapy objectives by setting goals, pertinent assignments, and therapeutic acts (see Fig. 10.3). A basic requirement mentioned by Wampold and Imel (2015) is the "initial therapeutic bond", because without mutual trust and understanding, without this alliance between the consultants and the adolescents, counseling would not happen and/or could not be effective.

Similar to the model by Wampold and Imel (2015), in "What should we expect from psychotherapy?", Goldfried (2013) summarizes the following general principles of change for therapy effectiveness:

a. facilitating expectations of positive results;
b. the therapeutic relationship;
c. facilitating the client's awareness of conditions that contribute to problems arising and persisting, as well as their influence on his/her feelings, thoughts, and behaviors, i.e. developing an explanatory model;
d. facilitating corrective experiences; and
e. encouragement to continually test these corrective experiences in the client's "reality", outside of the therapeutic setting.

Below, these general principles of change will be looked into one by one with a view to counseling adolescents.

Facilitating expectations of positive results: One key component of therapeutic effectiveness consists in the client's expectations and beliefs concerning the usefulness of counseling. When adolescents come to counseling, they have probably lived through several disappointments and frustrations already, and their behaviors have not enabled them to satisfy their basic needs. They have implicit or explicit explanations for how the problems started, but usually these explanations do not yield any suggestions on how to change the situation.

In counseling, therefore, one objective is to understand, together with the adolescents, why repeated attempts at coping have been unsuccessful so far. Another objective is working together on an explanatory model that generates alternative perspectives—thereby implying higher degrees of freedom—and that is, therefore, more open to new approaches to solutions. Feasible approaches to solutions include helping adolescents develop hope and modify their expectations about their chances to change things. They should realize that it makes sense for them to try out something new.

Studies show that expectations of positive results and hope have positive effects on the outcome of a therapy (e.g. Constantino, Ametrano, & Greenberg, 2012). An attitude of positive expectation is, therefore, also key to going into approach instead of sitting tight in avoidance. Thus, such an attitude is key to resilience as well.

Expectations of positive results can be supported by explicitly talking about them. In addition, they also develop due to consultants' faith in the adolescents' positive development potential. In counseling, this faith may be expressed explicitly or in other ways, e.g. nonverbally, and it is an important aspect of the therapeutic relationship.

The therapeutic relationship: It is undisputed that the relationship is a central factor in therapy and counseling (Orlinsky, Grawe, & Parks, 1994; Orlinsky, Roennestadt, & Willutzki, 2004). It is the relationship itself that leads to changes in counseling. It is not only the basis of the counseling process, and it does much more than create a good foundation.

The two-process consistency theory model introduced by Grawe (2004) shows how a positive relationship in counseling and therapy can lead to changes. When the adolescent gains positive relationship experiences in counseling or therapy, his or her need for attachment is nourished. This can happen through positive regard, appreciative feedback, and understanding, all of which reduces incongruence and thus leads to enhanced well-being (see Fig. 10.4).

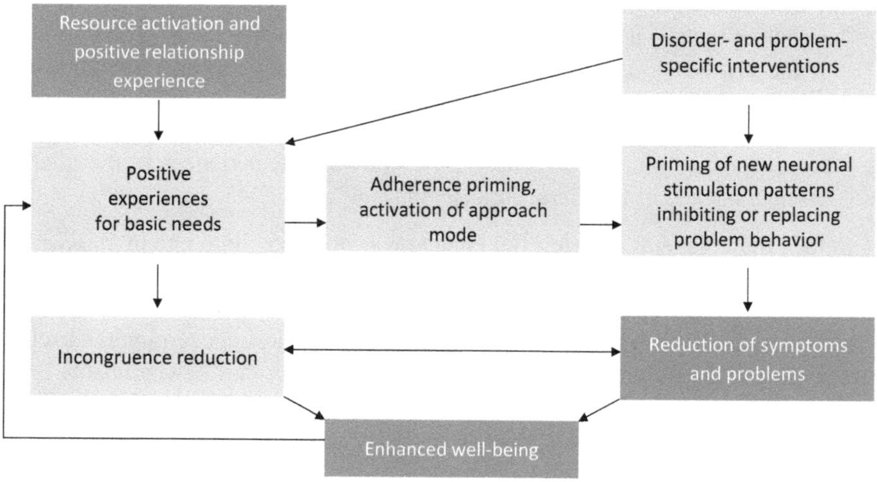

Fig. 10.4 Two-process consistency theory model following Grawe (2004)

At the same time, need-fulfilling experiences lead to mental activity being "rather positive and oriented towards approach instead of towards defense and avoidance" (Grawe, 2004, p. 409). Approach behavior is directed towards motivational objectives, i.e. satisfaction of basic needs. Positive experiences in the relationship with the counselor or therapist can strengthen adolescents and encourage them, for instance, to behave differently in other relationships and thus to gain new experiences, which can strengthen the need for attachment once more. In parallel, need-fulfilling relationships can encourage them or enable them to cooperate in problem- and disorder-specific interventions, which would result in a reduction of symptoms and problems, and thus enhance their well-being as well.

A good relationship in counseling also enables adolescents to change their negative assumptions about themselves, the others, and the future, so that the vicious circle described above can be broken. Thus, directly in and with counseling, they gain corrective experiences about themselves and others.

In his person-centered approach, Rogers (2004) postulates three core conditions: sensitive understanding (empathy), unconditioned acceptance (unconditional positive regard), and the principle of genuineness (congruence). The relationship as well as the entire therapeutic behavior should, therefore, follow from these fundamental attitudes. The counselor's accepting attitude should enable the adolescents to develop a similar attitude towards themselves. Sensitive understanding (empathy) and unconditioned acceptance (unconditional positive regard) improve their understanding of themselves, thus strengthening their trust in themselves and stabilizing their self-esteem. Grawe calls this factor "resource activation". The third core condition is the principle of genuineness (congruence). Genuineness lets the adolescents gain corrective relationship experiences within counseling (see 10.2.4). Thus, a good relationship is a fundamental precondition for changes in counseling, but it causes changes directly as well.

Another important aspect is that the adolescents need to understand why it would be worth it for them to go in for the approach process again. They need a plausible explanatory model that shows them how they can overcome their problems.

10.2.2 Developing an Explanatory Model

Adolescents become more autonomous, i.e. better able to decide and act, thanks to their growing understanding of the conditions that contribute to problems arising and persisting and of how such conditions influence feelings, thoughts, and behaviors, as well as by their greater congruence (Sachse, 1999). Awareness of how problems emerge and persist can be supported by sensitive understanding. A counselor's empathic understanding aims at getting to know and understanding the adolescent's represented experiences and feelings. In this way, the counselor should strive to empathize with the adolescent's perception of the world and thus help him or her to better understand that world. In his description of the factors of psychotherapy, Grawe, Donati, and Bernauer (1994) calls this "motivational clarification". Its aim is to clarify the feelings and needs that are problem-relevant, as well as their connection with thoughts, intentions, and behaviors. In order to clarify and better understand the adolescent's problems, however, these have to be activated first, so that the feelings connected with them can be experienced. In conversational psychotherapy, this is called "experience activation" (Finke, 2004), while Grawe et al. (1994) calls this factor "problem actualization".

Based on a better understanding of the persistence conditions, i.e. the reasons for the repeated failures of earlier attempts at coping, a new explanatory model should be developed. Its purpose is to change the adolescent's expectations by providing new and alternative perspectives and approaches to solutions.

According to Wampold and Imel (2015), the criteria for assessing the quality of such explanatory models are subjective. This means they have to be plausible for the adolescents (and their environment), i.e. compatible with their view of the world, and thus acceptable to them. Moreover, they should be open to new solutions and support the adolescents' self-effectiveness. So, the adolescents should understand and recognize that they can influence things. It is up to them to make the change. An important objective of counseling is to help the adolescents develop hope that their problems can be solved or handled. This also changes the adolescents' motivation to address their difficulties.

Interventions—which should be derivable from an explanatory model—must also be plausible and transparent not only for the adolescent and his/her environment, but also, of course, for the counselor. They should show which steps the adolescent could take towards satisfying his/her (basic) needs, thus increasing his/her expectations of positive results and generating hope.

10.2.3 Facilitating Corrective Experiences

In a good, stable relationship where the adolescent feels regarded and understood, corrective relationship experiences are possible in the course of counseling. With the third core principle according to Rogers—congruence or genuineness—the counselor gets actively involved in the relationship, confronting the adolescent if this is expedient, or clarifying the relationship with him or her. In this involvement, the counselor gives explicit opinions on specific subjects, ideas, or behaviors of the adolescent. In the clarification of the relationship, the counseling relationship is discussed explicitly, for instance by the counselor verbalizing fears or needs of the adolescent. This can help the adolescent to become aware of his or her relational patterns, understand them, and thus make them accessible in order to work on them (for more details and case examples, see Knafla, Schaer, & Steinebach, 2017). Confrontation, e.g. with contradictions between behaviors and statements, enables the adolescent to recognize them. This process of recognition can solve incongruences and change behaviors.

The aim is to synchronize the adolescents' experiences with their self-concept, i.e. congruence, and to enable them to adjust their behavior accordingly without contradictions.

10.2.4 Encouragement to Test Corrective Experiences in "Reality"

Support, encouragement, assistance, and positive reinforcement is needed for adolescents to find courage and bring themselves to venture into the approach mode again, and to try out new behaviors after unsuccessful and frustrating experiences. Therefore, it is important to give adolescents courage and confidence. Walter and Peller (1992) call this "cheerleading"—encouraging, reinforcing, and celebrating small steps forward. Testing new behaviors in the real world outside the counseling makes corrective experiences possible. If repeated, these, in turn, influence expectations and behaviors, causing a change of patterns.

In the face of setbacks, adolescents tend to lose courage quickly. Here, too, they need normalization, support, and help in order to learn how to deal with disappointments. Disappointments are part of everyday life for adolescents (and of course for adults). They cannot be avoided, but should be recognized as important experiences, without leading to deprecation of self or others. We, as counselors, also have to learn to endure these disappointments and frustrations with them. In this way, with the relationship and support by the counselor, adolescents become able to come back from avoidance to action (approach). Action means change processes in thoughts, behaviors, or feelings. In the approach mode, they serve to satisfy basic needs, and thus lead to enhanced well-being. Adolescents become more resilient when they find the courage for renewed approach—with the support of counseling.

10.3 Conclusion

Humans have an inherent tendency toward growth and development, but that does not happen automatically. Not only growth, but also well-being and health, arise only if different basic psychological needs are satisfied. One of the biggest challenges for young people is to fashion their living environment themselves for the fulfillment of their basic needs. On the one hand, they have to develop a variety of new strategies; on the other, they have to deal with frustrations with regard to their basic needs.

On the point of view of resilience, the main objective of counseling with adolescents is not to avoid the frustrations or to teach them *better* strategies to fulfill their basic needs. When adolescents are frustrated, demoralized, and hopeless, counseling should help them overcome the avoidance tendency and encourage them to try out and evaluate new and different strategies in order to gain new corrective experiences. And most of all, to help the adolescents integrate disappointments into their self-concept as a normal experiential reality, without deprecating oneself or others.

According to Frank and Frank (1991), clients mainly come to therapy or counseling not because of the suffering associated with their symptoms, but because of the hopelessness their symptoms cause them. Hopelessness develops when adolescents or their environment ascribe a morbid explanation to their experiences, feelings, and behaviors, and fight a losing battle against them. The transformation of meaning from demoralization to moralization is, therefore, a key process in therapy: overcoming hopelessness and then the symptoms themselves.

References

Abualkibash, S. K. A., & Lera, M. J. (2015). Psychological resilience among Palestinian school students: An exploratory study in the West Bank. *International Humanities Studies, 2*, 1–20.

Adler, A. (1920). *Praxis und Theorie der Individualpsychologie. Vorträge zur Einführung in die Psychotherapie für Ärzte, Psychologen und Lehrer*. München: Bergmann.

Bandura, A. (1977). Self-efficacy: Toward a unifying theory of behavioral change. *Psychological Review, 84*, 191–215.

Beardslee, W. R. (2009). *Hoffnung, Sinn und Kontinuität. Ein Programm für Familien depressiv erkrankter Eltern. Fortschritte der Gemeindepsychologie und Gesundheitsförderung* (Vol. 19). Tübingen: DGVT.

Berk, L. E. (2011). *Entwicklungspsychologie*. München: Pearson Studium.

Brazelton, T. B., & Greenspan, S. I. (2002). *Die sieben Grundbedürfnisse von Kindern. Was jedes Kind braucht, um gesund aufzuwachsen, gut zu lernen und glücklich zu sein*. Weinheim: Beltz.

Constantino, M. J., Ametrano, R. M., & Greenberg, R. P. (2012). Clinician interventions and participant characteristics that foster adaptive patient expectations for psychotherapy and psychotherapeutic change. *Psychotherapy, 49*(4), 557–569.

De Botton, A. (2001). *Trost der Philosophie. Eine Gebrauchsanweisung*. Frankfurt am Main: S. Fischer.

Deci, E. L., & Ryan, R. M. (2000). Self-determination theory and the facilitation of intrinsic motivation, social development, and well-being. *American Psychologist, 55*, 68–78.

Deci, E. L., & Ryan, R. M. (2004). *Handbook of self-determination research*. Rochester, NY: University of Rochester Press.

Epstein, S. (1990). Cognitive-experiential Self-theory. In L. Pervin (Ed.), *Handbook of personality theory and research: Theory and research* (pp. 165–192). New York, NY: Guilford.

Finke, J. (2004). *Gesprächspsychotherapie* (3rd ed.). Stuttgart: Thieme.

Frank, J. D. (1997). *Die Heiler. Wirkungsweise psychotherapeutischer Beeinflussung* (2nd ed.). Stuttgart: Klett-Cotta.

Frank, J. D., & Frank, J. B. (1991). *Persuasion and healing: A comparative study of psychotherapy* (3rd ed.). Baltimore, MD: Johns Hopkins University Press.

Goldfried, M. R. (2013). What should we expect from psychotherapy? *Clinical Psychology Review, 33*, 862–869.

Grawe, K. (2004). *Neuropsychotherapie*. Göttingen: Hogrefe.

Grawe, K., Donati, R., & Bernauer, F. (1994). *Psychotherapie im Wandel. Von der Konfession zur Profession*. Göttingen: Hogrefe.

Grosse Holtforth, M., & Grawe, K. (2004). Inkongruenz und Fallkonzeption in der Psychologischen Therapie. *Verhaltenstherapie und Psychosoziale Praxis, 36*, 9–21.

Heckhausen, J., & Heckhausen, H. (2010). *Motivation und Handeln*. Heidelberg: Springer.

Kaydkhorde, H., Moltafet, G., & Chinaveh, M. (2014). Relationship between satisfying psychological needs and resilience in high-school students in Dezful town. *Academic Journal of Psychological Studies, 3*(1), 57–62.

Knafla, I., Schaer, M., & Steinebach, C. (2017). *Jugendliche stärken. Wirkfaktoren in Beratung und Therapie*. Weinheim: Beltz.

Maslow, A. H. (1954). *Motivation und Persönlichkeit*. Reinbek: Rowohlt.

Orlinsky, D. E., Grawe, K., & Parks, B. K. (1994). Process and outcome in psychotherapy. In A. E. Bergin & S. L. Garfield (Eds.), *Handbook of psychotherapy and behavior change* (4th ed., pp. 270–376). New York, NY: Wiley.

Orlinsky, D., Roennestadt, M. H., & Willutzki, U. (2004). Fifty years of psychotherapy process-outcome research: Continuity and change. In M. J. Lambert (Ed.), *Bergin and Garfield's handbook of psychotherapy and behavior change* (pp. 307–390). New York, NY: Wiley.

Ryan, R. M., & Deci, E. L. (2017). *Self-determination theory: Basic psychological needs in motivation, development, and wellness*. New York: Guilford Publishing.

Rogers, C. R. (2004). *Entwicklung der Persönlichkeit* (15th ed.). Stuttgart: Klett-Cotta.

Rosenzweig, S. (1936). Some implicit common factors in diverse methods of psychotherapy. *American Journal of Orthopsychiatry, 6*, 412–415.

Rotter, J. (1966). Generalized expectancies for internal versus external control of reinforcement. *Psychological Monographs, 80* (609).

Sachse, R. (1999). *Lehrbuch der Gesprächspsychotherapie*. Göttingen: Hogrefe.

Schär, M. (2016). *Paarberatung und Paartherapie - Partnerschaft zwischen Problemen und Ressource*. Heidelberg: Springer.

Schär, M., & Steinebach, C. (2015). *Resilienzfördernde Psychotherapie bei Kindern, Jugendlichen und Familien: Erfüllte Grundbedürfnisse als Ressource*. Weinheim: Beltz.

Walter, J. L., & Peller, J. E. (1992). *Become solution-focused in brief therapy*. New York, NY: Brunner/Mazel.

Wampold, B. E., & Budge, S. L. (2011). The 2011 Leona Tyler award address: The relationship—And its relationship to the common and specific factors of psychotherapy. *The Counseling Psychologist, 40*(4), 601–623.

Wampold, B. E., & Imel, Z. E. (2015). *The great psychotherapy debate: Research evidence for what works in psychotherapy* (2nd ed.). New York, NY: Routledge.

Young, J. E., Klosko, J. S., & Weishaar, M. E. (2008). *Schematherapie. Ein praxisorientiertes Handbuch*. Paderborn: Junfermann.

Chapter 11
A Socio-affective, Developmentally Informed Perspective for Contemplative Practices in Adolescence: Towards Resilient Communities

Sebastián Medeiros and Simón Guendelman

Abstract In this chapter, we describe socio-emotional developmental psychological abilities such as self-regulation, mentalization, and empathy in childhood and adolescence and examine how contemplative practice may foster and enhance such capacities, contributing to building personal and social resilience. Development is understood as the result of biological (genetic) and environmental (cultural, social, interpersonal factors) interactions. The main notion at stake is the plasticity of people's socio-emotional capacities throughout developmental stages, from childhood to adolescence. In other words, from a dynamic systems approach, development is a state of flux led by multicausal interactions between the physical, environmental, and psychosocial domains. Such a complex process results in the emergence of variability regarding psychological and biological skills (e.g. self-regulation); within this context, other mental facets including the sense of self and personality develop as well (Smith and Thelen in Trends Cogn Sci 7(8):343–348, 2003). We describe the adolescent mind along with the psychological challenges and neurological developmental specificities of young people, speculating that contemplative practices, among other interventions, may lay the groundwork for self and social resilience by targeting specific psychological needs in connection with socio-emotional development. Furthermore, we refer to early parenting, psychotherapy, and educational interventions as social prevention strategies which open up new opportunities for family and children in this particularly sensitive context. Finally, we share some views and suggestions for future research regarding the integration of contemplative practices from an individual to a communal level.

S. Medeiros (✉)
Psychiatry Department, Pontificia Universidad Católica de Chile, Santiago, Chile
e-mail: smedeiro@uc.cl

S. Medeiros · S. Guendelman
Centro Mindfulness y Medicina, Santiago, Chile

S. Guendelman
Social Cognition Group, Berlin School of Mind and Brain, Humboldt Universität, Berlin, Germany

S. Medeiros
Millennium Institute for Research in Depression and Personality, Santiago, Chile

C. Steinebach and Á. I. Langer (eds.), *Enhancing Resilience in Youth*,
https://doi.org/10.1007/978-3-030-25513-8_11

Keywords Mentalization · Empathy · Genetic-environment interaction · Multicomponent interventions · Contemplative practices

11.1 Introduction

Socio-affective capacities are established early in life and continue to be developed throughout it in a dynamic, progressive, and relational way. They play a crucial role regarding copying and stress regulation. Research on the effect of early stress and trauma has shown its formative impact in the construction of socio-emotional capacities in children and adolescents, shaping dynamic phenotypic characters for vulnerability and resilience. In this chapter, we describe socio-emotional developmental psychological abilities such as self-regulation, mentalization, and empathy in childhood and adolescence and examine how contemplative practice may foster and enhance such capacities, contributing to building personal and social resilience.

Here we understand development as the result of biological (genetic) and environment (cultural, social, interpersonal factors) interactions. The main notion at stake is the plasticity of the socio-emotional capacities throughout developmental stages, from childhood to adolescence. In other words, from a dynamic systems approach, development is a state of flux lead by multicausal interactions between physical, environmental, and psychosocial domains. Such a complex process results in the emergence of variability regarding psychological and biological skills (e.g. self-regulation); within this context, other mental facets including the sense of self and personality develop as well (Smith & Thelen, 2003).

We describe the adolescent mind along with the psychological challenges and neurological developmental specificities of young people, speculating that contemplative practices, among other interventions, may lay the groundwork for self and social resilience by targeting specific psychological needs in connection with socio-emotional development. Furthermore, we refer to early parenting, psychotherapy, and educational interventions as social prevention strategies which open up new venues for family and children in this particularly sensitive context. Finally, we offer some comments and suggestions for future research regarding the integration of contemplative practices from an individual to a communal level.

11.2 Early Socio-affective Development as Terrain for Resilience

Current perspectives in psychology and psychiatry assume that self and social capacities emerge as the result of the dynamic interaction of genetic, environmental, and social factors. Less emphasis is given to conceive fix diagnostic categories instead it attempts to understand how social and biological aspects interact leading to the maturation of crucial socio-emotional capacities that constitute vulnerability and resilience factors (Pollak, 2015). For example, as in other studies, a longitudinal study conducted by Conway, Raposa, Hammen, and Brennan (2018) showed that social stressors early in life determine transdiagnostic psychopathological vulnerabilities later on.

Models of genetic-environment interaction highlight that early life stressful experiences can indeed alter genetic profiles in critical brain circuits devoted to emotion and cognition, determining a psychological foundation which will later on interact with novel social and life challenges, leading to a range of possible mental health levels (Daskalakis, Bagot, Parker, Vinkers, & de Kloet, 2013).

Another way to understand these socio-emotional resilience/vulnerability factors is through the motivational system model proposed by Paul Gilbert, which includes the threat detection system (linked to feelings such as anger, anxiety), the soothing-affiliative system (linked to feelings such as content and connectedness), and the incentive-reward system (linked to feelings such as desire, gain, and progress). These motivational systems correspond with brain circuits and can be differentially shaped throughout development, posing specific challenges during adolescence. In the case of trauma- or fear-related disorders in childhood, the threat system appears overactivated and capacities for self-soothing and connectedness are low (Gilbert, 2010). When intense threat is perceived and social support and consolation are not available, more primitive strategies for self-preservation are activated (i.e. fight/flight and freeze responses), leading to maladaptive behavior (Nesse, Bhatnagar, & Ellis, 2016; Porges, 2011). This may result in anxiety, dysfunctional cognitions, body dysregulation, and social dysfunctions, among other symptoms.

In the following, we describe three widely studied *socio-affective developmental functions: Self-regulation, mentalization, empathy and altruism*, as they have shown to be crucial in determining vulnerability and resilience factors, thus linking early development (stress) and subsequent good mental health and/or psychopathology.

Self-regulation refers to the ability to inhibit and/or modify cognitions, feelings, behavior, and desires in order to facilitate goal-oriented actions and respond optimally to demanding inner and outer stimuli (Baumeister & Heatherton, 1996; Posner, Rothbart, Sheese, & Tang, 2007; Zelazo & Lyons, 2012). In the context of early attachment relationships, affective experiences are crucial in the development of self-regulatory capacities and adjustment to stress contributing to well-being and resilience throughout life (Schore, 2012). According to Bucci (2007), when arousal is overwhelming for the child and/or the caregiver is dysfunctional, effective mechanisms of self-regulation are not fully developed. The organization of regulatory capacities is deeply affected, manifesting itself later through vulnerability to stress, anxiety, depression, aggression, and impulsivity (Lewis et al., 2008; Pagliaccio, Luby, Luking, Belden, & Barch, 2014).

Mentalization or reflective function refers to the ability to understand human behavior through inference of motivated intentional mental states (e.g. desires, memories, intentions) (Fonagy, Bateman, & Luyten, 2012). It occupies an essential place in developmental psychology and psychopathology, as it depends on the quality of early mother-child relationships, particularly on the development of a secure attachment system where maternal mentalizing abilities are present

(Fonagy, Target, Gergely, & Jurist, 2002). Mentalization is also sensitive to exposure to relational or developmental trauma; mentalization deficits, although not always causal, are associated with a wide range of psychopathologies including autism, schizophrenia, and borderline disorder (in Roffman, Gerber, & Flick, 2012).

Empathy is the ability to share affective states, whereby the person who perceives knows that a given emotion originates from the other (de Vignemont & Singer, 2006). From a felt sense of other people's experience, different responses can emerge in the observer, varying from rejection and stress to taking care of the other. For Rogers (1965), empathy is the emotional and cognitive ability to correctly perceive another person's internal frames of reference—in terms of their meanings and emotional components—as if one were the other or were in their own skin, but without losing the condition "as if", that is, without identifying oneself or losing the I—another differentiation. Siegel (2007) proposes that empathy is built from internal changes, the result of resonance circuits that translate the effect of the perception of other signals in the limbic system and their bodily manifestations. Altruism or prosociality, corresponds to a variety of feelings (such as compassion or sympathy) and behaviors (different helping actions) that actively target and intend to alleviate another person's mental state (like suffering). In simple words, an altruistic response can arise from empathy (feeling like the other) or mentalizing (understanding the other) (Davis, 2015). According to Halifax (2012), compassion and altruistic behavior arise from the interaction of *attentional-cognitive* (e.g. what we know from the other), *somatic-body* (e.g. physiological resonance), and *emotional* (e.g. what feelings we have and how much we care about the other) aspects in the observer. Interestingly, attentional and emotional aspects, as well as prosociality, are modeled throughout development and can be trained by contemplative interventions.

11.3 The Adolescent Mind and Brain

11.3.1 Psychological Context and Particular Needs

What is the psychology of adolescents? What are their particular conflicts, needs, and anxieties? What are their vulnerabilities and strengths? These questions help us reflect on the role of contemplative interventions interacting with complex developmental systems, in ongoing processes, where domains of identity and self-regulation are at play. Adolescence is a period filled with tensions between wanting to belong and finding out one's way; trying to be accepted by others and at the same developing one's own identity and self-worth. From a psychodynamic perspective, it can be said to include conflicts between the active need for care versus self-sufficiency and between independence/autarky and dependence (OPD Task Force, 2008). Moreover, for adolescents, the social world of peers is a crucial source of challenges, including the importance to fit in and the heightened relevance of social evaluation (Somerville, 2013).

Studies have shown that adolescents are prone to take risk in several domains, including health and recreation (Blakemore, 2018a). This aspect is related with what is known as novelty seeking and the creative exploration of relationships (see Table 11.1). A large-scale intercultural study showed that sensation-seeking behaviors increased between 10 and 20 years of age and decreased after the early twenties; in contrast, self-regulation markedly increased from early to late adolescence (Steinberg et al., 2017).

Coming back to Gilbert's evolutionary origins of emotion regulation, adolescence can be characterized by variable forms of threat detection (e.g. perhaps lower threat perception facilitates engagement in high risk behaviors), usually high drive (e.g. novelty seeking), and variable forms of self-soothing (e.g. diverse strategies for self-calming). In the case of early stress, these systems may undergo complex dysregulations. During adolescence, the soothing system may be enhanced through healthy interactions and practical strategies. When emotional experience becomes less threatening and a feeling of safety is present, social engagement is possible (Porges, 2011). According to Steinberg, (2007) and Steinberg et al. (2008), during late adolescence and early adulthood risk perception is refined and resistance to peer influence strengthened; moreover, anticipation of future consequences is improved and sensation seeking and impulsivity are lessened.

Table 11.1 summarizes specific tasks, psychological and brain mechanisms present during adolescence, and potential targets for contemplative practices. We suggest contemplative practices can foster the social engagement system through threat regulation and the cultivation of socio-cognitive abilities, facilitating more adaptive behavior. Thus, the creation and maintenance of supportive relationships with peers, which have been shown to be the best predictors of well-being, longevity, and happiness (Siegel, 2013), can be fostered.

11.3.2 The Adolescent Brain

During adolescence, the brain experiences several changes, one of the most important being the overall reduction in gray matter (neurons and synapses) and increase in white matter (different brain tracts and fibers) (Mills et al., 2016). These changes are the result of a complex maturational processes in brain organization, including a decrease in the number of synapses (synaptic pruning) and an increase in the myelination of neuronal fibers, which mainly occur in the pre-frontal, temporal, and parietal cortex (Petanjek et al., 2011). However, this does not mean the number of neurons is necessarily declining, but that the neuronal connections and tracts are going through a massive optimization of their functional architecture (Blakemore, 2018b).

These brain changes might be the substrate for the multiple psychological and social changes (e.g. increased self-regulation and mentalization) experienced during adolescence. Somerville (2013) points out the particular relevance of the maturation of the socio-affective circuits, highlighting the role of these regions in perceiv-

Table 11.1 Specific adolescence tasks, psychological and brain mechanisms, and potential targets for contemplative practices. Abbreviations: temporo parietal junction (TPJ), superior temporal sulcus (STS)

Drives	Psychological mechanism in adolescence	Referential brain system	Downside	Mindfulness and compassion—potential targets
Novelty seeking	Increased inner drive for rewards. Looking for and trying new experiences. Feeling more engaged and motivated with life	Reward system. Including nucleus accumbens and basal ganglia structures. Mediated by dopaminergic system	Sensation seeking, risk taking, impulsive decision making, "overemphasizing the thrill and downplaying the risk"	Self-regulation: increased capacity for regulation of intense affects. Delay of immediate gratification Self-soothing: capacity for cultivating positive emotions and engaging in healthy self-care strategies
Social connection	Creation and maintenance of supportive relationships with peers	Empathy (e.g. insula, anterior cingulate) and mentalizing (TPJ, Precuneus, STS) systems Vagal system Mediated by: Oxytocin among others	Overcommitment and over reliance of social relationships (loss of autonomy) Other people's necessities at the expense of one's own Lack of engagement and reliance on social relationships (isolation)	Altruistic and compassion dispositions: increasing social engagement and connection without losing personal autonomy Self-compassion: being aware of and fostering what is suitable for one's needs

(continued)

Table 11.1 (continued)

Drives	Psychological mechanism in adolescence	Referential brain system	Downside	Mindfulness and compassion—potential targets
Increased emotional intensity	Enhanced emotionally driven behaviors. Exacerbated emotional reactivity, for positive or negative situations	Emotion generation (amygdala, insula) and regulation (prefrontal and parietal cortex) systems	Intense and unmanageable emotional states. Impulsivity, moodiness, and unhelpful reactivity	Self-emotion regulation skills: affective tolerance, emotional awareness Self-soothing: capacity for cultivating positive emotions and engaging in healthy self-care strategies
Creative exploration, Self-development	Increased engagement in new activities (e.g. physical, intellectual, creative), new experiences (relationships, social groups, spirituality, etc.) and new ideas (e.g. questioning status quo, emergence of innovation)	Fronto-parietal and Default mode network systems	Challenges in the development of identity, vulnerability to peer pressure, and a lack of direction and purpose	Self-regulation skills: self-awareness, decentering/disengagement, self-acceptance Self-compassion in terms of being aware of and fostering what is suitable for one's needs

Adapted from Siegel "Brainstorm" (2013)

ing salient information, giving emotional value to perception (hedonic or aversive), engaging in social cognition (empathy and mentalization), and using this information for guiding learning and behavior. For example, a study inducing social emotions like shame and guilt showed that adolescents, compared to adults, had a higher activation in the dorsomedial part of the prefrontal cortex, a key area for mentalization (Burnett, Bird, Moll, Frith, & Blakemore, 2009).

11.4 Building Personal Resources in Childhood and Adolescence: Cultivating Resilience Through Mindfulness and Compassion

We have mentioned the relevance of early-life adversity and its impact on developmental capacities, altering psychological well-being in children and adolescents. Resilience has been defined as the process of negotiating, managing, and adapting to significant sources of stress or trauma, in which assets and resources within the individual, their life and environment facilitate this capacity for adaptation and 'bouncing back' in the face of adversity (Windle, 2011). Although resilience as a construct has different facets, it points out not only to the absence of pathology, but to the prevention of and recovery from different forms of adversities (Davydov, Stewart, Ritchie, & Chaudieu, 2010). Adolescence is a complex dynamic process in which developmental socio-affective abilities and attachment styles, evolved from early life experiences, are challenged and continuously remodeled. Importantly, in the context of adolescence and development, Rutten et al. (2013) highlight specific factors promoting resilience, mainly secure attachment, positive emotions, and purpose in life.

Contemplative practices such as mindfulness-based interventions (MBIs) and compassion-based interventions (CBIs), are structured programs that integrate mindfulness and compassion meditation practices into secular multicomponent interventions. Importantly, these diverse programs are designed to cultivate different psychological and socio-cognitive mental skills. In adult populations, MBIs have been shown to increase self-regulation, either by increasing attention regulation or emotion regulation capacities; correspondingly, MBIs might also increase activation of brain regions in affect regulation networks (Guendelman, Medeiros, & Rampes, 2017). CBIs have been shown to increase empathy and compassion dispositions (Kirby, Tellegen, & Steindl, 2017). Interestingly, in adults, mindfulness interventions have been shown to increase positive emotions and meaning in life (Goyal et al., 2014).

A large longitudinal study comparing a MBI and a CBI in adults found that both produced a differential effect on specific brain structures, with the MBI targeting regions associated with attention and body awareness and the CBI targeting regions associated with emotion, empathy, and affiliation/altruism (Valk et al., 2017). In sum, contemplative practices have been shown to target resilience factors such as self-regulation, empathy, and compassion; thus, they hold promise in serving to promote mental health benefits in adolescents. In this regard, as we summarized in Table 11.1, we speculate that MBIs and CBIs could target specific psychological processes during adolescence by developing or training particular socio-emotional skills. For example, the increased drive and proneness to seek novelty and its associated impulsive decision making could be balanced through the enhancement of self-regulation. A randomized controlled study in adolescents showed that a MBI led to decreased levels of impulsivity and aggressive behavior (Franco, Amutio, López-González, Oriol, & Martínez-Taboada, 2016). The increased intensity of emotional experience could be counterbalanced with emotion regulation and self-soothing strategies. Also, the enhanced drive for social connection and sensitivity to peer evaluations could be worked out with the balanced training of altruism (helping others) and self-compassion in terms of being aware of and fostering what is suitable for one's needs. In this line, another intervention study in preschoolers showed that a CBI increased self-regulation and prosociality using behavioral tasks (Flook, Goldberg, Pinger, & Davidson, 2015).

Despite the enthusiasm in the application of MBIs and CBIs in children and adolescents, this research field is only in its infancy. Although the initial output seems promising, there is a lack of studies evaluating neuronal correlates, and very few have used validated behavioral experiments to actually measure cognitive or social performances, precluding further understanding of psychological mechanisms linked to contemplative practices. Most studies are hindered by small sample sizes, a lack of active control groups, and reliance on self-reported questionnaires. New studies will need to overcome these methodological limitations to further demonstrate the effectiveness of contemplative practices in ameliorating mental health and facilitating the transition from personal self-regulation to social functioning.

11.4.1 Contemplative Practices in School Settings

As pointed out in earlier chapters, contemplative practices in school settings show promising results in fostering psychological health (see Andreu and Langer in this volume). We highlight the need to incorporate not only self-centered practices but also the cultivation of prosocial attitudes and compassion. Davidson et al. (2012) propose a model of cultivation of healthy educational contexts through the encouragement of individual changes (i.e. psychological functions and neural substrates), which are expected to result in positive behavioral and social outcomes. We suggest an integrated and horizontal approach in which not only teachers but all staff may share a common vision in order for sustained benefits to flourish. Moreover, by focusing on developmental aspects, educational interventions can be optimized to address specific needs in the prevention and management of relational stress and suffering.

11.4.2 Mindful Parenting

Even though it is beyond the scope of this chapter, we point to early parenting as a critical period where contemplative practices may be as fundamental in enhancing profound and long-term resilience. Bögels, Lehtonen, and Restifo (2010) describe how mindful parenting may foster parent–child interactions through mechanisms such as reducing parental stress, reactivity, and preoccupation, improving parental executive functioning and impulsivity, and increasing self-nourishing attention and co-parenting. Moreover, they suggest that this may help in breaking cycles of intergenerational transmission of trauma and dysfunctional styles. Regarding the role of parents and their engagement in a contemplative educational school context, we believe in the necessity of a shared and common vision on the values and socio-affective capacities to be enhanced in children. Ideally, parents should cultivate mindful and compassionate qualities in their own ongoing processes. This is especially relevant because parental difficulties in being present with their own experience during stressful interactions with their children probably translate the reactivation of their own traumas and vulnerabilities (Medeiros & Guendelman, 2016; Medeiros, 2017).

11.4.3 Psychotherapy

In western countries, the use of contemplative practices should not prevent patients from receiving psychotherapeutic help when they need it. Psychotherapy fosters self-regulation, which can be explicitly enhanced through specific skills learned in sessions (Cognitive Behavioral Therapy or CBT, Dialectical Behavior Therapy or DBT) or implicitly modeled through the therapeutic relation itself. Furthermore, given the interpersonal nature of psychotherapy, mentalizing abilities are key to the tasks to be fulfilled by the therapist (to work with the patient) and the patient (to develop in the treatment) (Fonagy & Bateman, 2006). Strengthening mentalization is considered a common factor and the basis of psychotherapeutic change in several clinical currents (for CBT, see Björgvinsson & Hart, 2006; for DBT, see Lewis, 2006).

In this context, it is necessary to determine how contemplative practices and psychotherapy can inform the work conducted at a social or community level. We believe in a synergy between contemplative approaches and psychotherapeutic interventions. Both offer the potential for integrating the psychological "work" at the individual level, but also offer a perspective for working at a social or communal level. Both can foster positive mental characteristics such as emotion regulation and social closeness while reducing psychopathology, thus contributing to social interactions and community building. In this vein, we suggest future research should also focus on interventions that not only develop attentional and cognitive facets of mindfulness, but that also explicitly cultivate socio-affective skills associated with compassion (empathy, assertiveness, prosociality, and altruism). Moreover, we suggest that contemplative interventions should target not only school students, but also teachers and the administrative body, thus contributing to a cultural and systemic change within the organization and community. Local idiosyncrasies and specific backgrounds and needs should also be considered when exploring the transition from personal to embedded cultural and community dimensions.

11.5 Conclusion

This chapter explores a dialogue between developmental, clinical, and neuroscientific aspects of the adolescent mind to reflect on the integration of contemplative practices in this population. Contemplative studies can be enriched by considering aspects of early affective dynamics for a more fruitful dialogue between research, prevention, and treatment. We propose that socio-affective capacities, self-regulation, mentalization, and empathy/prosociality act circularily as both *terrain* and target-mechanisms where contemplative practices build personal and social resilience. Given the critical role of early stress and the social environment in the later maturation of resilience systems, it is fundamental to acknowledge how developmental capacities are always plastic and can be modeled through experience. Contemplative practices offer potential benefits in targeting specific psychological challenges and socio-emotional capacities of adolescents, possibly subserving and ensuring resilience at a personal and relational level.

Funding This paper was supported by the Fund for Innovation and Competitiveness (FIC) of the Chilean Ministry of Economy, Development, and Tourism, through the Millennium Science Initiative, Grant No. IS130005.

References

Baumeister, R. F., & Heatherton, T. F. (1996). Self-regulation failure: An overview. *Psychological Inquiry, 7,* 1–15.
Björgvinsson, T., & Hart, J. (2006). Cognitive behavioral therapy promotes mentalizing. In J. G. Allen & P. Fonagy (Eds.), *The handbook of mentalization-based treatment* (pp. 157–170). Hoboken, NJ, USA: Wiley.
Blakemore, S. J. (2018a). Avoiding social risk in adolescence. *Current Directions in Psychological Science, 27*(2), 116–122.
Blakemore, S. J. (2018b). *Inventing ourselves*. New York: PublicAffairs.
Bögels, S. M., Lehtonen, A., & Restifo, K. (2010). Mindful parenting in mental health care. *Mindfulness, 1,* 107–120.
Bucci, W. (2007). Dissociation from the perspective of multiple code theory, part I: Psychological roots and implications for psychoanalytic treatment. *Contemporary Psychoanalysis, 43*(2), 165–184.

Burnett, S., Bird, G., Moll, J., Frith, C., & Blakemore, S. J. (2009). Development during adolescence of the neural processing of social emotion. *Journal of Cognitive Neuroscience, 21*(9), 1736–1750.
Conway, C. C., Raposa, E. B., Hammen, C., & Brennan, P. A. (2018). Transdiagnostic pathways from early social stress to psychopathology: A 20-year prospective study. *Journal of Child Psychology and Psychiatry, 59*(8), 855–862.
Daskalakis, N. P., Bagot, R. C., Parker, K. J., Vinkers, C. H., & de Kloet, E. R. (2013). The three-hit concept of vulnerability and resilience: Toward understanding adaptation to early-life adversity outcome. *Psychoneuroendocrinology, 38,* 1858–1873.
Davidson, R. J., Dunne, J. D., Eccles, J. S., Engle, A., Greenberg, M., Jennings, P., et al. (2012). Contemplative practices and mental training: Prospects for American education. *Child Development Perspectives, 6*(2), 146–153.
Davis, M. H. (2015). Empathy and prosocial behavior. In D. A. Schroeder & W. G. Graziano (Eds.), *The Oxford handbook of prosocial behavior* (pp. 282–306). New York: Oxford University Press.
Davydov, D. M., Stewart, R., Ritchie, K., & Chaudieu, I. (2010). Resilience and mental health. *Clinical Psychology Review, 30,* 479–495.
de Vignemont, F., & Singer, T. (2006). The empathic brain: How when and why? *Trends in Cognitive Sciences, 10,* 435–441.
Flook, L., Goldberg, S. B., Pinger, L., & Davidson, R. J. (2015). Promoting prosocial behavior and self-regulatory skills in preschool children through a mindfulness-based Kindness curriculum. *Developmental Psychology, 51*(1), 44–51.
Fonagy, P., Bateman, A., & Luyten, P. (2012). Introduction and overview. In A. Bateman & P. Fonagy (Eds.), *Handbook of mentalizing in mental health practice* (pp. 3–41). Arlington, VA: American Psychiatric Publishing.
Fonagy, P., & Bateman, A. W. (2006). Mechanisms of change in mentalization based treatment of BPD. *Journal of Clinical Psychology, 62,* 411–430.
Fonagy, P., Target, M., Gergely, G., & Jurist, E. L. (2002). *Affect regulation, mentalization, and the development of self.* New York: Other Press.
Franco, C., Amutio, A., López-González, L., Oriol, X., & Martínez-Taboada, C. (2016). Effect of a mindfulness training program on the impulsivity and aggression levels of adolescents with behavioral problems in the classroom. *Frontiers in Psychology, 7,* 1385.
Gilbert, P. (2010). *Compassion focused therapy: Distinctive features.* London: Routledge.
Goyal, M., Singh, S., Sibinga, E. M. S., Gould, N. F., Rowland-Seymour, A., Sharma, R., et al. (2014). Meditation programs for psychological stress and well-being: A systematic review and meta-analysis. *Journal of American Medical Association, Internal Medicine, 174*(3), 357–368.
Guendelman, S., Medeiros, S., & Rampes, H. (2017). Mindfulness and emotion regulation: Insights from neurobiological, psychological, and clinical studies. *Frontiers in Psychology, 8,* 220.
Halifax, J. (2012). A heuristic model of enactive compassion. *Current Opinnion in Supportive and Palliative Care, 6*(2), 228–235.
Kirby, J. N., Tellegen, C. L., & Steindl, S. R. (2017). A meta-analysis of compassion-based interventions: Current state of knowledge and future directions. *Behavior Therapy, 48*(6), 778–792.
Lewis, L. (2006). Enhancing mentalizing capacity through dialectical behavior therapy skills training and positive psychology. In J. G. Allen & P. Fonagy (Eds.), *Handbook of mentalization-based treatment* (pp. 171–182). Chichester: Wiley.
Lewis, M. D., Granic, I., Lamm, C., Zelazo, P. D., Stieben, J., Todd, R. M., et al. (2008). Changes in the neural bases of emotion regulation associated with clinical improvement in children with behavior problems. *Developmental Psychopathology, 20,* 913–939.
Medeiros, S. (2017). Holding mutual vulnerability in brilliant sanity. *Studies in Gender and Sexuality, 18*(4), 244–250.
Medeiros, S., & Guendelman, S. (2016). Developmental trauma from a Buddhist and relational inter-subjective perspective. *International Journal of Psychotherapy, 20,* 94–113.
Mills, K. L., Goddings, A. L., Herting, M. M., Meuwese, R., Blakemore, S.-J., Crone, E. A., et al. (2016). Structural brain development between childhood and adulthood: convergence across four longitudinal samples. *NeuroImage, 41,* 273–281.

Nesse, R. M., Bhatnagar, S., & Ellis, B. (2016). Evolutionary origins and functions of the stress response system. In G. Finck (Ed.), *Stress: Concepts, cognition, emotion, and behavior* (pp. 95–101). New York: Academic Press.

OPD Task Force. (2008). *Operationalized psychodynamic diagnosis OPD-2: Manual of diagnosis and treatment planning Opd Task Force*. Göttingen: Hogrefe.

Pagliaccio, D., Luby, J. L., Luking, K. R., Belden, A. C., & Barch, D. M. (2014). Brain–behavior relationships in the experience and regulation of negative emotion in healthy children: Implications for risk for childhood depression. *Developmental Psychopathology, 26,* 1289–1303.

Petanjek, Z., Judaš, M., Šimić, G., Roko, M. R., Uylings, H., Rakic, P., et al. (2011). Extraordinary neoteny of synaptic spines in the human prefrontal cortex. *Proceedings of the National Academy of Science of the United States of America, 108*(32), 13281–13286.

Pollak, S. D. (2015). Developmental psychopathology: Recent advances and future challenges. *World Psychiatry, 14,* 262–269.

Porges, S. (2011). *The polyvagal theory: Neurophysiological foundations of emotions, attachment, communication, self-regulation*. New York: Norton.

Posner, M. I., Rothbart, M. K., Sheese, B. E., & Tang, Y. (2007). The anterior cingulategyrus and the mechanism of self-regulation. *Cognitive. Affective Behavioral Neuroscience, 7,* 391–395.

Roffman, J. L., Gerber, A. J., & Flick, D. M. (2012). Neural models of psychodynamic concepts and treatments: Implications for psychodynamic psychotherapy. In R. A. Levy, J. S. Ablon, & H. Kächele (Eds.), *Psychodynamic psychotherapy research: Evidence-based practice and practice-based evidence* (pp. 193–218). New York: Springer.

Rogers, C. R. (1965). *Client-centered therapy: Its current practice, implications and theory*. Boston, MA: Houghton-Mifflin.

Rutten, B. P. F., Hammels, C., Geschwind, N., Menne-Lothmann, C., Pishva, E., Schruers, K., et al. (2013). Resilience in mental health: Linking psychological and neurobiological perspectives. *Acta Psychiatrica Scandinavica, 128,* 3–20.

Schore, A. N. (2012). *The science of the art of psychotherapy*. New York: W.W. Norton.

Siegel, D. J. (2007). *The mindful brain: Reflection and attunement in the cultivation of well-being*. New York, NY: Norton.

Siegel, D. J. (2013). *Brainstorm: The power and purpose of the teenage brain*. New York: Penguin.

Smith, L. B., & Thelen, E. (2003). Development as a dynamic system. *Trends in Cognitive Sciences, 7*(8), 343–348.

Somerville, L. (2013). The teenage brain: Sensitivity to social evaluation. *Current Directions in Psychological Science, 22,* 121–127.

Steinberg, L. (2007). Risk taking in adolescence: New perspectives from brain and behavioral science. *Current Directions in Psychological Science, 16*(2), 55–59.

Steinberg, L., Albert, D., Cauffman, E., Banich, M., Graham, S., & Woolard, J. (2008). Age differences in sensation seeking and impulsivity as indexed by behavior and self-report: Evidence for a dual systems model. *Developmental Psychology, 44*(6), 1764–1778.

Steinberg, L., Icenogle, G., Shulman, E. P., Breiner, K., Chein, J., Bacchini, D., et al. (2017). Around the world, adolescence is a time of heightened sensation seeking and immature self-regulation. *Developmental Science, 21,* 1–13.

Valk, S. L., Bernhardt, B. C., Trautwein, F.-M., Böckler, A., Kanske, P., Guizard, N., et al. (2017). Structural plasticity of the social brain: Differential change after socio-affective and cognitive mental training. *Science Advances, 3*(10), 1–11.

Windle, G. (2011). What is resilience? A review and concept analysis. *Reviews in Clinical Gerontology, 21*(2), 152–169.

Zelazo, P. D., & Lyons, K. E. (2012). The potential benefits of mindfulness training in early childhood: A developmental social cognitive neuroscience perspective. *Child Development Perspectives, 6,* 154–160.

Chapter 12
Education as the Key to Facing Today's Challenges: How We Can Generate a More Resilient Environment and Promote a Paradigm Shift in Economics

Vanessa Nowak and Felix Fuders

Abstract Nowadays, we are still trapped in a paradigm whose guiding principle is to increase intensity: higher, faster, further. Therefore, many still think that an ever-stronger exploitation of natural resources and increasing monetary profits would bring us wealth and make us happy. For this very reason, we still teach students the values of an 'elbow-society', in which everyone seems to think only of themselves first. In this chapter, we show why it is important to shape a paradigm shift from a material to an ethical focus in order to construct a sustainable (in an economic, social, and ecological sense) and resilient society. From this perspective, we outline the importance of setting cornerstones in the field of education, describe concrete competency models, and recommend their implementation through teaching methods like Social and Emotional Learning (SEL) and Project Based Learning (PBL). Moreover, we contrast the old paradigm and a possible new paradigm based on the values of love and respect that would foster resilience, as illustrated by the best practice example of Bhutan. The complexity of adaptive challenges results from the fact that people are part of both the problem and the solution and key factors such as habits, customs, and cultures come into play and have to be reconsidered.

Keywords Paradigm change · Resilient paradigm · Teaching · Love · Respect

---

V. Nowak (✉)
German Chilean Competency Center for Development, Valdivia, Chile
e-mail: vanessa.regina.nowak@gmail.com

Faculty of Engineering and Technology, Universidad San Sebastián, Valdivia, Chile

F. Fuders
Faculty of Economics and Administration, Economics Institute, Universidad Austral de Chile, Valdivia, Chile

C. Steinebach and Á. I. Langer (eds.), *Enhancing Resilience in Youth*,
https://doi.org/10.1007/978-3-030-25513-8_12

12.1 Why a Paradigm Shift?

Albert Einstein once said that “we cannot solve our problems with the same thinking we used when we created them” (FBIS Daily Report, 1995). This recommendation is more up-to-date than ever given the phenomena of our time such as globalization, climate change, and the so-called fourth industrial revolution. We are facing challenges that are forcing us to rethink our way of living, working, and educating. Automation, for instance, has increasingly replaced repetitive and analytical tasks, placing greater demand on jobs that require social skills (Deming, 2015). This means we will need a different type of preparation for life, new ways of thinking in order to solve our problems. Moreover, we must realize that sometimes our way of thinking even co-creates problems, such as constantly seeking more economic growth, which fosters the destruction of the natural environment (Daly & Farley, 2011). This moment of insight that our way of seeing things is the problem is called *Eureka* (Vitruvius, n.d.) and is key to a paradigm change.

However, a paradigm change is a considerable challenge as it requires a perspective transformation (Clark, 1940) that has three dimensions: psychological (changes in understanding of the self), convictional (revision of belief systems), and behavioral (changes in lifestyle). Many times, it requires that we rethink our patterns and routines, which is not easy. On the contrary: when people realize that a certain way of thinking and acting is not bringing the expected result, they tend to intensify the existing solution, which can be illustrated by Henry Ford’s statement: “If I had asked people what they wanted, they would have said faster horses” (Vlaskovits, 2011). This shows that, instead of an automobile, Ford’s clients were likely to have thought of a more powerful version of the old solution. Today we are still trapped in a paradigm whose guiding principle is to increase intensity: higher, faster, further. Therefore, many still think that an ever-stronger exploitation of natural resources and increasing monetary profits would bring us wealth and make us happy. For this very reason, we still teach students the values of an ‘elbow-society’, in which everyone seems to think only of themselves first.

However, higher forces such as natural disasters teach us that it is high time for a change of perspective. In the following, we would like to illustrate how impulses in education could lead to a paradigm shift towards more resilience and an economy whose driver is love instead of competition as proposed in Chap. 17.

12.2 How to Create a Resilient Paradigm?

The aforementioned change of mindset and behavior will, most probably, not eventuate on its own. However, it could be encouraged, developed, and supported through educational measures. If we want to create a paradigm shift from competition to love in the economic system (see Chap. 17), we should start with a shift in the competency model for all actors in the system. In other words, if our aim is to create an economy of love where people believe that their purpose in life is to contribute to society with their talents, then we must first allow and appreciate different kinds of talents and second, teach the actors of this economy to know and respect themselves and their environment. This means that the educational system and teaching methods should aim to develop broader skills in order to gear all social actors' attitudes, values, and ethics towards holistic ways of thinking, feeling and acting.

In this regard, we argue that the mission of education should be to prepare students for real life by generating resources that enable them to deal with themselves (i.e. identifying and developing one's talent and vocation) and their environment (becoming part of the social and ecological context). This would entail the application of a certain set of values. Such a reform has parallels with the sense of resilience established by Christoph Steinebach, which includes internal processes, the environment, and a value framework. For Steinebach, resilience means:

> The positive adaptation and sustainable development of a system to respond to short- or longer-term everyday challenges or severe stress. Based on internal system processes and through dealing with the environment, the system defines new reference values and develops required competencies, and the ability to cope with future stress improves. (Steinebach, 2015, p. 557)

Resilience is the result of a paradigm that aimed at constructing a strong, responsive, and sustainable system. Our hypothesis is that promoting a shift in our approach to education and the way we see the economy, based on the three dimensions identified by Steinebach (2015), will lead to more resilience on an individual level and eventually translate into a positive impact on the whole society and environment. Those three dimensions are the following:

(1) Learning to know and manage oneself
(2) Interacting with the environment
(3) Applying values.

12.3 Education as Key to a Paradigm Shift: Competency Models for a New Paradigm

In order to define the "new reference values" and develop the "required competencies" identified by Steinebach, it is necessary to constantly rethink and adapt competency models and teaching methodologies. Through new competency models and teaching methods, pupils acquire the necessary tools to develop self-awareness, fully understand their own abilities (in different roles and contexts), and identify their vocation, which enables them to face their environment differently. All of this will make individuals more *resilient* and produce active participants of an economic system based on love and respect, which is described more in detail in Chap. 17.

There are different competency models for education and lifelong learning that consider competencies beyond technical aspects and include social and emotional factors. This is in keeping with the idea that humans possess *multiple intelligences* (Gardner, 1993) and are not limited to the cognitive intelligence quantified by classic IQ testing. According to Gardner's model, there are seven different types of intelligence: linguistic, logical-mathematical, musical, spatial, bodily-kinesthetic, interpersonal, and intrapersonal.

Indeed, in many situations we need emotional intelligence to complement knowledge in order to take the right decision. Five key principles are seen as features of emotional intelligence. These are (i) being aware of one's emotions, (ii) being able to manage one's own emotions, (iii) being sensitive to the emotions of others, (iv) being able to respond to and negotiate with other people emotionally, (v) being able to use one's own emotions to motivate oneself (Salovey & Mayer, 1990: 313). Emotional intelligence includes, alongside other factors, empathy and ethical thinking. The psychologist and neuroscientist Howard Gardner goes as far as to claim that a "bad person can never be a good professional" (Amiguet, 2016). According to Gardner, to be "really good" we need to have an emotional investment in our work. This is something that many sources from both the educational and the economic domains agree with; therefore, a competency model outlining the skills required in the 21st century needs to include interpersonal competencies like communication and collaboration (Soffel, 2016), interacting in heterogeneous groups (OECD, 1998), and learning to live together. These all require broader aspects of emotional intelligence such as empathy and tolerance (Delors & UNESCO, 1996).

Within such a context, it is interesting to identify competency models which allow for the incorporation of both educational and economic disciplines. One example is Vocational Training. Note that vocation is at the heart of the term Vocational Training. Also, the German word for profession ('*Beruf*') is based on the root *Berufung* (vocation). In this field, the German Standing Conference of the Ministers of Education and Cultural Affairs (*Kultusministerkonferenz*, KMK) developed a model in 1996 whose purpose was to empower students/professionals to be able to act responsibly in a working context. This was termed *professional acting competency* (in German: *Berufliche Handlungskompetenz)*. Similarly, the German Qualifications Framework for Lifelong Learning (AK DQR, 2011) also provides a model of *professional acting competency,* composed of two triads that create two different dimensions. In one, there are three different types of competencies (technical, social, and personal), whereas the other comprises knowledge, abilities, and attitudes. According to this model, all of those aspects are necessary and equally important in the process of creating a holistic professional (Fig. 12.1).

Another model that goes beyond cognitive competence and integrates personal behavior in an environmental context is the "Four Pillars of Education" proposed by Jacques Delors in a report for the UNESCO (Delors & UNESCO, 1996). The first pillar is related to mental processes, and is entitled "learning to know". This requires acquiring tools of comprehension as well as training attention, memory, and intellect. The second pillar refers to the acquisition of skills and is entitled "learning to do". Here, the emphasis is on empowering students to influence their environment. This might require coaching to help negotiate real-world interactions and situations. The third pillar refers to social competence and is called "learning to live together".

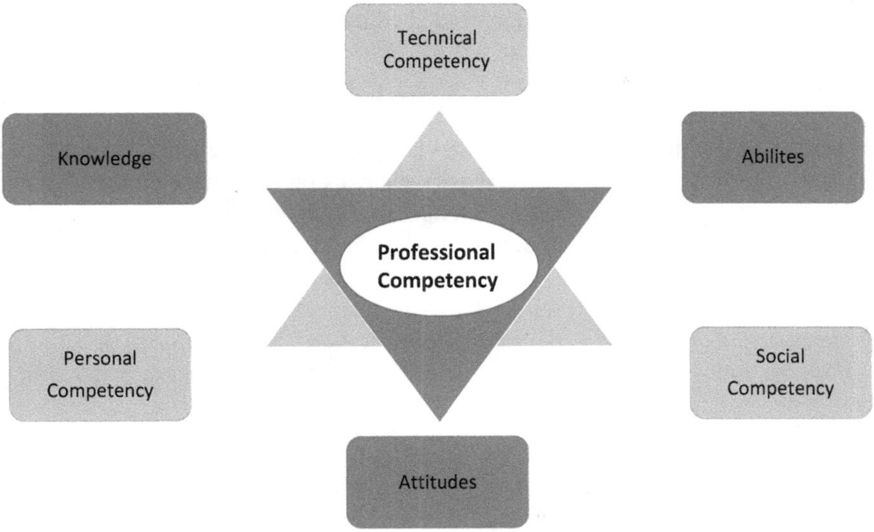

Fig. 12.1 Professional acting competency, cf. German Qualifications Framework for Lifelong Learning (2009)

A person who has acquired this competence is able to cooperate with others. This interdependence requires a level of mutual understanding (empathy) and compassion. The fourth and last pillar is called "learning to be" and refers to the integration of the three previous pillars. This final stage produces responsible, self-confident students.

One characteristic both models have in common is that they describe the components a person needs to develop in order to act responsibly and holistically within their environment. Both models also include the three dimensions mentioned above: (1) Learning to know and manage oneself, (2) Interacting with the environment, (3) Applying values (Steinebach, 2015) or, with the terminology suggested by CASEL, (1) Self-Awareness and Management, (2) Social Awareness and Relationship Skills, and (3) Responsible Decision Making (CASEL, 2017). The two models also illustrate that the concept of a holistic person, in a constructivist sense, is not recent but the product of decades of development. Nowadays, the real challenge is to determine how to translate these models into workable educational initiatives. Therefore, we propose teaching methods aimed at facilitating the shift toward this new paradigm.

12.4 New Teaching Methods for a New Paradigm

How can we best transfer the models outlined above to teaching practice so as to promote change and prepare individuals to be active and responsible actors in an economy based on love instead of competition? This is clearly an important question.

For such a task, teaching methods are needed which stimulate not only cognitive but emotional intelligence.

We now outline teaching methods that are part of a constructivist learning theory paradigm. This means that learning is the result of an active construction process by the learner and includes his or her previous knowledge and experience, among other elements. Furthermore, the constructivist view rests on the notion that the learner and his or her history and context are a central aspect in the learning process. Within this paradigm, the learner's autonomy, self-respect, and observational capacity are key concepts. In other words, the learning process is tailored to the student. This is certainly not a teacher-based process where the learner "suffers" passively, as might be the case using the framework of a structuralist paradigm.

For constructivist teaching, according to Dubs (1995), this means that learning should meet the following criteria:

- Learning is an active process
- Complex and holistic areas of concern, that are oriented around real-life situations
- Through collective, group learning, the individual interpretation is reflected and reconsidered
- Mistakes are regarded as part of the learning process
- Previous experience and interests of the learner are highly important
- Emotions and identification have to be included in the learning process
- Evaluation is not only concerned with the learning outcome, but also with the process, methods, and strategies used.

This makes it clear that the learner's talents and predispositions play an important role and that his or her intrinsic motivation is highly relevant for the learning process. This is possible as learning happens actively, not only as a result of extrinsic motivation. Both methods—'Social and Emotional Learning' and 'Project Based Learning'—have real potential to contribute to the necessary paradigm shift to achieve an *economy of love* and a more resilient society.

Social and emotional learning (SEL): Social and emotional learning integrates five different competencies that are commonly acquired at school. However, their impact goes far beyond the classroom: a number of studies have shown that they can influence the culture not only of the whole school, but also that of the students' homes and communities (Durlak, Weissberg, Dymnicki, Taylor, & Schellinger, 2011; Weissberg, Durlak, Domitrovich, & Gullotta, 2015). In other words, they impact the learners in the micro, meso, exo and macro contexts. The broad influence of this educational initiative has parallels with Steinebach's resilience model, whose resources can also be found in different contexts (Steinebach, 2013):

- Resources of the person and social competencies
- Resources of the family
- Resources of the school or vocational training institution (good climate, clear rules and models)
- Relation with peers (social and emotional support)
- Resources of society (availability of education and training offers).

Researchers generally agree upon five key competencies of SEL (Durlak et al., 2011; Weissberg et al., 2015). These competencies provide the foundations for high-quality social relationships and nurturing resilience to a variety of challenges. These core competencies of SEL are Self-Awareness, Self-Management, Social Awareness, Relationship Skills, and Responsible Decision Making. These competencies are in keeping with those we have already outlined as necessary to build up both *resilience* and an *economy of love*. In the following model, provided by CASEL (2017), the competencies are described more in detail with real-world examples of their application. Once again, one can conclude that those competencies (e.g. identifying problems, empathy or ethical responsibility) are key to a long-term paradigm shift in economics and society (Fig. 12.2).

Importantly, studies that have compared the learning outcomes of Social and Emotional Learning with those of traditional instruction methods have shown that SEL increases students' academic performance (Durlak et al., 2011). Furthermore, SEL programs have broader positive effects: they reduce aggression and emotional distress among students, increase helping behaviors in school, and improve positive attitudes towards oneself and others (Durlak et al., 2011). SEL also strengthens students' relationships with their peers, families, and teachers, meaning that it can help build a student's support base and therefore their resilience to challenges (Steinebach, 2013) and shows measurable benefits that exceed its costs, often by considerable amounts (Belfield et al., 2015). These characteristics make SEL a potentially valuable tool to achieve the suggested paradigm shift.

Project Based Learning (PBL): Project Based Learning is another example of a teaching method that, alongside fostering resilience (Barron & Darling-Hammond, 2008), develops competencies necessary for a paradigm shift in economics. PBL allows students to learn by experiencing and solving real-world problems, complement theoretical and practical learning, and integrate reflection into the learning environment. It promotes the autonomous learning process of students through com-

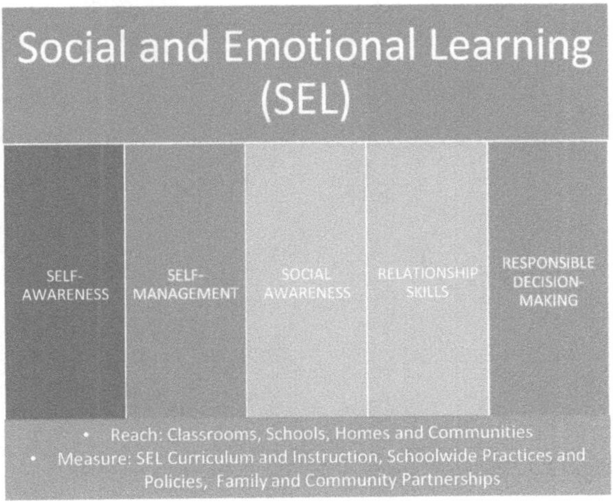

Fig. 12.2 Social and emotional learning, cf. framework for systemic social and emotional learning and contexts, Collaborative for Academic, Social, and Emotional Learning (2017)

plex tasks that have more than one solution. To complete these tasks, students usually work in pairs or groups while teachers act as coaches and facilitators to stimulate inquiry and reflection (Barron & Darling-Hammond, 2008; Thomas, 2000).

One of the unique aspects of the PBL method is that it purposefully includes the whole process of stages required to a complete action (Hacker, 1998). This can be viewed as a cycle where students plan an action, decide on specifics, execute their idea, and control the results before evaluating them and reapplying their knowledge to inform the whole circle again. This is conceptualized in Fig. 12.3.

This teaching method engages students in creating, questioning, and revising knowledge, while at the same time developing their skills in critical thinking, collaboration, communication, reasoning, synthesis, and resilience (Barron & Darling-Hammond, 2008). Studies comparing learning outcomes for students taught using PBL and those taught using traditional instruction show that PBL deepens long-term retention of content, improves problem-solving and collaboration skills, and improves students' attitudes towards learning (Strobel & van Barneveld, 2009; Walker & Leary, 2009). As with SEL, PBL goes beyond the school context and can be applied in learning contexts in a wider sense. This is illustrated with the example of GaiaEducation, an education project that contributes to the UNESCO Global Action Programme on Education for Sustainable Development. GaiaEducation applies PBL to prepare stakeholders with skills and tools for real-life solutions such as designing sustainable settlements in developing countries.

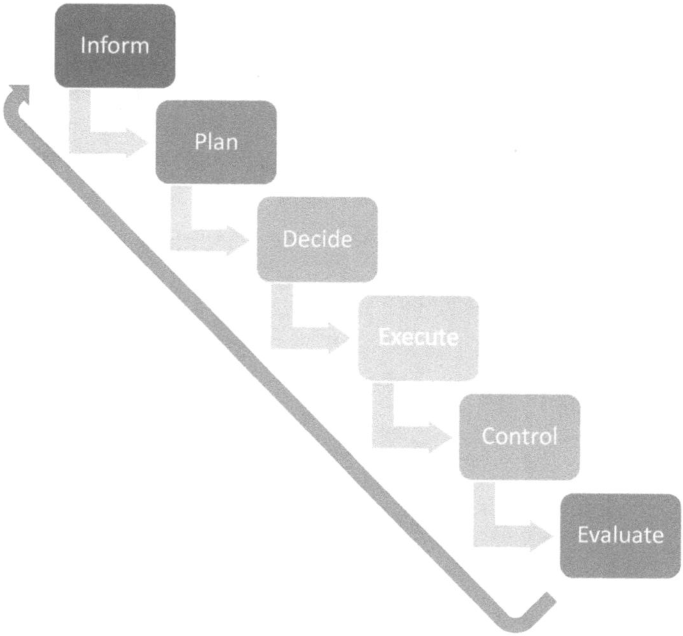

Fig. 12.3 Phases of a complete action, cf. Hacker (1998)

Both mentioned methods, SEL and PBL, foster interpersonal skills such as teamwork, coordination, and collaboration, as well as leadership skills such as responsibility, assertive communication, self-presentation, and social influence. These can be seen as essential tools to enhance consciousness and to promote the realization of a resilient society and economy. Moreover, in both examples, students are learning from and with peers while the teachers operate as facilitators. This suggests that we also need a new role distribution between teachers and learners for a paradigm shift. This fits into Haidt's interpretation of Jean Piaget's recommendation for moral development—for Haidt, "the best thing adults can do to foster moral development is to get out of the way" (Haidt, 2008, p. 66).

To illustrate the teacher's role, we can use the metaphor of how a gardener (the teacher) tends to his or her plants (the students). Here, in order to produce the best botanical specimens, the gardener knows he must give the plants space to grow and develop on their own. To continue the metaphor, conventional teaching can be seen more as a "sculptor" who limits his students and works with pressure like a craftsman producing a certain good. The role of the teacher as a gardener or facilitator also implies higher self-guidance by the students in the learning process (which has to be trained). This leads to different evaluation methods that are not only teacher-centered but also oriented toward self or group evaluations among the students. Through such activities, the students get trained to (i) reflect on and contextualize their learning process, (ii) identify their strengths and areas to develop, and (iii) recognize valuable resources and abilities in themselves and others that aid the achievement of a common goal. The suggestion that teaching is most efficient when a student is given an active role in the learning process has parallels with an ancient Chinese proverb, which again shows that even though the idea is not new, it is hard to implement:

> Tell me and I'll forget it,
> Show it to me and I may remember,
> Involve me and I will understand.

12.5 A Shift Towards Resilience: The Old and the New Paradigm

After having analyzed how educational measures could favor a paradigm shift, we would now like to introduce a simplified model that shows the contrast of the old to the new paradigm and what that means in the fields of education and economics. A more detailed analysis about the shift in the economy towards an economy based on the value of love is presented in Chap. 17 of this book.

Another objective of this table is to visualize that the cornerstones we set in education will later be reflected in the economic system. For instance, if a person was taught at school that the most important thing is to be the best and win in his or her work life, it will be challenging for this person to work within a team, as this requires a different mindset. However, for companies to be competitive, their employees needed to have experience sharing ideas and viewpoints with diverse groups of people. Such an acknowledgment highlights the importance of cross cultural and interdisciplinary thinking in societal advancement. This coincides with the experience of one of the most successful businessmen in China and founder of *Alibaba*, Jack Ma, who emphasized the importance of the triad of different quotients: the intelligence quotient (IQ), the emotional quotient (EQ), and the love quotient (LQ). In an interview given to the World Economic Forum, he made the following statement: "To gain success a person will need high EQ; if you don't want to lose quickly you will need a high IQ, and if you want to be respected you need high LQ—the IQ of love" (Flashman, 2018).

To achieve these competencies, it is extremely important to set a sound foundation within the education field and prepare people step by step for a new paradigm and their future challenges. Students have to be trained to work in a team, use their different intelligences, manage themselves, assume responsibility, and perceive mistakes as an opportunity to learn (Bradberry, 2017). If we educate young people this way, they will be more likely to apply those competencies in their adult lives and become valuable actors of a more resilient society and economy. This kind of education is the cornerstone of flexible, innovative, and empowered working people who are aware of their strengths and weaknesses and act in awareness of their environment, seek to contribute to the common good, and make responsible decisions.

In this regard, the kingdom of Bhutan, located in the Eastern Himalayas, can serve as best practice towards a new paradigm. Bhutan is a very interesting example, not only given the fact that its performance is measured by the Gross National Happiness (GNH) instead of the Gross Domestic Product (GDP) like in many other countries, but also because this paradigm shift was accompanied by educational measures. While the GDP is the final value of the goods and services produced within the geographic boundaries of a country during a specified period of time (The Economic Times, n.d.), the GNH consists of the following indicators: physical, mental, and spiritual health; time-balance; social and community vitality; cultural vitality; education; living standards; good governance; and ecological vitality (Ura et al., 2012).

This measuring shift from a material, quantitative production focus to an ethical approach that privileges the holistic well-being of the citizens and the environment was implemented alongside an educational initiative of the government called *Educating for GNH*. On an educational level, the measures to promote the GNH paradigm are twofold. First, values have been integrated in the curriculum: they inform the principal's and the teachers' actions and daily life practices at school (Drupka & Brien, 2018). Drupka and Brien summarized the following emphasized values: "deep critical and creative thinking, ecological literacy, practice of the country's profound ancient wisdom, contemplative learning, a holistic understanding of the world, genuine care for nature and for others, competency to deal effectively with the modern world, preparation for right livelihood, and informed civic engagement" (Drupka & Brien, 2018, p. 12).

Second, this was complemented by the *Green Schools for Green Bhutan* campaign, that understands "green" in a broad sense including both the ecological and the social environment (Hayward & Colman, 2010). Two of the central pillars of this initiative were promoting the involvement of parents and communities, which can be understood as an important source of resilience, as well as the creation of an atmosphere "that provides respect, care, warmth, and delight in the school" (Drupka & Brien, 2018, p. 13), values that are also the heart of an different economic paradigm as described in Chap. 17.

We can conclude that the GNH vision is strongly in line with a resilient paradigm, as we can presume that it promotes the pillars established by Steinebach and CASEL: (1) Learning to know and manage oneself (Self-Awareness and Management), (2) Interacting with the environment (Social Awareness and Relationship Skills), and (3) Applying values (Responsible Decision Making).

Another example that can be mentioned in the context of a paradigm shift in the education sector is Singapore, the leader of the 2015 PISA (Programme for International Student Asessment) ranking (Wood, 2018). After a solid track record of ranked exam results, the island state is adapting its educational system according to the future skills that will be required in working environments. Those skills will be less routine and memory oriented, instead focusing on typical human skills like creativity, leadership, and problem solving, according to the 2018 Future of Jobs report issued by the World Economic Forum (Wood, 2018), which is in line with the new paradigm detailed in Table 12.1.

12.6 Summary and Outlook

In this chapter, we have shown why it is important to shape a paradigm shift from a material to an ethical focus in order to construct a sustainable (in an economic, social, and ecological sense) and resilient society. Therefore, we have outlined the importance of setting cornerstones in the field of education, described concrete competency models, and recommended their implementation through teaching methods like SEL and PBL. To enhance a paradigm shift, we suggest that the highlighted educational measures are a vital resource in preparing for a perspective transformation and therefore build up abilities, values, and attitudes. Those measures would not only encourage more personal and societal resilience but also establish further innovation and entrepreneurial skills (i.e. stress management, self-discipline, self-motivation, goal setting, communication, relationship building, problem identification, and problem solving). These, in turn, would make the whole economy more flexible, resilient, and forwardthinking. Through such an initiative, sustainable economic development could also be fostered alongside improved ethics and values.

Moreover, we have contrasted the old paradigm and a possible new paradigm based on the values of love and respect that would foster resilience, as illustrated by the best practice example of Bhutan. Besides the measures mentioned in this chapter, for a future paradigm shift it would be equally important to consider new

Table 12.1 Comparison between the old and a possible new paradigm from an educational and economic point of view

Field	Dimension	Old paradigm	New paradigm
Education	Learning process	Knowledge-based	Integration of knowledge-based with social and emotional learning
	Measuring intelligence	Intelligence quotient	Multiple intelligences: Intelligence quotient Emotional quotient Learning quotient Among others
	Education focus	Teacher-focused approach, students compete	Pupil-focused approach, students work together
	Role of the student	Receives information	Creates knowledge, empowered
	Role of the teacher	Teacher as "sculptor"	Teacher as "gardener" (facilitator)
	Learning Motivation	Mainly extrinsic	Mainly intrinsic
	Mistakes are synonym for	Failure	Part of the learning process
	Monitoring	External control	Self-management
	Competency model	One-dimensional hierarchy of competencies	Competencies are multiple and complete each other
	Output	Discipline, applying orders	Creativity, Network Thinking, Decision Making, Responsibility
Economy	Goal	Exploitation, Maximize profit, Growth	Sustainability (social, economic and environmental)
	Way of relating with other actors of the system	Competition (only one actor can win)	Collaboration, respect, love (win win)
	Performance index	Gross Domestic Product (GDP) [1]	Gross National Happiness (GNH)
	Organization	Hierarchy	Network, Team
	Society model	Industrial Society	Knowledge Society
	Individual model	The individual is alone and therefore has to compete	The individual is part of the society and acts in awareness of its environment. It seeks to contribute to the common good
	Output	Repetition	Innovation

(continued)

Table 12.1 (continued)

Field	Dimension	Old paradigm	New paradigm
	Prepares for	Routine	Flexibility
	Relationship between person and system	Adapts person to a framework like an object	Promotes a persons' talents like a subject who creates the system
	Organizations focus	Internal	Context-sensitive, integrated in ecosystem
	Decision making	Egoistic	Ethical, based on the common good
	Motivation for career choice	Mainly extrinsic (e.g. prestige-, money-, security-based)	Mainly intrinsic (vocation- and talent-based)

leadership models, in analogy to the mentioned teaching models, which would lead to increased creativity, diversity, and resilience in the working world. It should be noted that studies have shown that the labor market increasingly rewards social skills as they permit to reduce coordination costs allowing workers to specialize and work together more efficiently (Deming, 2015). As we emphasized, paradigm shifts not only in general but also in every organization are complex processes which can be facilitated by external experts through training and consultancy. This can be especially helpful when the challenge is not only of a technical nature but also has an adaptive component (Heifetz, Grashow, & Linsky, 2009)—as is the case with most of the big and knotty phenomena mentioned at the beginning of the chapter such as global warming and digitization, among many others.

The latter applies to the models we highlighted above for both education and economy. The complexity of adaptive challenges results from the fact that people are part of both the problem and the solution and key factors such as habits, customs, and cultures come into play and have to be reconsidered. To put it once again in Albert Einstein's words: "We cannot solve our problems with the same thinking we used when we created them" (FBIS Daily Report, 1995).

References

AK DQR (Arbeitskreis Deutscher Qualifikationsrahmen) (2011). *Deutscher Qualifikationsrahmen für lebenslanges Lernen.* http://www.dqr.de/media/content/Der_Deutsche_Qualifikationsrahmen_fue_lebenslanges_Lernen.pdf. Accessed 1 October 2018.

Amiguet, L. (2016). *Una mala persona no llega nunca a ser buen profesional.* La Vanguardia. https://www.lavanguardia.com/lacontra/20160411/401021583313/una-mala-persona-no-llega-nunca-a-ser-buen-profesional.html. Accessed December 3, 2018.

Barron, B. (2003). When smart groups fail. *The Journal of the Learning Sciences, 12*(3), 307–359.

Barron, B., & Darling-Hammond, L. (2008). *Teaching for meaningful learning: A review of research on inquiry-based and cooperative learning. Powerful learning: What we know about teaching for understanding.* San Francisco, CA: Jossey-Bass.

Belfield, C., Bowden, B., Klapp, A., Levin, H., Shand, R., & Zander, S. (2015). *The economic value of social and emotional learning*. New York, NY: Center for Benefit-Cost Studies. in Education.
Bradberry, T. (2017). *Emotional Intelligence: What is it and why we need it*. World Economic Forum. https://www.weforum.org/agenda/2017/02/why-you-need-emotional-intelligence/. Accessed December 3, 2018.
CASEL (2017). Collaborative for Academic, Social, and Emotional Learning. https://casel.org. Accessed September 29, 2018.
Clark, J. (1940). Toward a concept of workable competition. *The American Economic Review*, 241–256.
Daly, H., & Farley, J. (2011). *Ecological economics—Prcinciples and applications* (2nd ed.). Washington, USA: Island Press.
Delors, J. (1994). Los cuatro pilares de la educación. *La educación encierra un tesoro*, 91–103.
Delors, J. (1997). *La educación encierra un tesoro: Informe a la UNESCO de la Comisión Internacional sobre la Educación para el Siglo XXI*. México: Correo de la Unesco.
Delors, J., & UNESCO. (1996). *International Commission on Education for the Twenty-first Century*. Learning, the treasure within: Report to UNESCO of the International Commission on Education for the Twenty-first Century.
Deming, D. J. (2015). The growing importance of social skills in the labor market. *The Quarterly Journal of Economics, 132*(4), 1593–1640.
Drupka, K., & Brien, K. (2018, November 15). Educating for Gross National Happiness: A new paradigm for education in Bhutan. *Antistasis* 3(2). https://journals.lib.unb.ca/index.php/antistasis/article/viewFile/21119/24379. Accessed January 12, 2019.
Dubs, R. (1995). Constructivism—Reflections from the perspective of the organization of instruction. *Zeitschrift für Pädagogik, 6*, 889–903.
Durlak, J., Weissberg, R. P., Dymnicki, A. B., Taylor, R. D., & Schellinger, K. B. (2011). The impact of enhancing students' social and emotional learning: A meta-analysis of school-based universal interventions. *Child Development, 82*(1), 405–432.
FBIS Daily Report. (1995). Einstein's famous saying in Copenhagen, p. 45". FBIS Daily Report, East Europe. https://libquotes.com/albert-einstein/quote/lbs1u5w. Accessed January 18, 2019.
Flashman, G. (2018). *Jack Ma on the IQ of love—and other top quotes from his Davos interview*. World Economic Forum Annual Meeting. https://www.weforum.org/agenda/2018/01/jack-ma-davos-top-quotes/. Accessed December 18, 2018.
Gardner, H. (1993). *Frames of mind: The theory of multiple intelligences*. New York, NY: BasicBooks.
Hacker, W. (1998). *Allgemeine Arbeitspsychologie*. Munich: Huber.
Haidt, J. (2008). Morality. *Perspectives on Psychological Science, 3*(1), 65–72.
Hayward, K., & Colman, R. (2010). *Educating for GNH*. Thimphu, Bhutan: GPI Atlantic. http://www.gpiatlantic.org/pdf/educatingforgnh/educating_for_gnh_proceedings.pdf. Accessed January 12, 2019.
Heifetz, R. A., Grashow, A., & Linsky, M. (2009). *The practice of adaptive leadership: Tools and tactics for changing your organization and the world*. Boston, MA: Harvard Business Press.
OECD (Organisation for Economic Co-operation and Development) (1998). Education at a Glance–OECD Indicators, OECD, Paris.
Piaget, J. (1932/1983). *Das moralische Urteil beim Kinde*. Stuttgart: Klett-Cotta.
Salovey, P., & Mayer, J. D. (1990). Emotional intelligence. *Imagination, Cognition, and Personality, 9*, 185–211.
Soffel, J. (2016). *What are the 21st-century skills every student needs?* World Economic Forum. Accessed 1 October 2018.
Steinebach, C. (2013). Beratung: Stärkenorientierte Gespräche. In C. Steinebach & K. Gharabaghi (Eds.), *Resilienzförderung im Jugendalter. Praxis und Perspektiven* (pp. 51–68). Springer.
Steinebach, C. (2015). Resilience. In J. D. Wright (Ed.), *International encyclopedia of the social & behavioral sciences* (2nd ed., Vol. 20, pp. 555–560). Oxford: Elsevier.

Steinebach, C., Schrenk, A., Steinebach, U., & Brendtro, L. (2018). *Positive Peer Culture. Manual für starke Gruppengespräche*. Weinheim: Beltz Juventa.
Strobel, J., & van Barneveld, A. (2009). When is PBL more effective? A meta-synthesis of meta-analyses comparing PBL to conventional classrooms. *The Interdisciplinary Journal of Problem-Based Learning, 3*(1), 44–58.
Taylor, R. D., Oberle, E., Durlak, J. A., & Weissberg, R. P. (2017). Promoting positive youth development through school-based social and emotional learning interventions: A meta-analysis of follow-up effects. *Child Development, 88*(4), 1156–1171.
The Economic Times. (n.d.). Definition of 'Gross Domestic Product'. *The Economic Times*. https://economictimes.indiatimes.com/definition/gross-domestic-product. Accessed December 4, 2018.
Thomas, J. W. (2000). *A review of research on project-based learning*. http://www.bie.org/images/uploads/general/9d06758fd346969cb63653d00dca55c0.pdf. Accessed January 18, 2019.
Tippelt, R., & Lindemann, H. (2001). *El Método de Proyecto*. https://www.uaa.mx/direcciones/dgdp/defaa/descargas/el_metodo_de_proyectos.pdf. Accessed January 18, 2019.
Ura, K., Alkire, S., Zangmo, T., & Wangdi, K. (2012). *A short guide to gross national happiness index*. Thimphu: The Centre of Bhutan Studies.
Vitruvius, M. P. (n.d.). *De Architectura, Book IX, paragraphs 9–12*. http://penelope.uchicago.edu/Thayer/E/Roman/Texts/Vitruvius/9*.html. Accessed December 4, 2018.
Vlaskovits, P. (2011). Henry Ford, innovation and that "Faster Horse" quote. *Harvard Business Review*. https://hbr.org/2011/08/henry-ford-never-said-the-fast. Accessed December 4, 2018.
Walker, A., & Leary, H. (2009). A problem-based learning meta analysis: Differences across problem types, implementation types, disciplines, and assessment levels. *Interdisciplinary Journal of Problem-based Learning, 3*(1), 12–43.
Weissberg, R. P., Durlak, J. A., Domitrovich, C. E., & Gullotta, T. P. (Eds.) (2015). Social and emotional learning: Past, present, and future. In J. A. Durlak, C. E. Domitrovich, R. P. Weissberg, & T. P. Gullotta (Eds.), *Handbook of social and emotional learning: Research and practice* (pp. 3–19). New York, NY, US: The Guilford Press.
Wood, J. (2018). *Children in Singapore will no longer be ranked by exam results. Here's why*. World Economic Forum. https://www.weforum.org/agenda/2018/10/singapore-has-abolished-school-exam-rankings-here-s-why. Accessed December 4, 2018.

Part IV
Further Perspectives

Chapter 13
A Framework for Relational Mindfulness: Implications for Human Development

Roberto Arístegui and Claudio Araya-Véliz

Abstract Mindfulness has traditionally been understood from an individual perspective, without necessarily reviewing or questioning the conception of the self involved, an understanding that has consequences at a practical level, derived from its different applications. In response to this trend, we develop an understanding perspective of Mindfulness in a relational setting. There is a contrast between the suppositions of the delimited being and those of the relational being. The delimited being carries a modern vision, typical of a representational cognitivism, which we question in this article. To have clarity in the field of the self, and following the distinction advanced by Ricoeur, we describe two modes of use of the term *identity*: identity as sameness and identity as ipseity. In this article, we review these different notions of identity and then apply them to the field of mindfulness, where an individual and delimited notion of self has historically prevailed. In contrast, the alternative of a relational perspective grants access to the mindfulness moments of the relationship with oneself and others. In this context, we propose developing a relational perspective to understand mindfulness, which is characterized by being embodied in the world of life with others. Arguing from the perspective of the relational self, the article details the consequences of sustaining a non-individualistic conception of human development.

Keywords Relational perspective · Co-creation · Conscience · Broadening · Relational self

Mindfulness has traditionally been understood from an individual perspective, without necessarily reviewing or questioning the conception of the self involved, an understanding that has consequences at a practical level, derived from its different applications. Alternatively, we develop an understanding perspective of mindfulness in a relational setting. There is a contrast of the suppositions of being delimited with those of the relational being. The delimited being carries a modern vision, typical of a representational cognitivism, which is questioned in the present article. To have clarity in the field of the self, two modes of use of the term identity are described,

R. Arístegui (✉) · C. Araya-Véliz
Escuela de Psicología, Universidad Adolfo Ibáñez, Santiago de Chile, Chile
e-mail: Roberto.aristegui@uai.cl

C. Steinebach and Á. I. Langer (eds.), *Enhancing Resilience in Youth*,
https://doi.org/10.1007/978-3-030-25513-8_13

following the distinction of Ricouer, which are: Identity as sameness, and identity as Ipseity. In the present article, the different notions of itself are reviewed, and then applied to the field of mindfulness. Historically in the field of mindfulness, an individual and delimited notion of self has prevailed; in contrast, the alternative of a relational perspective allows access to the mindfulness moments of relationship with oneself and others. It is proposed to develop a relational perspective to understand mindfulness, which is characterized by being embodied in the world of life with others. Arguing from the perspective of the relational self, the article deepens the consequences of sustaining a non-individualistic conception of human development.

13.1 Introduction

13.1.1 The Problem of Translation-Interpretation of Mindfulness as an Individual Being Delimited

Mindfulness is applied in a variety of interventions, both in physical health and in mental health. His presence has been on the rise in recent years, where he has highlighted the evidence that shows its effectiveness for treating multiple disorders, making it a powerful tool (Black, 2015). The mindfulness-based interventions (MBIs) are recognized, as they follow the basic structure of the model given by the mindfulness-based stress reduction program (MBSR), introduced by Kabat-Zinn (1982, 1990) in the clinical setting and scientific.

Within the context of mindfulness applications, the problem of comprehension (of translation-interpretation) of mindfulness, reduced to the individual framework or individual knowledge (Kwee, 2010; Kwee et al. 2006) has recently been mentioned. In the same sense, four definitions of mindfulness are recognized within the currents of investigation that approach it, that include versions of scientific definition, of social psychology, of Buddhist root and a wide range of comprehensions from the neurosciences, the human development and the Attachment theory (McCown, 2013; McCown et al. 2015). Even so, although different types of mindfulness definitions have been proposed, they all emphasize the dimension of the conceptualization of the practice of mindfulness in a framework of the individual being. Conceived and described the latter, according to the vocabulary of mental terms used as a subject, which in its interior reflects the world with its representational mind. This is how state studies as traits presuppose the perspective of an individual and delimited being.

As an alternative to the previous perspective, the relational perspective has been proposed (Kwee, 2010, Kwee et al. 2006; McCown, 2013) establishing a qualitative change with respect to the formal definitions of mindfulness in use. We coincide in the direction that points to the co-creation of mindfulness moments in the space of sharing that is offered each time after the practice (McCown, 2013). However, although the individual dimension at stake in the usual interpretation has been pointed out, the assumptions of the self implied in these definitions are not made explicit.

Which compromises the scope of the understanding of mindfulness practice, as a valid way for human development, as forms of transformational action and not only of representation.

When it is assumed that meditating or collecting is equivalent to a certain way of departing from the world, or of suppressing the self (Tugendhat, 2004), we are not in the field of human development; rather one enters into the pre-judgment of the assumptions of being individual delimited.

What guides us in the following writing is to consider the sense of unity in the multiplicity of daily life, by assuming the commitment of being-in-the-world with others as a background (Heidegger, 1926/2013), for interaction of experience and reflection.

Applied to mindfulness, the above raised adds a problem in terms of modern translation-interpretation regarding the suppression of the self, by the centrality of the notion of self in the context of psychological well-being and health.

Assuming from the outset a relational perspective (Gergen, 2015), we propose that it is relevant to develop an understanding or elucidation about the commitment of the individual conception to the epistemological (meta-theoretical) assumptions of the discourse of being delimited. At the same time, examine the changes that come with the notion of the self and the understanding of the practice, choosing a conception of the relational being in mindfulness (Arístegui, 2017a).

To address our purpose we will follow a storyline that will consecutively develop the following three themes:

(1) Notions of the self.
(2) Being delimited in mindfulness.
(3) Being relational versus being delimited in mindfulness.

13.1.1.1 Notions of the Self

Notions of the self at the philosophical level, in the subject-object distinction: In an early essay, Sartre (1968) radically questioned the notion of a self, when examining the flux of consciousness phenomenologically, there does not appear a self there, nor is it necessary to be placed outside as a unifying pole. By understanding all consciousness as consciousness of, the self that appears would be an object for the consciousness to reflect, but not for whom (the subject) pre-reflexively experiences its lived consciousness. Sartre's vision makes it possible to understand this vision, which has recently been revealed by philosophers and neuroscientists (Gallagher and Zahavi, 2013) and who also proposes that the self appears as transcendent to himself

This leads to the need to explain certain notions of the self, which are implicit in the discussion and critique of the self, especially in the domain of research and practices of mindfulness, as we pointed out.

Different notions of the self: We will develop a brief exposition of some notions of the ego at stake in the discussion, which contrast the idea of the classic ego as an ego, with recent formulations of experiential and narrative type (Gallagehr & Zahavi, 2013)

a. I as pure identity: the notion of the self is distinguished as pure identity, to refer to the self as "myself", which remains one and identical through time. It comes to be a pure subject, the pole-self, as a structure that is presupposed to know the objects. It is a necessary condition of possibility for experience. It does not appear, because if it did (as an object) it would stop being a me.
b. I as a narrative: a contemporary perspective that conceives the self as a narrative construction through which we interpret ourselves. Establishing the distinction between being as a thing and being a subject that is understood, as a who. This understanding of the self emphasizes the temporal dimension of who we are and rejects the idea of a pre-linguistic existence of the self. The temporal dimension of the self and the unity of the self is emphasized in the unity of the narrative.
c. Experiential: in the experiential dimension of selfhood, the sense of self is conceived, or self-consciousness with a sense of self. A distinction is made between a central consciousness and an extended consciousness, related to the central self and the autobiographical self, respectively.

13.1.1.2 The Individual Being in Mindfulness

Being delimited presupposes the modern Subject-Object scheme mediated by internal representation: The step from the understanding of mindfulness from an individual setting to a framing or relational perspective supposes to ask first about the notion of the individual delimited underlying, as an assumption not necessarily examined, coming from the modern subject-object scheme, mediated by the internal representation. In this conception the mind-world relation is posed in terms of conceiving the world as an objective reality, independent of the individual subjective mind. It is what is called an epistemological dualism. It is conceived that there is an Inside/Outside, where in a pole is the subject and in front of the object (Dreyfus and Taylor, 2016). The way to access the world is representation. It is a mediation scheme, indirect.

In the modern tradition it is thought that the proper form of knowledge consists in the exact representation of external reality. The mind is considered a mirror of reality. The individual subject, possessing a subjective mind, can represent objective reality if he accesses true knowledge, understood as a reflex. This means that it should not tarnish the image or exact representation of external reality with its subjectivity.

The modern philosophical tradition is prolonged in the theory of knowledge as a reflection in the philosophy of science, giving rise as an objective response, the notion of an epistemology without the knowing subject (Popper, 1972). The imperative of objectivity is raised above the subject and his conscience. The ideal of knowledge is at the level of the function of propositional language, in an ideal language.

If this perspective is deepened, epistemological assumptions appear that connect with the theory of knowledge as a reflection, of the mind as a mirror and of language as reflection or correspondence.

The representational perspective is based on the modern dualism, which starts from the basis that the subject and the object are separated, from this look knowing is synonymous with observing the object and representing us. The observer and the observed remain in different areas of understanding. This conception called representational cognitive uses as a predominant metaphor the computer, which operate symbols, and these symbols are analogous to logical-formal representations. There is thus a symmetry between the thought that occurs outside the mind.

Varela, Thompson and Rosch (1991) discuss and criticize the 3 presuppositions that would be at the base of this representation perspective, being these: 1. That we inhabit a world with particular and defined properties, that is, that we live in a world composed of objects that clearly differ from each other and that has clear and distinct properties. 2. The second assumption states that the subject can effectively capture the properties of objects and create mental representations of them, thus assuming a symmetry between mental representation and logical-formal representation. 3. Finally, the third assumption is that there would be a subjective "we", separate from who does things, that is, there is an independent knower and separated from objects and the known world.

Varela (1999, 2006) proposes that precisely the dualism is the artificial, the separation between mind and body are the illusion, since we never know decontextualized or disembodied.

In the tradition of modern psychology, this representational perspective has been translated into the development of behavioral and cognitivist paradigms. In that direction also appears the commitment with the tradition of the modern subject, subjected. In this tradition the subject is conceived epistemically as someone capable of knowing reality with his mind-mirror, passively, but not subjectively. It is therefore possible to eliminate the subjective dimension if one takes the step of knowing as objectivity.

In the context of the distinction between subject-object and representational mind, it is important to account for the object "as it is". The idea of an exact reflection, or of an objective correspondence with reality, is translated into the notion of correspondence-reference in science. The proposition with meaning reflects reality insofar as it can establish the reference unequivocally. What grounds this position is the conception of language as a reflection.

In conceiving the relation of the individual mind with the external objective reality, which also raises the problem of self-consciousness in the schema of representation of the subject-object model, the notion of correspondence to refer to the world and the self appears again (in a mechanism, where cognitivism accesses formal representation). By reversing the direction and bringing the words back to the interior of the subject that states them, by virtue of the reflex tradition, it is proposed that the words with which the modern subject describes itself and its states, the mental terms with which describe your experience, reflect your inner mental reality.

The mental vocabulary used constitutes the vocabulary of a delimited being, independent of the world. This tradition is linked to the logical atomism and goes back to the modern philosophical empiricism.

Previously, the romantic vocabulary allowed conceiving a supposed essence inside people. Subsequently, the modern descriptions led to conceive a mechanical self, equivalent to the product of operationalized descriptions, through tests, applied massively to detect the features and profiles prone to the best performance during the war. Currently, this mechanical perspective of the self is reflected in the discourse of the deficit, where descriptions of disorders or mental illness increase and multiply. Through psychological consultation, a procedure was established that leads from self-reference to psychological states according to a use of ordinary language to a translation in a formal language, in which the referential correspondence is specified with an internal psychological state. Words thus denote mental states, according to a pictorial context for the understanding of mental terms. The indeterminacy of the reference undermined the solidity of this tradition. The complication of this approach lies in the absence of criteria for the grounding of mental terms and the supposed reality of denoted internal properties (Arístegui, 2015; Rorty, 1979).

What can be considered in this space is if and how the relationship with the world and with itself is established, the individual mind is in a mindfulness state, or rather, if it is necessary to reformulate the traditional subject-object conception, anchored in the representation, which raises a reformulation of the epistemological assumptions of the mirror minds and of the relationship established with the world and with itself, looking for alternatives outside a subject-object framework. In other words, the question that emerges is whether the delimited individual being committed to the subject-object schema or paradigm reproduces the idea of a subject with an individual mind, representing objects. Asking how the translation of mindfulness has adhered to such a scheme will respond to the aporias of knowledge as a reflex and of the mirror mind in modernity, committed to the discourse and mental vocabulary in a pictorial or correspondence-reference scheme (which operates also in the speech of mental illness).

It will be considered as a valid alternative to reformulate the context of pictorial comprehension of self-referential mental terms, in the direction of a pragmatic context of understanding of vocabulary and mental terms. In other words, consider a re-description of mindfulness practice in a pragmatic context, as a joint action, coordinated action in a consensual space in the world with others and not within the individual mind according to the pictorial context used until now. Understanding self-referential mental terms as indicators of action in a context of action coordination situates mindfulness practice in an incarnated and relational contact space, not separated. In front of the delimitation a confluence appears in the horizon in the practice of full consciousness understood as a joint action.

13.1.1.3 Being Relational Versus Being Delimited in Mindfulness

We will approach the position of the relational being, in order to investigate and question the assumptions and notions of the self implicit in the individual being delimited. To clarify a context of the understanding of the assumptions of the self in the practice of mindfulness, we will focus first on establishing a difference in the problematic raised from the traditional and contemporary identity.

We refer to the distinction in the conception of identity to two forms or modalities of identity, understood as sameness (identical identity) or as ipseity (identity Ipse). This distinction is established as the key theme in the work of Ricoeur (1995), "Oneself as Another"; where both traditions are thematized and a solution is proposed through the development of the notion of narrative identity.

The confrontation of both uses of the concept of identity problematizes how to understand the permanence in time.

In the specific field of the study of mindfulness, to make explicit the previous meanings is necessary in the consideration of the relational being in front of the individual being delimited. The permanence in time gives place, in the context of the distinction to the permanence of the character, in the confusion of sameness-ipseity, and to the maintenance of oneself in the promise, in the ipseity, detached the identity of the sameness. The narrative identity oscillates then, between two limits. If the distinction between idem and ipse is not addressed, identity theory poses paradoxes that are difficult to solve.

When addressing these two forms of Identity, the need to differentiate in what sense the problem of identity in mindfulness appears.

In a first approach, it should be noted that the traditional in differentiation between identity and sameness, gives rise to the assumption of the self as identical with itself. Therefore to the permanence in the time as permanence of the character. By examining in the Buddhist root of mindfulness the suffering, and the attachment that leads to self, we can understand the non-self referred to this necessary distancing to overcome self-centeredness. It is precisely here that the sameness is introduced as an assumption to deny, in order to make possible the disidentification with the position of the self, ego or pre-given and substantial ego. It is the opening to the experience of impermanence in time, which is proposed to us.

When we look at practice mindfulness with the assumption of identity as sameness, we confront the aporias of how to understand that there is no "I", from the atomistic translation-interpretation. When accessing a consideration of ipseity, in an experiential, phenomenological framework, an exit begins to appear.

Ipseity allows us to address the opening to the world, to others and also to the experience of the self as another. In this line, mindfulness is not confined to the delimited individual self, nor to the denial of the self (not-self), but it opens a dimension of experience of otherness as constitutive of experience, both in the world and with others and with itself, modifying the assemblage point or adjustment from the egocentric ego towards an eccentric self, in the everyday factual existence (the formulation of the being-in-the-world, accessing the clearing of the forest, according to Heidegger (1926/2013) Nor does it imply that the self-reference is to a self as an object The dimension of pre-reflective awareness with itself proposes a non-objectual presence.

Phenomenologists (Sartre, Merleau-Ponty, Husserl, Henry) focus on the ipseity or self referential structure open to the pre-reflective experience of consciousness, in the direction of the central self, in the first person. Emphasizing the subjective character, "mine" of experience, the how and not just the what. Self-experience occurs in a corporeal being immersed in the world, not isolated or in the mind.

We recognize in the dimension of ipseity the openness to being-in-the-world with others in the context of mindfulness practice. If the practice of mindfulness is not confined to the domain of the experience of a punctual ego, in the direction of the crossing between generative phenomenology (late Husserl) and hermeneutical phenomenology (Heidegger) we find the way for the articulation of experience in language, without having to establish a step to a conception of a self circumscribed to the dimension of the narrative. Rather, in the developments of ipseity along the lines of Heidegger, Sartre and Ricoeur we find a way from pre-reflective experience and the use of language in the pre-conceptual saying, in the present moment, in the "mindfulness moments".

We propose that the relational being provides context to understand the insertion of mindfulness as a relational practice, which allows to articulate the pre-reflective experience as a dimension of consciousness as incarnated and relational cognition.

At the confluence of mindfulness moments, as a contact, in the community of practice, corresponds to a Gestalt holism, experienced and expressed in the pre-conceptual saying (Arístegui, 2017b). The choice of practice as a way of life with others is a commitment, the dimension of promise of mutuality shared reciprocally.

It is precisely in this dimension of embodied relational cognition, where we see that the relational framework of mindfulness opens up a possibility of understanding the life cycle in a novel way.

Especially in the field of adolescence, which has usually been understood from the normative and role perspective (Erikson, 1998). The relational perspective would make it possible to understand this stage of the life cycle by broadening the view of roles and including the dimension of the world of adolescent social life, connecting with their relational being. In this area we highlight the possibility of reflecting identity from the embodied relational dimension.

This allows us to establish a bridge with what has been called integrative communication (Siegel, 2012) that brings the connection between neuropsychological dimensions and the dimension of social cognition at hand.

This new embodied relational perspective, understood as a framework for understanding adolescence, would contribute to overcoming the definition of the delimited being of the adolescent, in order to understand the identity of the adolescent from the perspective of relational being (Gergen, 2015), transcending the conception of the isolated self, integrating the dimension of the self understood relationally.

13.2 Understanding Mindfulness from the Relational Self

We propose to understand mindfulness as a relational and embodied practice, where mindfulness moments are co-constructed with a potential to reformulate the implications of the individual mirror mind and the description mediated by the mental vocabulary of a delimited individual mind. When mindfulness is conceived as inherently relational, it proposes and promotes an experience and re-description of being-in-the-world-with-others, which allows to live in an embodied process of relational presence (Araya-Véliz, Arístegui, & Fossa, 2017).

The relational being develops the being-in-the-world assuming some relevant expositions, such as:

a. The relationship with experience is not addressed primarily with representation, but is presented from the pre-reflective.
b. The objects are not pre-existing, but arise in the experience of a breakdown of availability at hand.
c. The presence before the eyes of an object, is a possible direction to take after a break, where derivatively arises the notion of a subject in front of the world, separated, and that represents "what there is". It corresponds to the reflection after the break, and constitutes the traditional vision in which the delimited being emerges, in the origin of being conceived as individual.
d. In availability at hand, self-reliance on the experience of the self does not imply a "fact of the matter", but a congruence with the experience of being like another.

Alternatively, it is possible to connect with the situation outside of representational mediation, with a bodily sensation understood as a direct referent of experience, without having to access it through conceptualization oriented to a priori sense. It is a pre-conceptual practical knowledge, without the need for a prior sense, meaning generally lived as ineffective in the contingency of a decoupling of the world of life and of the system. It is precisely here that the possibility of a contact with experience with itself and with others in the world of life arises, through a practical and experiential way of entry, such as the space of the methodology of relational mindfulness. Accessing the dimension of meaning in the background implies a dimension of experience understood as a direct referent.

When understanding the consciousness from a phenomenological perspective, we do not refer to the meaning given by an individual mind, it is the social activity the ultimate foundation, where the relational process is presented, which provides sustenance and opens the field of possibilities for the emergence of the being in relation.

Mindfulness then arises in that relational space, as a relational and ethical dimension of caring for oneself and others. The orientation of the practice of mindfulness towards the cultivation of well-being in the field of human development (and also of mental health) is neither individual nor collective (Araya-Véliz & Arístegui, 2016), but operates in the meeting space, of the development of human capacities through joint action (not of conceptual representations).

13.3 Implications in the Field of Human Development

From the conception of the self of modernity itself also emerges a specific conception of human development, characterized by an individualist emphasis, here the notion of progress is put into play in the development of the subjective dimension, without necessarily taking into account the context and the inter-subjective scope. This modern perspective is influenced by how mindfulness is understood, where it has been understood as a practice of human development limited to the individual, emphasizing the conception of a self understood as independent and separated from the context, thus generating an understanding of development in our opinion partial or at least self-centered (egocentric perspective). We postulate that from what is described in this article the possibility of establishing a perspective of human development based on a relational perspective is opened, which offers a renewed alternative of human development, especially in this context, referred to the stage of adolescence. Since it opens the possibility of articulating the personal scope, including the context and the meeting space and the relationship with other people. This relational perspective can contribute to a broader understanding of human development, not falling either in the purely individual or in the purely collective, proposing a space of development and relational welfare.

References

Araya-Véliz, C., Arístegui, R., & Fossa, P. (2017). Pasos hacia una enacción relacional. Aporte, ambigüedades y limitaciones del concepto embodied mind en Francisco Varela: un análisis meta-teórico. *Mindfulness & Compassion, 2*(1), 41–46.

Araya-Véliz, C. & Arístegui, R., (2016). Pasos hacia un bienestar relacional: Mindfulness como un espacio de relación con otros. In Daniel Duhart y David Sirlopú (Ed.), *Bienestar y Espiritualidad: Diálogos desde la psicología, la filosofía y la sociología* (pp. 61–72). Santiago: UDD Ediciones.

Arístegui, R. (2017a). Enaction and neurophenomenology in language. In A. Ibáñez, L. Sedeño, & A. García (Eds.), *Neuroscience and social science: The Missing Link* (pp. 471–500). Switzerland: Springer.

Arístegui, R. (2017b). Fenomenología Hermenéutica, Análisis Existencial, Mindfulness. https://www.researchgate.net/publications/314405001. Accessed January 30, 2019.

Arístegui, R. (2015). *Construccionismo social y Discusión de Paradigmas en Psicología.* USA: The Taos Institute Publications/WorldShare Books.

Black, D. (2015). *American mindfulness research association-AMRA-Data base.* https://goamra.org/resources/. Accessed January 30, 2019.

Dreyfus, H. L., & Taylor, C. (2016). *Recuperar el realismo.* Madrid: Rialp.

Erikson, E. H. (1998). *The life cycle completed.* London: W.W. Norton & Co.

Gallagher, S., & Zahavi, D. (2013). *La mente fenomenológica.* Madrid: Alianza.

Gergen, K. (2015). *El ser relacional.* Bilbao: Editorial Desclée De Brouwer, S.A.

Heidegger, M. (1926/2013). Being and time. Malden: Blackwell.

Kabat-Zinn, J. (1982). An outpatient program in behavioral medicine for chronic pain patients based on the practice of mindfulness meditation: Theoretical considerations and preliminary results. *General Hospital Psychiatry, 4*(1), 33–47.

Kabat-Zinn, J. (1990). *Full catastrophe living: Using the wisdom of your body and mind to face stress, pain and illness.* New York: Delacorte.

Kwee, M. G. T. (Ed.). (2010). *New horizons in Buddhist psychology.* Chagrin Falls: Taos Institute Publications.

Kwee, M. G. T., Gergen, K. J., & Koshikawa, F. (Eds.). (2006). *Horizons in Buddhist psychology: Practice, research & theory.* Taos, NM: Taos Institute Publications.

McCown, D. (2013). The Ethical space of mindfulness in clinical practice. https://research.tilburguniversity.edu/en/publications/the-ethical-space-of-mindfulness-in-clinical-practice. Accessed January 30, 2019.

McCown, D., Reibel, D., & Micozzi, M. (2015). *Teaching mindfulness*. New York: Springer.

Popper, K. R. (1972). *Conjeturas y refutaciones: El desarrollo del conocimiento cientifico*. Spain: Paidós.

Ricœur, P. (1995). *Oneself as another*. Chicago: Unioversity of Chicago Press.

Rorty, R. (1979). *Philosophy and the mirror of nature*. Princeton, NJ: Princeton University Press.

Sartre, J. P. (1968). *La trascendencia del ego*. Buenos Aires: Calden.

Siegel, D. J. (2012). *Pocket guide to interpersonal neurobiology: An integrative handbook of the mind*. New York: W.W. Norton & Co.

Tugendhat, E. (2004). *Egocentricidad y Mística*. Barcelona: Editorial Gedisa.

Varela, F. J. (1999). *Ethical know-how: Action, wisdom, and cognition*. Stanford, Calif: Stanford University Press.

Varela, F. J. (2006). *Conocer: Las ciencias cognitivas; tendencias y perspectivas cartografía de las ideas actuales*. Spain: Editorial Gedisa.

Varela, F. J., Thompson, E., & Rosch, E. (1991). *The embodied mind: Cognitive science and human experience*. Cambridge, Massachusetts: MIT Press.

Chapter 14
Psychotherapy for Adolescents: Mindfulness and Compassion in Individual and Group Settings

Nathania Klauser and Philipp Steinebach

Abstract Mindfulness-based interventions (MBIs) focus on introducing non-judgmental awareness of the present moment. The positive effects of MBIs on symptom reduction, well-being, and quality of life in adults have been reported extensively. MBIs are increasingly implemented in diverse psychotherapy approaches for adolescents. Given the focus of manuals and studies on group psychotherapy, group processes are considered in detail in the present chapter. Specifically, we briefly describe current treatment manuals which focus on mindfulness and self-compassion as an intervention. We review manuals based on the form of intervention (group vs. individual) and on theoretical considerations that led to the versions for adolescents. We briefly present MBIs in other manualized therapeutic approaches. In a second step, we propose specific aspects of psychotherapy in adolescents and review the level of consideration in mindfulness-based treatment manuals for adolescents. In a third step, we discuss specific aspects of group delivered mindfulness-based psychotherapy in youth. Adaptation processes of treatment manuals, which were originally designed for adults should be revised considering their underlying understanding of youth-specific aspects in psychotherapy. Whereas motivation and the cognitive level of adolescents is widely considered in most adapted manuals, important steps in the identity development of adolescents, such as comparison toward others, shame, and autonomy have been neglected. Further research efforts should focus on the topic of application and implementation of mindfulness in psychotherapy, especially in groups and with adolescents.

Keywords Compassion-based interventions · Adaptations · Therapeutic approaches · Psychotherapy · Group psychotherapy

---

N. Klauser
Psychological Institute, University of Heidelberg, Heidelberg, Germany

P. Steinebach (✉)
Department of Psychiatry and Psychotherapy, University Medical Center Göttingen, Göttingen, Germany
e-mail: p.steinebach@posteo.de

C. Steinebach and Á. I. Langer (eds.), *Enhancing Resilience in Youth*,
https://doi.org/10.1007/978-3-030-25513-8_14

14.1 Introduction

In the present chapter, we will briefly describe current treatment manuals which focus on mindfulness and self-compassion as an intervention. Manuals are reviewed based on the form of intervention (group vs. individual) and on theoretical considerations that led to the versions for adolescents. MBIs in other manualized therapeutic approaches are briefly presented.

In a second step, specific aspects of psychotherapy in adolescents are proposed and the level of consideration in mindfulness-based treatment manuals for adolescents reviewed.

In a third step, specific aspects of group delivered mindfulness-based psychotherapy in youth are discussed.

14.2 Theoretical Background

Mindfulness-based interventions (MBIs) focus on introducing non-judgmental awareness of the present moment (Baer, 2003). The positive effects of MBIs on symptom reduction, well-being, and quality of life in adults have been reported extensively (Baer, 2003; Hofmann, Sawyer, Witt, & Oh, 2010; Khoury, Sharma, Rush, & Fournier, 2015). Reviews also describe neurological and biological evidence of its efficacy (Chiesa & Serretti, 2010; Tang, Hölzel, & Posner, 2015). However, reviews also point to the lack of high quality studies and to open questions regarding working mechanisms of MBIs (e.g. Davidson & Kaszniak, 2015). An extensive body of literature addresses mindfulness and MBIS, contributing to the ongoing debate on the definition, key conceptual aspects, working mechanisms, and origins of mindfulness (Brown, Creswell, & Ryan, 2016). More importantly, continuing research studies report evidence about the effectiveness of MBIs also in children and youth in clinical and non-clinical samples. A recent meta-analysis reports a small to moderate omnibus effect size (Zoogman, Goldberg, Hoyt, & Miller, 2015). The authors find higher effect sizes in clinical samples compared to generally healthy participants and higher effects on psychological symptoms compared to other outcome measures, such as somatic symptoms or mindfulness related measures.

These promising findings have further supported the development of mindfulness-based treatment manuals for adults which were then adapted for psychotherapy with adolescents (Wisner, 2017).

Compassion-based interventions (CBIs) aim at the establishment of a mindful attitude and a compassionate stance, which includes the awareness of the suffering of another person or oneself and the desire to alleviate the suffering (Goetz, Keltner, & Simon-Thomas, 2010). Though reported in the literature to a lesser degree, compassion-based interventions have shown promising outcomes in adults (Kirby, 2016) and have been proposed as important pathways to mental health in children and youth (Roeser & Pinela, 2014). To date, most interventions have focused on self-compassion or compassion towards the self as an intervention in psychotherapy and mental health prevention (Bluth, Gaylord, Campo, Mullarkey, & Hobbs, 2016).

14.3 Manualized Mindfulness-Based-Interventions in Psychotherapy with Adolescents

Many manualized psychotherapeutic approaches in adolescents predominately concentrate on MBIs or self-compassion as interventions. The most cited approaches in the literature have been adapted from an adult version of the psychotherapy manual (O'Brien, Larson, & Murrell, 2008). Given the lack of common adaptation mechanisms for the work with youth, it appears necessary to review manualized MBI psychotherapy approaches regarding their adaptation process. Since MBIs have been manualized for a broad range of clients and disorders, our present considerations focus on a few common psychotherapy approaches.

14.3.1 Mindfulness-Based Stress Reduction for Teens (MBSR; Biegel, Brown, Shapiro, & Schubert, 2009)

The MBSR for Teens program was one of the first intervention about mindfulness in young people. Though not being a specific psychotherapy manual, moderate effects on reduction of depressive symptoms have been reported for MBSR in adolescents (Chi, Bo, Liu, Zhang, & Chi, 2018). MBSR for Teens is a group-based program and its development was guided by the adult version of the program. Adaptation of the program for children includes considerations regarding the attention span of young people as well as a focus on experiential and body exercises (Saltzman & Goldin, 2008). In the adolescent program, which was designed for participants at the age of 14–18 years, mindfulness practices at home were shorter and there was no full day session. Issues common in adolescence were also discussed with the group, including self-image, life transitions, self-harming behaviors, and problems in interpersonal relationships (Biegel et al., 2009).

14.3.2 Dialectical Behavioral Therapy for Adolescents (DBT-A & DBT Skills for Adolescents; Miller, Rathus, & Linehan, 2007; Rathus, Linehan, & Miller, 2015)

Dialectical behavioral therapy was initially designed for the treatment of borderline-personality disorder but is now applied in the work with various patient and client groups (Linehan, 1993). DBT uses MBIs as a skill to reduce confusion about the self which is continuously practiced throughout the skill training groups. Skill training typically is a group-based program, but individual psychotherapy and skill groups are combined in DBT. DBT-A also includes parents in the treatment groups and has specific family sessions. The program was reduced, simplified, and a module for the dialectic view on dilemmas was implemented ("walking the middle path"; Fleischhaker, Sixt, & Schulz, 2011). Regarding assessment and diagnosis, DBT-A encourages therapists to include school and family contexts in their understanding of the case (Miller, Rathus, Linehan, Wetzler, & Leigh, 1997).

14.3.3 Mindfulness-Based Cognitive Therapy for Children (MBCT-C & MBCT for Depression in Adolescents; Ames, Richardson, Payne, Smith, & Leigh, 2014; Semple, Lee, & Miller, 2006)

A genuine mindfulness focused psychotherapy program is the MBCT for adults, which was initially designed for the treatment of chronic depression (MBCT; Segal, Williams, & Teasdale, 2002). It has also been conceptualized as a manual for children at the age of 9–12 and most studies apply it in a group setting. Adaptations for child-friendly interventions include reduction of number of exercises, the reduction of the length of exercises, and the reduction of group size. Also included is a focus on body sensations and physical perceptions during the exercises. Parents are actively included in the program by attending sessions at the beginning and the end of the program, and by assisting exercises at home (Semple et al., 2006). The program has been administered in adolescents with a focus on depression but its conceptualization has not received as much attention as the version for children (Ames et al., 2014).

14.3.4 Making Friends with Yourself (MFY; Bluth et al., 2016)

MFY is a manualized psychotherapeutic program for children and youth at the age of 11–17 years to help them deal with depression and anxiety. The program was developed based on the mindful self-compassion program for adults (Neff & Germer, 2013), which aims at preventing mental disorders by establishing resilience through self-compassion. In comparison to the program for adults, MFY has reduced length of sessions, and includes more activity-based exercises and specific information on the adolescent brain. Studies on MFY are mainly administered in groups (Bluth et al., 2016).

14.3.5 Acceptance and Commitment Therapy for Adolescents (ACT-A; Turrell & Bell, 2016)

ACT is a manualized program which was developed for various contexts such as specific individual psychotherapy, psychotherapeutic groups, as well as general mental health prevention in schools. MBIs are seen as a way to implement an accepting stance (Turrell & Bell, 2016). The version for psychotherapy in adolescents is based on the assumption that acceptance and commitment are essential approaches in developmental challenges, such as identity development, and it also includes a functional analysis of the family and school context. Furthermore, the general style of ACT, which uses metaphors, a less directive approach and experiential exercises, is thought to especially suit young people (O'Brien et al., 2008).

14.3.6 Metacognitive Therapy (MCT; Wells, 2011)

MCT focusses on the change of metacognitions, which are controlling and judging thoughts about thoughts, in the therapy of depression and anxiety (Wells & Matthews, 1995). A central part of MCT is the teaching of detached mindfulness, a conceptualization of mindfulness, which is based on information processing ideas. Detached mindfulness aims at facilitating metacognitive states and de-centered relationships with thoughts (Wells, 2005). Detached mindfulness is introduced using cognitive exercises and experiments. Few studies have adapted MCT for the work with adolescents but there is initial evidence that adolescents are capable of metacognitive thinking (see Simons, 2016). A manualized treatment for children with generalized anxiety disorder exists, which proposes extensive ideas for the work with children. MTC for children teaches detached mindfulness, using a focus on guided practical exercises, metaphors, cue cards and parent workshops (Esbjørn, Normann, & Reinholdt-Dunne, 2015).

14.3.7 Common Adaptations

In summary, manualized mindfulness and compassion approaches all derive from treatment programs for adults and focus mainly on the group setting. Furthermore, the adaptation of an adult program to a program for adolescents is rarely described in full detail and was to a lesser degree based on theoretical considerations regarding psychotherapy in adolescents. However, a few common processes are inferable. Most adaptations include (1) a reduction of practice time (e.g. meditation exercises) and simplification of the program (e.g. via metaphors) to guarantee understanding, (2) a focus on experiential or physical exercises to take into account the reduced attention span, and, (3) the involvement or consideration of parents, families or schools to establish a contextual view or implement changes in the adolescents' context.

14.4 Mindfulness-Based-Interventions in Other Therapeutic Approaches

Before manualized programs focusing on MBIs were developed for psychotherapy with adolescents, practitioners tried to integrate MBIs and comparable exercises into their sessions as part of their usual psychotherapeutic treatment. The original definition of mindfulness with its four foundations of mindfulness proposes being mindful of body, feelings, mind/thoughts and others/surroundings (Cullen, 2011; Kabat-Zinn, 1994). These four different aspects of human experiences can in some way be found in behavior therapy as well. The treatment of mental disorders in behavior therapy is the observation of thoughts, feelings, body reactions and behaviors in different situations (compare the SORKC-model; Kanfer & Saslow, 1969). These so-called behavior analyses focus on reactions which are related to problematic symptoms and therefore are more focused than the general observant and non-judgmental openness for experiences described by mindfulness.

More similarities and differences between mindfulness and former cognitive behavior therapy emerge regarding the way MBIs have already been integrated in established therapeutic approaches. On the one hand, collections of mindfulness exercises have been published and are being used in psychotherapies. On the other hand, behavioral manuals contain exercises that are similar to MBIs, and are presented without necessarily explaining the concept of mindfulness at all. Several examples of these integrative approaches are presented in the following passages.

14.4.1 Collections of Mindfulness Exercises for Individual and Group Psychotherapy

One use of integrating mindfulness in established therapeutic approaches is the general use of stand-alone MBIs which have been adapted for children and youth and focus on the beginner spirit (Greco & Hayes, 2011; Geisler & Muttenhammer, 2016). Hereby, mindfulness is introduced through different exercises that can be used by practitioners as one part of the overall treatment of typical mental disorders. Most of these exercises are based on MBIs that are commonly used in adult psychotherapy, only content and length is adapted to children and youth's context. A general introduction to mindfulness is suggested, yet it is optional. In addition, these collections of MBIs also contain exercises which focus on self-compassion and meta-cognition (detached mindfulness) by learning how to recognize thoughts and actions, and to observe them instead of starting to immediately value or change them.

14.4.2 MBIs as Parts of Other Therapeutic Manuals

In addition to these collections of mindfulness exercises, which are labeled as MBIs, other manualized intervention programs for different mental disorders use comparable exercises without using the word "mindfulness" in their descriptions. One of these examples in the German context is the "training of emotional competences" (Training emotionaler Kompetenzen; Berking, 2017), which was developed for adults and young adults at 16 years of age or older. One of the competences taught in this training is the difference between "evaluation and reaction" and "awareness without evaluation". It must be noted that the word "mindfulness" is not used in the description for patients and only included in the practitioner's manual. However, the taught and practiced competence is one major aspect of mindfulness.

Another example is the body image therapy for eating disorders (Vocks & Legenbauer, 2010). In individual or group settings, patients are confronted with their body image and are introduced to exercises focusing on pleasure and body experiences without immediately evaluating them. By focusing on pleasant aspects of their body, they should learn to view their body from another perspective, treat it well, start to enjoy it, and so change their negative body image. These exercises known as "pleasure exercises" are general awareness exercises, but calling them positive experiences is biased in a way which is incompatible with mindfulness.

Such pleasure exercises which focus on developing a better feeling about oneself and establishing a routine of pleasurable and self-enjoyment enhancing activities, have a conceptual overlap with self-compassion exercises and can also be found in manuals for anxiety (Traub & In-Albon, 2017) and depression (Groen & Petermann, 2015).

14.5 Specific Aspects of Psychotherapy in Adolescents

Apart from general challenges connected with mindfulness, a closer look at specific challenges during adolescence must now follow.

14.5.1 Developmental Aspects and Challenges

Adolescence is defined as the time of transition from childhood to adulthood, beginning at the start of puberty and ending at the time of adult responsibilities (Levesque, 2011). Not only a physical but also a social transition takes place during this period: Peer relationships become more complex and important, self-consciousness is heightened, and comparison with others is one major aspect of identity development (Steinberg & Morris, 2001). Havighurst (1972) conceptualized the various challenges adolescents face in different developmental tasks, which can be summarized as achieving new and mature relationships, accepting sexual roles and one's body, emotional independence of parents, preparing for occupation and adult family life, and acquiring values as a guide to socially responsible behavior.

14.5.2 Implications for Therapy

Regarding psychotherapy with adolescents and their developmental tasks at this stage of development, it is obvious that the four foundations of mindfulness are challenges in general. Being mindful of their own body, feelings, minds, and the world around them is not easy for adolescents who experience changes in all areas. MBIs and similar exercises need to be adapted to meet these challenges. The following age-related aspects should be considered:

Cognitive level: The newly gained ability to think on a meta-cognitive level starts during adolescence and opens up new possibilities for psychotherapeutic treatment: meta-cognitive strategies are usable and first manuals for specific mental disorders are published (for example OCD, Simons, 2012). Meta-cognitive therapy (MCT) is adapted to be specifically experience based by using a lot of metaphors (Simons, 2018).

Motivation: Commitment is one of the major concerns of child and youth psychotherapists, because most adolescents are rather forced to see a therapist by parents, friends or teachers. Especially the DBT-A program described above has as strong emphasis on commitment strategies (Miller, Rathus, & Linehan, 2007). Commitment is necessary for MBIs as well, that's why token systems for children (Van der Oord, Bögels, & Peijnenburg, 2012) and encouragement for adolescents is proposed as a technique (Geisler & Muttenhammer, 2016).

Comparison with others: Due to the high pressure for better achievements in school and the typical challenges during adolescence, most of the adolescents form their identities by comparing themselves and their achievements with their peers. This is one important part of identity formation, but also significant for psychotherapy. Especially group settings lead to possible comparisons with others, which can be self-esteem enhancing or diminishing. Some MBIs rely on the feedback and exchange with others afterwards. In youth group settings it should therefore be considered to practice these exercises individually and silently, with minimal and directed feedback, described for example in Geisler and Muttenhammer (2016). In that way the evaluative comparisons between participants can be held at a minimum. However, as discussed in the next section, the positive effects of group therapy partially rely on an extensive exchange of experiences.

Shame: Shame is usually evoked when failure is recognized, when expectations cannot be met, but also when something is very intimate. Recognizing shame in patients is very important for psychotherapy because it can be crucial to symptoms and can lead to therapy termination by the patient (Dearing & Tangney, 2011). For adolescents, shame is likely to be triggered by focusing on their body or becoming aware of thoughts and feelings they would like to forget in the present moment in order to feel "at ease". Mindfulness could help to deal with shame (Hooker & Fodor, 2008). However, it could also increase the momentarily experienced shame (e.g. due to feelings of failure) and practitioners should be aware of this possible effect.

Autonomy: One major developmental challenge during adolescence is the achievement of emotional independence from parents. As mentioned above, peers and their opinion become more important. As a result, adolescents strive for autonomy and distance themselves from their parents during that time (Levesque, 2011). This can be one explanation for the often experienced personal resistance towards mindfulness exercises by the adolescent, which are introduced by other adults and regarded positively by peers.

14.5.3 Specific Aspects of Group Psychotherapy in Adolescents

Given the focus of most manualized mindfulness and self-compassion programs on the group setting, therapeutic working mechanisms in group therapy with adolescents should be discussed. Challenges in group therapy with adolescents are partially overlapping with developmental challenges in the transition to adulthood, as described above. However, they offer an alternative perspective on the therapeutic process. Like group therapy for adults, many group programs for adolescents focus on specific interventions (e.g. psychoeducation, practicing of new behavior) as working mechanisms. Apart from that, general working mechanisms of group therapy have been proposed and discussed regarding their importance for working with adolescents. Haen and Aronson discuss several group working mechanisms, initially proposed by Yalom and Leszcz for adult groups with regard to their role in working with adolescents (Haen & Aronson, 2017; Yalom & Leszcz, 2005). These include universality, imparting information, recapitulation of the family experience, altruism, socializing techniques, cohesion, installing a sense of hope, and importance of interpersonal relations.

Working mechanisms for MBIs in groups could draw upon these considerations to improve outcomes. For example, mindfulness exercises and the sharing of individual experiences during the exercises can create a feeling of universality regarding the nature of attention and cognitions. However, especially in adolescents, the sharing of personal or intimate thoughts might be shameful and connected to the fear of being judged by others. Therefore, establishing a sense of cohesion and trust in the group appears to be a necessary first step in MBIs in group settings. Furthermore, a sense of belonging and trust in the group is possibly a new experience for troubled adolescents and can play an important role in the reinstallation of a positive view on the self, given the identification with the group (Haen & Aronson, 2017).

Compassion-based interventions, which aim at altering compassionate feelings towards the suffering of others, could in turn lead to altruism (Leiberg, Klimecki, &

Singer, 2011). Also in a group setting, an attitude of altruism can be implemented by fostering helping behavior in peers. Therefore, not only the work with parents but also with peers should be considered in group therapy (Rubin, Bukowski, & Laursen, 2009). Examples of group programs, which especially work with peer relations, can be found in social work with troubled youth. For example, Positive Peer Culture (PPC, Vorrath, & Brendtro, 1985) aims at the implementation of generosity and prosocial helping behavior in peers in a strongly group-guided program. Other examples are the training of social competencies for adolescents, which include role plays in the group and the discussion of interpersonal behavior (for example Petermann & Petermann, 2010).

14.6 Conclusion and Challenges for the Field

MBIs are increasingly implemented in diverse psychotherapy approaches for adolescents. Given the focus of manuals and studies on group psychotherapy, group processes are considered in detail in the present chapter. Various questions remain unanswered and should be addressed in future studies.

First of all, adaptation processes of treatment manuals, which were originally designed for adults should be revised regarding their underlying understanding of youth specific aspects in psychotherapy. Whereas motivation and the cognitive level of adolescents is widely considered in most adapted manuals, important steps in the identity formation of adolescents, such as comparison with others, shame, and autonomy have been neglected.

For example, resistance towards MBIs can be heightened in group settings, given the setting of permanent possible comparison with others. This could be diminished with preparation. In other manuals which combine individual and group setting, relaxation exercises are learned and practiced individually and only then become part of group sessions (compare THAV, Görtz-Dorten & Döpfner, 2010). More familiarity with the exercises, will reduce the occurrence of shame in the group setting. In addition, knowing the exercises helps participants in group settings to stay focused on themselves instead of comparing their behavior to others' behaviors. Also, a tailored approach of the introduction to mindfulness is possible in individual therapy. Exercises can be shortened and adapted to the patient's level of understanding and mastery. If questions arise, they can be addressed immediately and the training can proceed, whereas questions during exercises in a group setting can lead to lengthy discussions and significantly interrupt the training sessions. Consequently, future MBIs could combine individual and group training to improve the practice of exercises in groups. Future studies should compare the effects of MBIs and their acceptance by adolescents when they are learned in individual versus group settings.

The integration of peer-guided exercises in group psychotherapy can be considered to address issues of autonomy and resistance towards new ideas, that are introduced by adults. Adolescents who already know an exercise could teach their peer group members. This is one way to strengthen the adolescent teacher's self-esteem and could lead to more model learning. If their peers support them, even shy or timid adolescents could try to introduce short MBIs or lead the training of well-known exercises, thus gain more mastery and trust their own competences.

These considerations are closely linked with fostering peer interaction and establishing positive peer values such as trust and cohesion. Given the importance of peer relations in adolescence, peer interactions should not only be seen as problematic dynamics that complicate the training of mindfulness in groups. Though being outside of the mainstream research, establishing positive values in groups, has been shown to have positive implications for troubled youth (Rubin et al., 2009).

One way of looking at peer processes in therapy, and considering its possible detrimental effects, is the integration of working mechanisms of group psychotherapy. Especially interpersonal mechanisms such as group cohesion, universality or altruism could add to existing group programs of MBIs. Furthermore, interpersonal values such as compassion could be pathways to altering group dynamics regarding prosocial behavior (Roeser & Pinela, 2014).

In general, working mechanisms of group therapy in adolescents should be addressed in future studies to answer open questions regarding the use of MBIs in groups.

In sum, further research efforts should focus on the topic of application and implementation of mindfulness in psychotherapy, especially in groups and with adolescents. It should be asked, whether the constant struggle and debate about the origins and nature of mindfulness as a concept has led to the neglection of these practical considerations.

References

Ames, C. S., Richardson, J., Payne, S., Smith, P., & Leigh, E. (2014). Mindfulness-based cognitive therapy for depression in adolescents. *Child and Adolescent Mental Health, 19*(1), 74–78. https://doi.org/10.1111/camh.12034.

Baer, R. A. (2003). Mindfulness training as a clinical intervention: A conceptual and empirical review. *Clinical Psychology: Science and Practice, 10*(2), 125–143. https://doi.org/10.1093/clipsy/bpg015.

Berking, M. (2017). *Training emotionaler Kompetenzen*. Berlin: Springer-Verlag.

Biegel, G. M., Brown, K. W., Shapiro, S. L., & Schubert, C. M. (2009). Mindfulness-based stress reduction for the treatment of adolescent psychiatric outpatients: A randomized clinical trial. *Journal of Consulting and Clinical Psychology, 77*(5), 855–866. https://doi.org/10.1037/a0016241.

Bluth, K., Gaylord, S. A., Campo, R. A., Mullarkey, M. C., & Hobbs, L. (2016). Making friends with yourself: A mixed methods pilot study of a mindful self-compassion program for adolescents. *Mindfulness, 7*(2), 479–492. https://doi.org/10.1007/s12671-015-0476-6.

Brown, K. W., Creswell, J. D., & Ryan, R. M. (Eds.). (2016). *Handbook of mindfulness: Theory, research, and practice* (Paperback ed.). New York, London: The Guilford Press.

Chi, X., Bo, A., Liu, T., Zhang, P., & Chi, I. (2018). Effects of mindfulness-based stress reduction on depression in adolescents and young adults: A systematic review and meta-analysis. *Frontiers in Psychology, 9,* 1034.

Chiesa, A., & Serretti, A. (2010). A systematic review of neurobiological and clinical features of mindfulness meditations. *Psychological Medicine, 40*(8), 1239–1252. https://doi.org/10.1017/S0033291709991747.

Cullen, M. (2011). Mindfulness-based interventions: An emerging phenomenon. *Mindfulness, 2*(3), 186–193. https://doi.org/10.1007/s12671-011-0058-1.

Davidson, R. J., & Kaszniak, A. W. (2015). Conceptual and methodological issues in research on mindfulness and meditation. *The American Psychologist, 70*(7), 581–592. https://doi.org/10.1037/a0039512.

Dearing, R. L. & Tangney, J. P. E. (2011). *Shame in the therapy hour.* American Psychological Association.

Esbjørn, B. H., Normann, N., & Reinholdt-Dunne, M. L. (2015). Adapting metacognitive therapy to children with generalised anxiety disorder: Suggestions for a manual. *Journal of Contemporary Psychotherapy, 45*(3), 159–166. https://doi.org/10.1007/s10879-015-9294-3.

Fleischhaker, C., Sixt, B. & Schulz, E. (2011). *DBT-A Dialektisch-behaviorale Therapie für Jugendliche: Ein Therapiemanual mit Arbeitsbuch auf CD.* Berlin, Heidelberg: Springer Berlin Heidelberg. http://dx.doi.org/10.1007/978-3-642-13008-3. Accessed January 12, 2019.

Geisler, U., & Muttenhammer, J. (2016). *Achtsamkeitsübungen mit Kindern und Jugendlichen in der Psychotherapie.* Paderborn: Junfermann Verlag.

Goetz, J. L., Keltner, D., & Simon-Thomas, E. (2010). Compassion: An evolutionary analysis and empirical review. *Psychological Bulletin, 136*(3), 351–374. https://doi.org/10.1037/a0018807.

Görtz-Dorten, A., & Döpfner, M. (2010). *Therapieprogramm für Kinder mit aggressivem Verhalten (THAV).* Göttingen: Hogrefe Verlag.

Greco, L., & Hayes, S. (Eds.). (2011). *Akzeptanz und Achtsamkeit in der Kinder-und Jugendlichenpsychotherapie.* Weinheim: Beltz.

Groen, G., & Petermann, F. (2015). *Therapie-Tools Depression im Kindes-und Jugendalter.* Weinheim: Beltz.

Haen, C., & Aronson, S. (Eds.). (2017). *Handbook of child and adolescent group therapy: A practitioner's reference.* New York: Routledge.

Havighurst, R. J. (1972). *Developmental tasks and education* (3rd ed.). New York: McKay.

Hofmann, S. G., Sawyer, A. T., Witt, A. A., & Oh, D. (2010). The effect of mindfulness-based therapy on anxiety and depression: A meta-analytic review. *Journal of Consulting and Clinical Psychology, 78*(2), 169–183. https://doi.org/10.1037/a0018555.

Hooker, K. E., & Fodor, I. E. (2008). Teaching mindfulness to children. *Gestalt Review, 12*(1), 75–91.

Kabat-Zinn, J. (1994). *Wherever you go, there you are.* New York: Hyperion.

Kanfer, F. H., & Saslow, G. (1969). Behavioral diagnosis. In C. M. Franks (Ed.), *Behavior therapy: Appraisal and status.* New York: McGraw-Hill.

Khoury, B., Sharma, M., Rush, S. E. & Fournier, C. (2015). Mindfulness-based stress reduction for healthy individuals: A meta-analysis. *Journal of Psychosomatic Research, 78*(6), 519–528. https://doi.org/10.1016/j.jpsychores.2015.03.009. Accessed January 12, 2019.

Kirby, J. N. (2016). Compassion interventions: The programmes, the evidence, and implications for research and practice. *Psychology and Psychotherapy.* Advance online publication. https://doi.org/10.1111/papt.12104. Accessed January 12, 2019.

Leiberg, S., Klimecki, O., & Singer, T. (2011). Short-term compassion training increases prosocial behavior in a newly developed prosocial game. *PLoS ONE, 6*(3), e17798. https://doi.org/10.1371/journal.pone.0017798.

Levesque, R. J. (Ed.). (2011). *Encyclopedia of adolescence.* New York: Springer Science & Business Media.

Linehan, M. (1993). *Cognitive-behavioral treatment of borderline personality disorder. Diagnosis and treatment of mental disorders.* New York: Guilford Press. http://site.ebrary.com/lib/alltitles/docDetail.action?docID=10215368. Accessed January 12, 2019.

Miller, A. L., Rathus, J. H., & Linehan, M. (2007). *Dialectical behavior therapy with suicidal adolescents.* New York: Guilford Press.

Miller, A. L., Rathus, J. H., Linehan, M. M., Wetzler, S. & Leigh, E. (1997). Dialectical behavior therapy adapted for suicidal adolescents. *Journal of Psychiatric Practice,* 78, 1–10. https://www.ncbi.nlm.nih.gov/pmc/articles/PMC3820084/pdf/PSYJ2013-145219.pdf. Accessed January 12, 2019.

Neff, K. D. & Germer, C. K. (2013). A pilot study and randomized controlled trial of the mindful self-compassion program. *Journal of Clinical Psychology, 69*(1), 28–44. https://doi.org/10.1002/jclp.21923. Accessed January 12, 2019.

O'Brien, K. M., Larson, C. M., & Murrell, A. R. (2008). Third-wave behavior therapies for children and adolescents: Progress, challenges, and future directions. In L. A. Greco & S. C. Hayes (Eds.), *Acceptance & mindfulness treatments for children & adolescents: A practitioner's guide* (pp. 15–36). Oakland, CA: Context Press; New Harbinger Publications.

Petermann, F., & Petermann, U. (2010). *Training mit Jugendlichen. Förderung von Arbeits-und Sozialverhalten*. Göttingen: Hogrefe.

Rathus, J. H., Linehan, M. M., & Miller, A. L. (2015). *DBT skills manual for adolescents*. New York: Guilford Press.

Roeser, R. W. & Pinela, C. (2014). Mindfulness and compassion training in adolescence: A developmental contemplative science perspective. *New Directions for Youth Development,* 142, 9–30. https://doi.org/10.1002/yd.20094. Accessed January 12, 2019.

Rubin, K. H., Bukowski, W. M. & Laursen, B. P. (2009). *Handbook of peer interactions, relationships, and groups (Pbk. ed.). Social, emotional, and personality development in context.* New York: The Guilford Press.

Saltzman, A. & Goldin, P. (2008). Mindfulness-based stress reduction for school-age children. In L. A. Greco & S. C. Hayes (Eds.), *Acceptance & mindfulness treatments for children & adolescents: A practitioner's guide* (pp. 139–161). Reno, Nev., Ann Arbor, Michigan: Context Press; ProQuest.

Segal, Z. V., Williams, J. M. G. & Teasdale, J. D. (2002). *Mindfulness-based cognitive therapy for depression: A new approach to preventing relapse.* New York: Guilford Press. Retrieved from http://www.loc.gov/catdir/description/guilford051/2001045051.html. Accessed January 12, 2019.

Semple, R. J., Lee, J. & Miller, L. F. (2006). Mindfulness-Based Cognitive Therapy for Children. In R. A. Baer (Ed.), *Practical resources for the mental health professional. Mindfulness-based treatment approaches: Clinician's guide to evidence base and applications* (pp. 143–166). San Diego, Calif.: Academic Press.

Simons, M. (2012). Anders denken–Metakognitive Therapie für Kinder und Jugendliche mit Zwangsstörung: Ein Behandlungsplan. *Verhaltenstherapie, 22*(4), 259–267.

Simons, M. (2016). Die Ohnmacht der Gedanken—Metakognitive Therapie für Kinder und Jugendliche [The powerlessness of thoughts—metacognitive therapy for children and adolescents]. *Zeitschrift Für Kinder-Und Jugendpsychiatrie Und Psychotherapie, 44*(6), 423–431. https://doi.org/10.1024/1422-4917/a000438.

Simons, M. (2018). *Metakognitive Therapie mit Kindern und Jugendlichen.* Weinheim: Beltz.

Steinberg, L., & Morris, A. S. (2001). Adolescent development. *Annual Review of Psychology, 52*(1), 83–110.

Tang, Y.-Y., Hölzel, B. K. & Posner, M. I. (2015). The neuroscience of mindfulness meditation. Nature Reviews. *Neuroscience, 16*(4), 213–225. https://doi.org/10.1038/nrn3916. Accessed January 12, 2019.

Traub, J., & In-Albon, T. (2017). *Therapie-Tools Angststörungen im Kindes-und Jugendalter*. Weinheim: Beltz.

Turrell, S. L., & Bell, M. (2016). *ACT for adolescents: Treating teens and adolescents in individual and group therapy*. Oakland, CA: Context Press.

Van der Oord, S., Bögels, S. M., & Peijnenburg, D. (2012). The effectiveness of mindfulness training for children with ADHD and mindful parenting for their parents. *Journal of Child and Family Studies, 21*(1), 139–147.

Vocks, S. & Legenbauer, T. (2010). *Körperbildtherapie bei Anorexia und Bulimia nervosa. Ein kognitiv-verhaltenstherapeutisches Behandlungsprogramm.* Göttingen: Hogrefe.

Vorrath, H. H., & Brendtro, L. K. (1985). *Positive peer culture* (2nd ed.). New York: Aldine.
Wells, A. (2005). Detached mindfulness in cognitive therapy: A metacognitive analysis and ten techniques. *Journal of Rational-Emotive & Cognitive-Behavior Therapy, 23*(4), 337–355. https://doi.org/10.1007/s10942-005-0018-6. Accessed January 12, 2019.
Wells, A. (2011). *Metacognitive therapy for anxiety and depression*. New york: Guilford.
Wells, A., & Matthews, G. (1995). *Attention and emotion: A clinical perspective*. London: Psychology Press.
Wisner, B. L. (2017). *Mindfulness and meditation for adolescents: Practices and programs*. New York, NY, U.S.A.: Palgrave Macmillan.
Yalom, I. D., & Leszcz, M. (2005). *The theory and practice of group psychotherapy* (5th ed.). New York: Basic Books.
Zoogman, S., Goldberg, S. B., Hoyt, W. T. & Miller, L. (2015). Mindfulness interventions with youth: A meta-analysis. *Mindfulness, 6*(2), 290–302. https://doi.org/10.1007/s12671-013-0260-4. Accessed January 12, 2019.

Chapter 15
Mental Health, New Technologies, and Wellbeing for Adolescents

Adolfo J. Cangas, María José Fínez, Consuelo Morán, Noelia Navarro and Petra Moldes

Abstract An aspect which characterizes young people of today is their ability and familiarity with new technologies. They were born in the digital age, making social networks and a wide array of applications something natural and common in their lives. The main appeal of new technologies for young people, and in particular social networks, lies in the accessibility, availability, privacy, intense stimulation, interactive website format, and anonymity that they offer. Thus, it is evident we are living in a digital world and it is more practical to seek out allies in new technologies than to reject their potential. Nonetheless, these tools must be considered in a global context, including both personal and social aspects, and we cannot forget that using them improperly can prove problematic. Thus, the objective would be to educate young people about responsible use, promote interests and relationships beyond technology, and make them aware of the risks involved (e.g. abuse). In such cases, it would be advisable to evaluate the individual's use of technology and, if necessary, intervene. In contrast, when properly used, new technologies serve as an additional resource that favors resilience and trains young individuals to cope with difficulties that may arise either online or offline. With this approach, we would be preparing responsible citizens, ready for the challenges that exist in a globalized digital world, with both electronic tools to help them and social/community resources which must also be reinforced during this formative stage in life.

Keywords New technologies · Internet · Technology abuse · Multitaskers · Digital world

It is well known that adolescence is a period of changes, both physical and emotional, that is accompanied by the arrival of new responsibilities, abilities and personal relationships. During this time, young people develop a heightened sense of identity and acquire a greater degree of autonomy. Thus, adolescence represents a pivotal stage in our society when preparation for entry into the adult world begins. It is also

A. J. Cangas (✉) · N. Navarro · P. Moldes
University of Almería, Almería, Spain
e-mail: ajcangas@ual.es

M. J. Fínez · C. Morán
University of León, León, Spain

C. Steinebach and Á. I. Langer (eds.), *Enhancing Resilience in Youth*,
https://doi.org/10.1007/978-3-030-25513-8_15

a time marked by pressure to overcome challenges in various aspects of life, both at an academic level and in terms of socio-personal development.

Traditionally, the literature has focused more on the risks of this period, such as those associated with substance abuse, violence, and sexual relations without protection. However, an increasing number of studies stress that it is a period of learning and developing important social values (e.g., solidarity, social recognition) (Giménez, Vázquez, & Hervás, 2010).

In regard to mental health, there exists a possibility that some individuals will suffer from different mental illnesses at a young age. Indeed, it is estimated that between 10 and 20% of young people may develop some type of mental illness during adolescence, such as mood disorder, impulse control or anxiety (Kieling et al., 2011). In addition, this is the period when severe mental disorders typically begin, as in the cases of schizophrenia, anorexia, and substance abuse. It is also known that half of the population that suffers from a mental disorder for longer than one year will develop their condition before the age of 14, and 70% will do so before the age of 24 (Kessler, Chiu, Demler, Merikangas, & Walters, 2005). Therefore, it is a critical stage of personal development in which the promotion of mental health should be a priority.

15.1 Adolescents and New Technologies

An aspect which characterizes young people of today is their ability and familiarity with new technologies. They were born in the digital age, making social networks and a wide array of applications something *natural* and common in their lives. The main appeal of new technologies for young people, and in particular social networks, lies in the accessibility, availability, privacy, intense stimulation, interactive website format, and anonymity that they offer (Borzekowski & Rickert, 2001).

The youngest generations have made activities like playing on the computer, surfing the Internet, communicating on social networks, and sending e-mails everyday parts of life. Consequently, they have been named the "interactive generation" (Del Río-Pérez, Sádava-Chalezquer, & Bringué-Sala, 2010). Indeed, Internet use is nearly absolute among young people between 16 and 24. With regard to social networks, according to the report 'Digital in 2018' published by Hootsuite, a social media management platform, use among adolescents is also highly widespread. As for cell phones, young people today are one of the first generations to have access to such devices and 98% use them regularly (Jiménez, Piqueras, Mateu, Carballo, Orgilés, & Espada, 2012). Studies reveal that adolescents are hardly ever without their cell phones, with 78% of the young people surveyed declaring that they spend at least 2 h every day using the Internet on their mobile devices (Wartella, Rideout, Montague, Beaudoin-Ryan, & Lauricella, 2016).

Moreover, 60% of young people state they have met a new friend through applications such as Facebook, Instagram or online video games (Luthar, Cicchetti, & Becker, 2015). Similarly, various online applications and programs offer rapid and convenient access to a wide array of information on problematic issues for young people, such as information and advice on addictions and sexuality, which again proves much easier to do than through direct contact (Aguilera & Muench, 2012; Weinstein et al., 2016).

In addition to the Internet, an increasing number of electronic applications are developed each day which seek to improve various aspects of personal wellbeing and healthy lifestyles (Khazaal, Favrod, Sort, Borgeat, & Bouchard, 2018). Thus, new technologies facilitate access to information and monitor wide cross sections of the population. In addition, they are easy to use and feature appealing designs that appeal to the esthetic and musical tastes of different sectors of the young population. Overall, the factors mentioned create an environment in which these technologies have a growing presence in the daily lives of young people (Carmona, Cangas, & Langer, 2012; Johnson et al., 2016).

15.2 Problems Associated with Abuse of New Technologies Among Young People

This access to electronic resources does have certain advantages, such as the possibility to communicate with other people, but it also poses a number of risks, including overexposure, sleep deprivation and cyberbullying (Best, Manktelow, & Taylor, 2014). *Technology abuse can also cause young people to "disconnect" from offline interaction. In fact, one third of young people* (34%) *recognize their social network use has reduced the time they could devote to real personal interaction. Therefore, it is advisable to seek out a "balance" and be aware of how these resources are abused* (Rideout, 2015). It must also be remembered that relationships through digital technology may not produce the same satisfaction as offline relationships, not to mention the conflicts that can arise due to the "unreal" image that another individual may present, which could become a source of bullying, deception, etc. (Gardner & Davis, 2013). For this reason, it is essential that the use of these resources be accompanied by education and prudence.

Additionally, there is growing concern for the abuse of video games among young people, the time they dedicate to them, and the dependence these games produce. This problem has become so prominent that it has been identified as a diagnostic characteristic in the latest edition of the International Classification of Diseases (ICD-11). Another topic to take into consideration is the severe social isolation of many adolescents in their homes. This behavior most commonly occurs in highly competitive and technologically advanced societies, such as Japan, but it is present in other parts of the world as well. While this problem tends to be brought on by poor academic performance, work or personal issues, or family pressure, isolation can to a great extent be linked to the easy access that young people have to the virtual world from their homes. Thus, they are able to isolate themselves from other people, producing a phenomenon referred to as "Hikikomori" (Teo, et al, 2018).

This abuse tends to arise when behavior starts to noticeably interfere with other aspects of life, such as academic performance, relationships with peers, and family communication. This conduct manifests not only due to the characteristics of electronic resources themselves (e.g., whether they allow interaction with others or not, are easy to use), but a number of other factors also prove influential: (1) the personal characteristics of the individual (e.g., gender, in which case boys are more prone than girls); (2) psychopathological problems related to social anxiety, depression or stress; and, (3) other aspects of personality related to impulsiveness, self-control, hostility, or self-esteem. Furthermore, abuse of technology has also been linked to family environment (e.g., poor parental communication and family relationships) and poor relationships with peers (e.g., lack of social support and quality friendships) (Anderson, Steen, & Stavropoulos, 2017; Harris Hyun-soo, 2017).

In relation to this issue, numerous studies have revealed how the abuse of new technologies implies decreased personal wellbeing which translates to a decrease in satisfaction with life, an internalization of negative experiences, and psychological problems such as depression, anxiety, stress, and attention deficit (Clifton, Goodhall, Ban, & Birks, 2013). Similarly, research has linked the use of new technologies to a rather common characteristic in today's society—narcissism (Liu & Baumeister, 2016), albeit a connection has also been found with increased empathy as well, particularly among young people (Best et al., 2014).

In this respect it is essential to understand the characteristics of new technologies, adolescents' motivation for using them, the context in which they are used, and the way young people utilize them. Therefore, this analysis by no means seeks to "demonize" electronic resources; instead, it aims to identify both the advantages they offer and the risks they pose in order for responsible use of these technologies to exist, with all its possible benefits (e.g., motivation, learning, interaction with others, creativity) and minimal potential risks (Stavropoulos, Burleigh, Beard, Gomez, & Griffiths, 2018).

Additionally, whether we like it or not, as a society we must accept that the switch from analogical to digital is a present-day reality. For adults, this change may imply venturing into "unknown territory" as there is a degree of uncertainty and fear involved in addressing the "pros and cons" of technology. However, for adolescents, "the digital natives", this reality simply constitutes another tool that forms part of their daily lives. This "digital gap" clearly underscores the communication breakdown between generations (Serrano & Martínez, 2003).

15.3 Resilience and New Technologies Among Young People

A key aspect of modern-day psychology is resilience. Essentially, this concept refers to individuals that manage to adequately overcome adverse situations without suffering any negative aftereffects. We believe it is practical to consider the concept of "resilient processes" as opposed to only one individual "capacity", primarily because the former encompasses various factors of the individual and also their capacities (Luthar, Cicchetti, & Becker, 2000).

The absence of behavior problems is one of the most commonly-used indicators when measuring the adaptation or adjustment of resilient adolescents (Luthar et al., 2000). However, other authors highlight the importance of measuring other indices (e.g., life satisfaction, functional capacity, social skills, sound mental health) since some studies have found high levels of emotional distress among resilient young people with strong behavioral adjustment (Luthar, 1991).

When dealing with adolescents, social support and good family environment constitute protective factors (Masten, 2001), along with the support present in one's surroundings, a sound network of casual, social relationships, education, and spiritual or religious commitment in the form of group participation (Guedeney, 1998). In addition to these external factors we must include the specific characteristics of the individual adolescent, such as self-esteem or their strategies for coping with problems. Therefore, no single factor of personality stimulates resilience alone; instead, it is the interrelationship among them (i.e., personal and social resources) that ultimately helps an individual to overcome the adversities they encounter.

In this context, it could be said that risk and protection are forces constantly at work. That is, risk is somewhat inherent to life, but, if a safe environment exists, protection presents itself as a way of counteracting any difficulties. Thus, if an individual experiences a trauma, it does not necessarily dictate their future because two individuals can face said adversity in very different ways, so much so that in many cases people have even emerged stronger following the experience. In fact, after enduring an adversity it is impossible for a person to recover their previous state, which means that in the case of the resilient individual they assimilate the pain as a learning experience. According to Vanistendael and Lecomte (2002), this framework of past suffering and present resilience creates a peculiar mixture of fragility and strength, where the former comes from an experience endured and the latter from a challenge overcome.

New technologies can also prove to be a useful tool in the aforementioned process. More specifically, they allow adolescents to approach learning in a new way. Thus, they absorb a great deal of multimedia information, utilize and consume multiple data sources simultaneously, expect instant responses, remain in contact permanently, and perform better as part of a network, and even create their own content. It could be said that these young individuals are *multitaskers*.

On a pedagogical level, new technologies are being incorporated into the classroom, enjoying a growing presence in teaching-learning processes. Their use provides substantial benefits as a source of connection and communication infused with a key component of fun, which makes the presentation of content more appealing. Also, these technologies indeed constitute an important medium for learning and spreading intellectual information (Castellana, Sánchez-Carbonell, Graner, & Beranuy, 2006).

For example, a study by Sitzmann (2011) found that students whose studies were complemented with educational video games obtained better results than others who did not use this medium. In this case, the first group improved their knowledge of facts by 11%, their ability-based knowledge by 14%, and they retained knowledge 9% better.

In addition to their entertaining characteristics and overall ability to make the learning of theory and lessons more fun, the implementation of new technologies is also useful for instilling values like empathy, prosocial behavior, and the pursuit of better personal wellbeing (e.g., doing physical exercise or planning daily tasks). There is also growth in the use of applications that allow them to comment on their feelings by contacting others who have had similar experiences or who offer advice (Consolvo, Klasnja, McDonald, & Landay, 2012; Slovák & Fitzpatrick, 2015).

Regarding different types of applications, there is also a rising trend in the use of programs that help to reinforce "potentials", including artistic abilities (crucial for expression and facing difficulties), and others that educate on different problem solving tools, such as mindfulness techniques, yoga and relaxation (e.g. Baker & Khan, 2019; Van Emmerik, Berings, & Lancee, 2018) which make it possible, for example, to lower levels of stress and anxiety (i.e., *Mindfulness Focus Now, Calm or Mindfulness Focus Now*).

In the case of mindfulness, Mani, Kavanagh, Hides and Stoyanov (2015) identified the existence of more than 600 apps on iTunes and Google Apps. However, after further analysis, it was determined that very few offered a complete training experience. As for other results, Tunney, Cooney, Coyle, and O'Reilly (2017) compared a face to face mindfulness procedure with a digital one, observing that hardly any differences could be detected. Thus, these authors concluded that apps represented a sound complement to the daily practice of these techniques, particularly when used by young people, among whom notable results can be achieved for depression, anxiety, stress, and improvement of resilience (Flett, Hayne, Riordan, Thompson, & Conner, 2018). This by no means implies, however, that both procedures are the same, but rather than they can complement one another. Moreover, electronic devices can be used as a tool in the teaching of these abilities, providing support at home or serving as an alternative in situations when real interaction is simply not possible.

Furthermore, this does not mean that no additional changes are needed in the social or family surroundings of the individual. Instead, they can serve as a sound complement that offers adolescents access to resources for coping with difficulties, which constitutes a fundamental aspect of resilience.

In this same line, many programs that resort to the use of virtual reality are becoming more common for the purpose of addressing various clinical problems. One of the main advantages of this technology, along with improved motivation, is that it allows the development of abilities without the same level of worry for the possible consequences. In other words, these tools offer more freedom to experiment without the worry that making a mistake in real life would involve. Moreover, this technology achieves high levels of emotional implication (de Freitas & Maharg, 2011).

Regarding the latter, it is worth mentioning that since 2016, when the first Oculus Rift goggles went on the market, the field of virtual reality has expanded and reduced its prices tremendously. Forecasts predict that in the years to come virtual reality devices will become as common for young people as video game consoles or cell phones (Perry, 2016). These resources offer several advantages over other informative and/or preventative strategies; for example, they offer immediate feedback, which stimulates greater motivation among users, they are also user-friendly and inexpensive once developed, and they have an enormous potential to reach vast audiences. Moreover, virtual reality gives users the opportunity to put themselves in an "almost real" world where emotional involvement is at a maximum. This technology also allows us to interact in said surroundings, meaning we can experience and learn with our own actions in a "safe environment". These features are the reasons why treatments based on virtual reality have proven to be effective in treating various psychological disorders, such as phobias (Rothbaum, Hodges, Smith, Lee, & Price, 2000), obsessive compulsive disorder (Mataix-Cols & Marks, 2006), addictive behaviors (Lee, Kwon, Choi, & Yang, 2007), sexual disorders (Optale et al., 1997), among others.

The aforementioned technology is also being used with individuals who have recently been diagnosed with a severe illness. Some of these platforms include, in the treatment of cancer, *Re-Mission* and *Make a wish*, and, in AIDS treatment, *I'm Positive*, which strengthens the resilience of the partner of the HIV patient. These video games directly affect the user's resilience and place emphasize on promoting a positive outlook with regard to the resources and capacities available for facing the challenge that their illness represents. Furthermore, they propose active coping strategies that allow users to overcome and effectively manage fear. Additionally, they address the process of cognitive reevaluation with the objective of giving meaning to such negative experiences.

Similarly, prosocial video games constitute a fine example of how to promote empathy and gain perspective, which are essential components for the resolution of any type of conflict. Indeed, and contrary to games that may be violent or sexist, video games that are aware of social problems (e.g., the game *Peacemaker*), foster learning about the cultures or lives of other groups.

Continuing in this line, our research group developed a serious game, or educational video game, to raise awareness among young people about mental health problems. This particular demographic lacks sufficient information about what mental disorders are, what treatments exist, whether there are cures or not, how to respond when dealing with afflicted individuals, and so on. Moreover, young people do not realize that they can seek help if they suspect they themselves are suffering from some type of mental health issue and, additionally, that they can learn how to help peers who are dealing with problems of their own.

Stigma Stop, which is the name of the serious game, takes place in a non-immersive virtual reality environment and initially seeks to provide young people with information about problems related to mental health, most of which are either unknown to the public or misunderstood due to a great deal of erroneous information. Additionally, the game offers users a better understanding of individuals who suffer from such difficulties, thereby fostering empathy and reducing social isolation. *Stigma Stop* teaches users they must be aware that everyone is prone to suffering from a mental disorder (to a greater or lesser degree) at some point in our lives, which makes it fundamental to have access to accurate information and to know how to respond accordingly. In the case of *Stigma Stop*, the most important aspect is for young people to learn that problems in mental health can affect anyone, that the support of others is essential (e.g., peers, family and professionals), and, of course, that our attitude can prove vital for overcoming said problems.

We must bear in mind that the stigma associated with mental illness is currently one of the most alarming concerns. Said stigma is commonly responsible for delaying the search for professional help in an attempt to hide the issue, which only succeeds in prolonging the subsequent period of intervention. This stigma is mainly the result of disinformation about illnesses themselves and the aid available to treat them. Furthermore, not only does stigma affect the young people who are suffering but their parents as well, who quite often feel overwhelmed and at a loss for how to handle the situation (O'Reilly et al., 2018).

The first version of *Stigma Stop* is available for computer use in a 3D simulation program, and a new version is currently being developed in virtual reality format.

The results obtained with *Stigma Stop* until now have been very positive. Young people give highly favorable assessments of the information provided, which is of utmost importance considering it is the information itself that contributes to changing attitudes about mental health problems (Cangas et al., 2017). Similarly, in a study with university psychology students, the game proved to be similar in efficacy to face-to-face meetings with mental health patients and somewhat superior to a talk with a professional (Mullor, Sayans, Cangas, & Navarro, 2019).

Stigma Stop is also a tool that can be combined with other intervention methods (e.g., contact with mental health patients through first-hand testimonials or associations). It may also prove to be a quick and convenient method for young people to become familiar with mental health problems and acquire more accurate and honest information about them.

Summarizing, it is evident we are living in a digital world and it is more practical to seek out allies in new technologies than to reject their potential. Nonetheless, these tools must be considered in a global context, including both personal and social aspects, and we cannot forget that using them improperly can prove problematic. Thus, the objective would be to educate young people about responsible use, promote interests and relationships beyond technology, and make them aware of the risks involved (e.g., abuse). In such cases, it would be advisable to evaluate the individual's use of technology and, if necessary, intervene. In contrast, when properly used, new technologies serve as an additional resource that favors resilience and trains young individuals to cope with difficulties that may arise either online or offline. With this approach, we would be preparing responsible citizens, ready for the challenges that exist in a globalized digital world, with both electronic tools to help them and social/community resources which must also be reinforced during this formative stage in life.

Acknowledgements This work was supported by the Spanish Ministry of Science, Innovation and Universities (grant: PSI2017-84961-R AEI/FEDER, UE).

References

Aguilera, A., & Muench, F. (2012). There's an app for that: information technology applications for cognitive behavioral practitioners. *Behaviour Therapy, 35*(4), 65–73.

Anderson, E. L., Steen, E., & Stavropoulos, V. (2017). Internet use and problematic internet use: A systematic review of longitudinal research trends in adolescence and emergent adulthood. *International Journal of Adolescence and Youth, 22*(4), 430–454.

Baker, A., & Khan, M. (2019). Relax player app with relaxation melodies and different sounds. In S. Umair & M. Y. Shah (Eds.), *Mobile devices and smart gadgets in human rights* (pp. 237–253). Hershey: IGI Global.

Best, P., Manktelow, R., & Taylor, B. (2014). Online communication, social media and adolescent wellbeing: A systematic narrative review. *Children and Youth Services Review, 41,* 27–36.

Borzekowski, D. L. G., & Rickert, V. I. (2001). Adolescent cybersurfing for health information. *Archives of Pediatric Adolescence Medicine, 155,* 813–817.

Cangas, A. J., Navarro, N., Parra, J., Ojeda, J. J., Cangas, D., Piedra, J. A. … Gallego, J. (2017). Stigma-Stop: A Serious Game against the Stigma toward Mental Health in Educational Settings. *Frontiers in psychology, 8,* 1385.

Carmona, L. A., Cangas, A. J., & Langer, A. (2012). Applications of 3D simulation in mental health: Utilities and new developments. In L. Labate (Ed.), *Mental illness. Evaluation, treatment and implications* (vol. II., pp. 37–56). Rijeka: Intech.

Castellana, M., Sánchez-Carbonell, X., Graner, C., & Beranuy, M. (2006). El adolescente ante las tecnologías de la información y la comunicación: Internet, móvil y videojuegos. *Papeles del Psicólogo, 28*(3), 196–204.

Clifton, A., Goodhall, D. L., Ban, S., & Birks, S. (2013). New perspectives on the contribution of digital technology and social media use to improve the mental wellbeing of children and young people: a state of the art review. *Neonatal, Paediatric and Child Health Nursing, 16*(1), 19–26.

Consolvo, S., Klasnja, P., McDonald, D. W., & Landay, J. (2012). Designing for healthy lifestyles: Design considerations for mobile technologies to encourage consumer health and wellness. *Foundations and Trends in Human-Computer Interaction, 6,* 167–315.

Del Río-Pérez, J., Sádava-Chalezquer, C., & Bringué-Sala, X. (2010). Menores y redes ¿sociales?: de la amistad al cyberbullying. *Revista de Estudios de Juventud, 88,* 115–129.

Flett, J. A., Hayne, H., Riordan, B. C., Thompson, L. M. & Conner, T. S. (2018). Mobile mindfulness meditation: A randomised controlled trial of the effect of two popular apps on mental health. *Mindfulness*, 1–14.

de Freitas, S., & Maharg, P. (2011). *Digital games and learning*. New York: Continuum International Publication Group.

Gardner, H., & Davis, K. (2013). *The app generation: How today's youth navigate identity, intimacy, and imagination in a digital world.* New Haven, CT: Yale University Press.

Giménez, M., Vázquez, C., & Hervás, G. (2010). El análisis de las fortalezas psicológicas en la adolescencia: Más allá de los modelos de vulnerabilidad. *Psychology Society & Education, 2,* 97–116.

Guedeney, A. (1998). Les determinants précoces de la resilience. In B. Cyrulnik (Ed.), *Ces enfants qui tiennent le coup* (pp. 13–26). Revigny-sur-Ornain: Hommes et Perspectives.

Hyun-soo Harris, K. (2017). The impact of online social networking on adolescent psychological well-being (WB): A population-level analysis of Korean school-aged children. *International Journal of Adolescence and Youth, 22*(3), 364–376.

Jiménez, M., Piqueras, J., Mateu, O., Carballo, J., Orgilés, M., & Espada, J. (2012). Diferencias de sexo, características de personalidad y afrontamiento en el uso de Internet, el móvil y los videojuegos en la adolescencia. *Health and Addictions, 12*(1), 57–78.

Johnson, D., Deterding, S., Kuhn, K. A., Staneva, A., Stoyanov, S., & Hides, L. (2016). Gamification for health and wellbeing: A systematic review of the literature. *Internet Interventions, 6,* 89–106.

Kessler, R. C., Chiu, W. T., Demler, O., Merikangas, K. R., & Walters, E. E. (2005). Prevalence, severity, and comorbidity of 12-month DSM-IV disorders in the National Comorbidity Survey Replication. *Archives of General Psychiatry, 62*(6), 617–627.

Khazaal, Y., Favrod, J., Sort, A., Borgeat, F., & Bouchard, S. (2018). Computers and games for mental health and well-being. *Frontiers in Psychiatry, 9,* 141.

Kieling, C., Baker-Henningham, H., Belfer, M., Conti, G., Ertem, I., Omigbodun, O., … Srinath, S. (2011). Child and adolescent mental health worldwide: Evidence for action. *Lancet,* 378, 1515-1525.

Lee, J. H., Kwon, H., Choi, J., & Yang, B. H. (2007). Cue-exposure therapy to decrease alcohol craving in virtual environment. *Cyberpsychology & Behavior, 10,* 617–623.

Lenhart, A., Smith, A., Anderson, M., Duggan, M. & Perrin, A. (2015). Teens, technology and friendships. Pew Research Center Website. http://assets.pewresearch.org/wp-content/uploads/sites/14/2015/08/Teens-and-Friendships-FINAL2.pdf. Accessed January 19, 2019.

Liu, D., & Baumeister, R. (2016). Social networking online and personality of self-worth: A meta-analysis. *Journal of Research in Personality, 64,* 79–89.

Luthar, S. (1991). Vulnerability and resilience: A study of high-risk adolescents. *Child Development, 62,* 600–616.

Luthar, S. S., Cicchetti, D., & Becker, B. (2000). Research on resilience: Response to commentaries. *Child Development, 71*(3), 573–575.

Mani, M., Kavanagh, D. J., Hides, L. & Stoyanov, S. R. (2015). Review and evaluation of mindfulness-based iPhone apps. *JMIR mHealth and uHealth, 3*(3).

Masten, A. S. (2001). Ordinary magic: Resilience processes in development. *American Psychologist, 56,* 227–238.

Mataix-Cols, D., & Marks, I. M. (2006). Self-help with minimal therapist contact for obsessiv-compulsive disorder: A review. *European Psychiatry, 21,* 75–80.

Mullor, D., Sayans, P., Cangas, A. J., & Navarro, N. (2019). An empirical study on the Serious Game stigma-stop and its impact of reducing stigma in mental illness: A comparative study on psychology students. *Cyberpsychology, Behavior, and Social Networking, 22*, 205–211.

O'Reilly, M., Dogra, N., Whiteman, N., Hughes, J., Eruyar, S., & Reilly, P. (2018). Is social media bad for mental health and wellbeing? Exploring the perspectives of adolescents. *Clinical child psychology and psychiatry, 23*(4), 601–613.

Optale, G., Munari, A., Nasta, A., Pianon, C., Baldaro Verde, J., … Viggiano, G. (1997). Multimedia and virtual reality techniques in the treatment of male erectile disorders. *International Journal of Impotence Research, 9*, 197–203.

Perry, T. S. (2016). Virtual reality goes social. *IEEE Spectrum, 53*(1), 56–57.

Rideout, V. (2015). *The common sense census: Media use by tweens and teens.* https://www.commonsensemedia.org/research/the-common-sense-census-media-use-by-tweens-and-teens. Accessed January 19, 2019.

Rothbaum, B. O., Hodges, L., Smith, S., Lee, J. H., & Price, L. (2000). A controlled study of virtual reality exposure therapy for the fear of flying. *Journal of Consulting and Clinical Psychology, 68,* 1020–1026.

Serrano, A., & Martínez, E. (2003). *La Brecha Digital: Mitos y Realidades*. México: Editorial UABC.

Sitzmann, T. (2011). A meta-analytic examination of the instructional effectiveness of computer-based simulation games. *Personnel Psychology, 64,* 489–528.

Slovak, P., & Fitzpatrick, G. (2015). Teaching and developing social and emotional skills with technology. *ACM Transactions on Computer-Human Interaction, 22*(4), 1–34.

Stavropoulos, V., Burleigh, T. L., Beard, C. Gomez, R. & Griffiths, M.D. (2018). Being there: A preliminary study examining the role of presence in Internet Gaming Disorder. *International Journal of Mental Health and Addictions,* https://slidept.net/view-doc.html?utm_source=stavropoulos-v-burleigh-t-l-beard-c-gomez-r-griffiths-m-d-2018-being-there-a-preliminary-study-examining-the-role-of-presence-in-internet-gaming-disorder-international-journal-of-mental-health-and-addictions-in-press&utm_campaign=download. Accessed January 19, 2019.

Teo, A. R., Chen, J. I., Kubo, H., Katsuki, R., Sato-Kasai, M., Shimokawa, N., … Kato, T. A. (2018). Development and Validation of the 25-item Hikikomori Questionnaire (HQ-25). *Psychiatry and clinical neurosciences, 72*(10), 780-788.

Tunney, C., Cooney, P., Coyle, D. & O'Reilly, G. (2017). Comparing young people's experience of technology-delivered v. face-to-face mindfulness and relaxation: Two-armed qualitative focus group study. *British Journal of Psychiatry, 210*(4), 284–289.

Van Emmerik, A. A., Berings, F., & Lancee, J. (2018). Efficacy of a mindfulness-based mobile application: a randomized waiting-list controlled trial. *Mindfulness, 9,* 187–198.

Vanistendael, S., & Lecomte, J. (2002). *La felicidad es posible. Despertar en niños maltratados la confianza en sí mismos: construir la resiliencia.* Barcelona: Gedisa.

Wartella, E., Rideout, V., Montague, H., Beaudoin-Ryan, L., & Lauricella, A. (2016). Teens, health and technology: A national survey. *Media and Communication, 4,* 13–23.

Weinstein, E. C., Selman, R. L., Thomas, S., Kim, J. E., White, A. E., & Dinakar, K. (2016). How to cope with digital stress: the recommendations adolescents offer their peers online. *Journal of Adolescent Research, 31*(4), 415–441.

Chapter 16
Transformations of Social Bonds and Mental Health: How Can Mindfulness Counter Individualization and the Influence of Communication Technologies?

Mariane Krause

Abstract This study focuses on the effect of social transformations—including those connected to information and communication technologies—on interpersonal bonds and community building. I describe and problematize said transformations, discuss the threats and opportunities that they can entail in terms of mental health, and suggest how contemplative practices such as mindfulness can buffer threats by fostering healthy bonds at both the individual and community levels, which should help improve psychological well-being. The conclusion of this analysis is that, over the last decades, humanity (at least in Western societies) has been witness to a weakening of traditional bonds, compounded by a growing individualization process and the dissolution of traditional and stable communities. This process results in individuals who are more reliant on themselves (and less dependent on prescribed social norms) when it comes to constructing their lives. Practicing mindfulness, especially those varieties that include acceptance and compassion, makes it possible to buffer the negative effect that the transformations discussed can have on mental health. Contemplative practices such as mindfulness can teach the stressed inhabitants of technologically-mediated relationships to pay attention to their experience in the present moment, learn to know and accept their own thoughts and emotions, be kind to themselves, and maintain an attitude of empathetic and accepting openness toward others.

Keywords Personal bonds · Community bonds · Hyperconnectivity · Transformation of communities · Contemplative practices

M. Krause (✉)
School of Psychology, Pontificia Universidad Católica de Chile, Santiago, Chile
e-mail: mkrause@uc.cl

Millennium Institute for Research in Depression and Personality, MIDAP, Santiago, Chile

C. Steinebach and Á. I. Langer (eds.), *Enhancing Resilience in Youth*,
https://doi.org/10.1007/978-3-030-25513-8_16

16.1 Social Bonds and Mental Health

16.1.1 Importance of Personal Bonds

The importance of personal bonds for mental health, particularly those formed in early childhood, is arguably one of the most robust findings of psychology research (Olhaberry et al., 2014). Even before birth, the affective processes involved in the attachment relationship between the caregiver and the infant are essential for the development of the self and of the affective and social resources that make relationships with others possible. Developing as an individual—which entails differentiating oneself from the rest—and establishing nourishing relationships with others are among the fundamental tasks that every human being must complete. For both tasks, the bonds developed early in life are crucial (Cierpka, 2016). This relational matrix is necessary for our mind to develop; also, these affective networks support us emotionally and socially all through our lives.

Growing up in a protective environment with significant people is therefore essential for achieving mental health. Failings in these environments entail a burden, since they determine a psychological vulnerability when addressing future developmental challenges. Attachment insecurities, in general, increase the risk of suffering psychological disorders (Mikulincer & Shaver, 2007). Vulnerability is greater when attachment insecurities are linked to low perceived social support in the person's broader context (Dagnino, Pérez, C., Gómez, A., Gloger, S. & Krause, 2017). Particularly, early attachment trauma has been found to be connected with future mental health problems (McLeod, 1991; McLeod & Shanahan, 1993), especially when these adverse conditions are cumulative (McLeod & Shanahan, 1996).

Nevertheless, corrective experiences exist that can be helpful in later developmental stages such as adolescence, a period during which the relation with oneself and others acquires special importance. And given that post-childhood stressors are relevant as well (Heim & Nemeroff, 2001), it is also possible to conduct preventive actions in later stages of life. Unfortunately, evidence also shows that unhealthy attachment styles can be intergenerationally transmitted, which increases the likelihood of mental health problems in new generations (Gómez & Jaén, 2011). This underscores the importance of curative actions aimed at personal bonds and those intended to prevent their deterioration in various stages of life.

In brief, interpersonal affective relationships are fundamental for human development from early childhood to old age, and therefore constitute the main protective factor of our mental and physical health.

16.1.2 Importance of Community Bonds

As previously noted, relations with others are highly relevant not only in early childhood or adolescence, but throughout a person's life. Consequently, psychosocial research has provided evidence of the importance of community bonds for mental health (Castonguay, 2011; Krause & Montenegro, 2016). A long tradition of research has shown the association between stressful life events, low social support, and mental health (Brown, Sklair, Harris & Birley, 1986). The social support provided by relations with others is the main protective factor when dealing with stressful life events causally associated with mental health problems (Brown et al., 1973). This effect of social support on mental health has been observed across cultures (Kessler & Bromet, 2013).

The importance of bonds throughout one's life results from the fact that humans are essentially social beings, and this social nature is expressed precisely through the permanent construction of communities (Krause & Montenegro, 2016).

Taking into account classical elements of the concept of community and acknowledging their current transformations (Veinot & Williams, 2012), community can be defined as "a human group that develops upon shared meanings and a common identity, whose members define themselves as such and are linked to each other by a sense of belonging and a relationship sustained through communication, shared goals, and joint actions which occur in a variable material and temporal space" (Krause & Montenegro, 2016, p. 291). Through the relationship between their members, communities construct a sense of community (McMillan & Chavis, 1986), expressed through shared interpretations, values, symbols, and rituals. These common aspects support their capacity for acting as a group, contributing to the social and subjective integration of their members (Bessant, 2011) and becoming "a relational and affective universe" (Mannarini & Fedi, 2009, p. 223).

The link between community and mental health is well supported by research. Several characteristics of communities can explain their positive impact on their members' health. For example, communities increase the well-being of their members through the establishment of interpersonal bonds, mostly when expressed through mutual support (Sarason, 1974) that is perceived as such (Cohen, 2004). Health is also promoted through common identification (Campbell & McLean, 2003; McMillan & Chavis, 1986) and through the feeling that one is a valuable or meaningful person for others in the community (Sarason, 1974). Other important health promoting aspects include emotional connection and security (Colclough & Sitaraman, 2005).

An additional health related aspect of communities is their effectiveness in attaining shared goals, which leads to the experience of social competence and empowerment, the latter being directly related to health and psychological well-being (Rappaport, 1984; Turró & Krause, 2008; UNDP, 2004).

Given the solid evidence for the relationship between social and community bonds and general and mental health, it is particularly relevant to analyze the transformations that these elements have undergone over the last decades.

16.2 The Transformation of Social Bonds

16.2.1 The Shift Toward Individualization

Over the last decades, modern Western societies have experienced major transformations in the way in which bonds with others are constructed and preserved. These transformations include the weakening of the traditional forms of collective action along with changes in social consciousness and in the ways of belonging to a community.

As social and community points of reference become relativized, individuals depend increasingly more on themselves (Hodgetts, Bolam, & Stephens, 2005) for constructing their identities and life plans (Araujo & Martuccelli, 2010; Beck & Beck-Gersheim, 2002; Krause et al., 2015). This has been conceptualized as a growing individualization process (Beck & Beck-Gersheim, 2002; Güell, Peters, & Morales, 2012). Thus, these sociocultural changes have a profound impact on people's subjectivities and forms of sociability (Bauman, 2007; Beck & Beck-Gersheim, 2002; Castells, 2001, Castel, 2011; Sennett, 2006).

For Bessant (2011), modernity has weakened traditional social bonds, resulting in a social world that is fragmented, isolated, and atomized. In this context, sociocultural changes have influenced individuals' relationship with themselves and others, which means that this modernization process can threaten mental health due to the resulting increase in impersonality, moral neutrality, and individualism (Nisbet, [1953]1967). In this context, we can conceptualize the weakening of social bonds and communities as a mediating variable between sociocultural changes and illness (Campbell & Murray, 2004; Cornish, 2004).

Empirical evidence exists which links these changes in social and community embeddedness with one of the world's most prevalent mental health problems: depression. This sociocultural hypothesis of depression holds that the disorder is more prevalent in countries with more individualistic sociocultural characteristics, with the relationship also depending on biological factors via "culture-gene co-evolution" (Chiao & Blizinsky, 2010), which involves interactions between culture, stress, emotion regulation, and genetic polymorphisms (Kim et al., 2011; Way & Lieberman, 2010). Based on these findings, Luyten and Blatt (2013, p. 179) proposed, for societies that are more sensitive to the social environment, that "as many of these societies shift toward a greater emphasis on achievement and self-definition (individualism), with less emphasis on social bonds and social support, it can be expected that the prevalence of psychopathology will increase as the moderating influence of social support and collectivistic attitudes [...] in these socially sensitive populations decreases".

Over the last two decades, the social changes described above have been complemented by a new dimension of everyday life that strongly impacts interpersonal relations: the hyperpresence of information and communication technologies.

16.2.2 *Relations Mediated by Information and Communication Technologies*

The current era, characterized by the hyperconnectivity and hyperinformation granted by information and communication technologies (ICTs), has intensified the change process described, which entails both threats and opportunities in terms of mental health.

16.2.2.1 The Transformation of Personal Bonds

The mediation of ICTs has transformed both the number and form of people's bonds with others. The most prominent characteristic of this transformation is immediacy, which affects information and relations. The former effect has certainly transformed our relationship with knowledge by simplifying access to it, which has the potential to lessen educational and cultural differences. Authors speak of a democratization in access to information (Tolosa, 2013). Nevertheless, at a psychological level, the omnipresence of information also entails the threat of attentional saturation (due to the excessive amount of information available) and confusion (due to the excessive number of ways of accessing it). For people, it is a challenge to weigh and identify differences between the types of information that each source provides (Tolosa, 2013).

As for the immediacy of relations, it would appear to eliminate the threat of loneliness, enabling us to establish close relationships even across large geographical distances; however, this can generate confusion regarding the levels of intimacy involved, which is compounded by the supplementation of nonverbal cues with simple and homogenized graphical elements used to express emotions (emojis).

In psychosocial terms, multiple memberships and participation in Internet-mediated social networks involve a new step in the individualization process, particularly regarding the self-construction of identity or of multiple identities deployed in each virtual context. These new possibilities of existence in each person's relational world can be considered to be enriching, but they can also be regarded as a threat to mental health, especially when associated with "perfectionism", materialized through signs of approval (such as the "likes" that can be obtained in virtual social networks). For Curran and Hill (2017, p. 1), "neoliberalism has succeeded in shifting cultural values so to now emphasize competitiveness, individualism, and irrational ideals of the perfectible self (...) [that] are systemic within contemporary language patterns, the media, and social and civic institutions, and are evident in the rise of competitive and individualistic traits, materialistic behavior, and presentational anxieties among recent generations of young people". Thus, increased opportunities for self-construction (either real or imagined) can go hand in hand with a (culturally mediated) increase in perfectionism. This has been labeled Multidimensional Perfectionism (Curran & Hill, 2017) and is characterized by an exacerbation of the desire to be perfect, with unrealistic expectations of oneself and punitive self-assessment or context-blaming. In the latter case, the context is regarded as excessively demanding and judgmental, which causes the person to feel that he/she requires perfection to ensure other people's approval. In addition, the individual can project perfectionism on his/her social environment. "When perfectionistic expectations are directed toward others, individuals impose unrealistic standards on those around them and evaluate others critically (other-oriented perfectionism)" (Curran & Hill, 2017, p. 1).

16.2.2.2 The Transformation of Communities

Current changes brought about by new communication technologies have not caused communities to disappear. However, they have transformed them, which can hinder their contribution to mental health. At present, individuals belong to multiple communities characterized by their transience and the fact that they are often disconnected from a shared physical or geographical space (Krause & Montenegro, 2016; UNDP, 2004).

Current communities have been described as having undergone four major transformations affecting as many dimensions: space, structure, time, and permanence.

With respect to space, communities are currently less embedded in geographical locations and have fewer face-to-face interactions. ICTs, especially the Internet, have detached communication from territorial and physical co-presence, which has opened up new community building opportunities (Krause and Montenegro, 2016). Early in this century, Castells (2001, p. 126) had already noted that "'place-based sociability' and 'territorially defined community' … certainly play a minor role in structuring social relationships for the majority of the population in developed societies". It is interesting to reflect on the possibilities derived from digitally mediated interaction, the most evident of which may be the creation of virtual communities, defined by Chambers as "online networks that display the psychological and cultural qualities of strong community with little or no physical proximity". Thus, ICTs generate a different kind of space for the emergence of communities.

In terms of their structure, new forms of community are characterized by lower social network density and greater flexibility of roles and hierarchies (Tolosa, 2013). Furthermore, their external boundaries are fuzzier.

As for their temporality, these new forms of community frequently have a shorter lifespan. Communities can rapidly be created around shared interests and affinities, with no need for a long common history. On the other hand, this also means that these Internet-mediated communities depend on the ongoing efforts of their members to sustain them (Krause and Montenegro, 2016). The result is that multiple communities are being generated and discontinued all the time.

As for transformations affecting affiliation, Internet-mediated social relationships have made it easier to belong to various groups and networks simultaneously (UNDP, 2004). This can result in fragmented and specialized social relations, which has been labeled "networked individualism". ICTs have multiplied relations and coordinations among persons, but hinder a unified sense of belonging and a stable identity among the members of a community (Krause & Montenegro, 2016). "High levels of personal mobility fracture the maintenance of relationships with fixed communities and favor the formation of 'new' groups of people with similarly fluid characteristics" (Findlay, Hoy, & Stockdale, 2004, p. 61).

In sum, Internet-mediated communities bring forth a new format of communication, a different definition of space, a new temporality, and scattered and multifaceted identifications. A relevant question for the present chapter is how do these changes affect their functions related to mental health?

The above transformations in communities have a potential impact on well-being because they alter several of the psychosocial and psychological determinants of health (Kulkarni, 2012), such as social support, attachment, and identity, and may even interact with genetic conditions (Luyten & Blatt, 2013).

For example, current transformations have altered the density of social relations within communities, reducing the availability of social support, a community function that is essential for mental health. Also, belonging to multiple communities simultaneously may hinder their identity-defining function.

The new, more "circumstantial" communities can be very empowered and politically effective (Tolosa, 2013) but their shorter lifespan may impede the healthy effect of empowerment on individual participants. In the long run, their ephemeral nature could even increase hopelessness, causing a negative impact on mental health.

Nevertheless, these changes in communities can also be regarded as an opportunity, because they involve a flexibility and dynamism that might benefit health. In contrast, while traditional communities, particularly those with clear geographical roots, were almost imposed on individual persons, the more dynamic communities of today, especially those mediated by communication technology, may open up spaces for individual freedom, thus promoting well-being. The possibility of having multiple memberships grants more opportunities to community members, enabling them to establish new connections, take up new roles, and develop their skills.

However, some empirical studies and conceptual analyses have linked the transformation of communities to mental health problems (e.g. depression) that are becoming increasingly common around the world (Gotlib & Hammen, 2002). It has been hypothesized that the weakening of communities and social bonds operates as a mediating variable between sociocultural changes and mental health problems (Campbell & Murray, 2004; Cornish, 2004). In 1989, Seligman had already pointed out that increasing levels of depression may have to do with "environmental determinants", noting the contrast between its prevalence among the general US population and some "non-modern" cultures. He considered that the growth in individualism to the detriment of the common good was the factor causing increased depression rates in some societies. This argument is still current: for Castonguay (2011, p. 132), "the lack of commitment to common projects, one could suggest, has robbed individuals of buffers against depression when they are confronted with personal difficulties or failures. Our over-involvement in activities aimed at increasing our individualistic accomplishments, wealth, and comfort might well make it more difficult to reach out for and obtain help and support from others when we experience serious difficulties in our lives".

16.3 Mindfulness Within the Context of Transforming Bonds

This section discusses how mindfulness provides an alternative for countering some negative effects that current social transformations can have on mental health.

Compared to past decades, information and communication technologies have enabled people to gain more immediate access to information, thus increasing interpersonal contact opportunities. The increased amount of available information and the growing number of potential bonds represent major opportunities for individuals, but can also threaten their mental health. The informational aspect of our technological era challenges our attentional capacities, which are left exposed to hyperstimulation and thus to the threats of losing focus and developing stress. Regarding ties with others, ours is a world characterized by a degree of hyperconnectivity that can leave individuals feeling dissatisfied due to their superficial, incomplete, or even fictional relationships, established by scattered selves with a non-integrated psychological functioning. Adolescents, hungry for information and contacts with their peers due to specific characteristics of their stage of development, are especially vulnerable to this threat.

In this context of immediacy that technologically mediated human relationships entail, practicing mindfulness can help people establish a deeper connection with themselves and others, thus gaining protection from the threat of superficiality. Mindfulness can also protect people from "networked individualism" and the exacerbation of perfectionism, discussed in prior sections. In consequence, it is not surprising to find that mindfulness and other meditative techniques have increasingly been integrated into psychotherapeutic (Kirmayer, 2015) and preventive interventions (Langer, Ulloa-Jiménez, Cangas, Rojas, & Krause, 2015).

16.3.1 Mindfulness for Contact with Oneself

Mindfulness, as "a mode of awareness that is present-centered and nonevaluative" (Kirmayer, 2015, p. 447), is a practice that lessens the stressful impact of the "hyperreality" of information and communication technologies and their attendant self-demands (Kirmayer, 2015). It heightens our perception of our own bodily and mental states, and therefore of our own needs and desires, within the context of a self-compassionate and accepting attitude. By helping us stay focused on ourselves, practicing mindfulness fosters psychological integration and the experience of a cohesive identity. With respect to its use for preventing psychological problems, it has been found to be an effective antidote to stress (Kirmayer, 2015), which is one of the main precursors of mental health issues. Systematic reviews and meta-analyses have provided extensive evidence of the efficacy of mindfulness-based interventions for a variety of mental health problems (Chiesa & Serretti, 2011; Keng, Smoski, & Robins, 2011).

16.3.2 *Mindfulness for Bonding with Others*

In a world where maintaining deep bonds with others is at risk, it is relevant to consider the potential of mindfulness practices as tools to foster empathy and, consequently, prosocial behaviors. The latter encourage civic commitment and social cohesion, because they involve focusing on a more general common good: that of the community. Empirical research has shown evidence for the positive effect of interventions aimed at strengthening bonds in social or community contexts, since contact reduces prejudice toward others, decreases anxiety, and increases empathy (Pettigrew, 2018). Increased contact with people from a variety of cultures, such as migrants, extends one's knowledge about others and helps one trust them (González et al., 2017). Studies belonging to this line of research show that prosociality is associated with high levels of empathy (Abrams, Van de Vyver, Pelletier, & Cameron, 2015).

From this perspective, mindfulness-based interventions can lead to greater openness toward others and a less anxious and prejudiced attitude, which should foster the establishment of personal bonds. It has even been demonstrated that greater openness toward one's own psychological states, trained through mindfulness practices, increases people's ability to represent and infer others' mental states. In other words, understanding ourselves helps us understand others (Böckler, Herrmann, Trautwein, Holmes, & Singer, 2017).

These findings open up interesting possibilities for preventive interventions aimed at young people, which should be able to foster both their contact with themselves and their empathy toward others. In this regard, a study conducted by Langer et al. (2015)—which sought to analyze the subjective experience of a group of adolescents after a mindfulness-based intervention developed for school contexts—represents a valuable precedent. Results published by Langer et al. (2015) reveal that adolescents report cognitive effects such as increased attention and concentration and improvements in their ability to solve problematic situations, along with emotional effects such as better mood, tranquility, and reduced stress symptoms, which have a positive effect on interactions with others by lessening aggressive behaviors. The young people interviewed also reported more self-acceptance, increased kindness and gratitude, and decreased self-criticism.

However, given the variety of mindfulness training methods available, in order to achieve an impact on empathy and thus strengthen bonds with others, it is important to consider research that shows that compassion-based practices are especially effective in producing ethical-motivational changes like a nonjudgmental attitude, compassion, and self-compassion (Hildebrandt, McCall, & Singer, 2017).

16.4 Conclusions

In this chapter, I described social transformations, particularly those affecting interpersonal and community bonds, analyzed their impact on mental health, and reflected on how mindfulness-based intervention strategies can contribute in this context.

The conclusion of this analysis is that, over the last decades, humanity (at least in Western societies) has been witness to a weakening of traditional bonds, compounded by a growing individualization process (Beck & Beck-Gernsheim, 2002) and the dissolution of traditional and stable communities (Bessant, 2011). This process results in individuals who are more reliant on themselves (and less dependent on prescribed social norms) when it comes to constructing their lives.

In a context marked by individualization and the weakening of community bonds, contemplative practices can shield us from potential reductions in well-being, which may be one of the reasons behind their growing popularity in Western cultures (Kirmayer, 2015). However, we need to include in this analysis a reflection on the impact of the largest transformation of the last decades: the widespread growth of information and communication technologies.

The social transformation of social bonds that took place in past decades has now been overcome by an explosion of technologically-mediated relationships, which have created a sort of "hyper-reality" of social bonds, now omnipresent and instantaneous. This new reality can be subjectively experienced as an exacerbation of the present: "it's all there, at our fingertips". A person living in today's world is potentially able to access all of the world's information and can follow every Internet link; also, by experimenting with a variety of characters, he/she has all the possible ways of "being" at his/her disposal. Amid this sea of possibilities, identifying our own defining characteristics and those of others can be a major challenge. Mindfulness and other contemplative practices precisely enable us to experience what is "true" in our contact with ourselves and others, thus preventing our own identity and our bonds with others from vanishing in a superficial "as if" world, where it is possible to construct multiple "false selves" subjected to extreme perfectionist demands. Practicing mindfulness, especially those varieties that include acceptance and compassion (Hildebrandt et al., 2017), makes it possible to buffer the negative effect that the transformations discussed can have on mental health. Contemplative practices such as mindfulness can teach the stressed inhabitants of technologically-mediated relationships to pay attention to their experience in the present moment, learn to know and accept their own thoughts and emotions, be kind to themselves, and maintain an attitude of empathetic and accepting openness toward others. By improving the relation with ourselves and others, contemplative practices can protect mental health while also giving us a chance to revert the impact of past adverse situations on our social bonds (Davidson and Begley, 2012).

References

Abrams, D., Van de Vyver, J., Pelletier, J., & Cameron, L. (2015). Children's prosocial behavioural intentions towards outgroup members. *British Journal of Developmental Psychology, 33*(3), 277–294.

Araujo, K., & Martuccelli, D. (2010). Individuation and the work of individuals. *Educação e Pesquisa, 36,* 77–91.

Bauman, Z. (2007). *Consuming life*. Cambridge: Polity Press.

Beck, U., & Beck-Gernsheim, E. (2002). *Individualization: institutionalized individualism and its social and political consequences*. London: Sage.

Bessant, K. (2011). Authenticity, community, and modernity. *Journal for the Theory of Social Behaviour, 41*(1), 2–32.

Böckler, A., Herrmann, L., Trautwein, F.-M., Holmes, T., & Singer, T. (2017). Know thy selves: Learning to understand oneself increases the ability to understand others. *Journal of Cognitive Enhancement, 1,* 197–209.

Brown, G. W., Andrews, B., Harris, T. O., Adler, Z., & Bridge, L. (1986). Social Support, self-esteem and depression. *Psychological Medicine, 6,* 813–831.

Brown, G. W., Sklair, F., Harris, T. O., & Birley, J. L. (1973). Life events and psychiatric disorders, Part I: Some methodological issues. *Psychological Medicine, 3,* 74–87.

Campbell, C., & McLean, C. (2003). Social capital, local community participation and the construction of Pakistani identities in England: Implications for health inequalities policies. *Journal of Health Psychology, 8*(2), 247–262.

Campbell, C., & Murray, M. (2004). Community health psychology: Promoting analysis and action for social change. *Journal of Health Psychology, 9*(2), 187–195.

Castonguay, L. G. (2011). Psychotherapy, psychopathology, research and practice. Pathways of connection and integration. *Psychotherapy Research, 21,* 125–140.

Castel, R. (2011). *Die Krise der Arbeit. Neue Unsicherheiten und die Zukunft des Individuums*. Hamburg: Hamburger Institut für Sozialforschung.

Castells, M. (2001). *Das Informationszeitalter*. Opladen: Leske & Budrich.

Chiao, J. Y., & Blizinsky, K. D. (2010). Culture—gene coevolution of individualism-collectivism and the serotonin transporter gene. *Proceedings of the Royal Society B: Biological Sciences, 277*(1681), 529–537.

Chiesa, A., & Serretti, A. (2011). Mindfulness based cognitive therapy for psychiatric disorders: A systematic review and meta-analysis. *Psychiatry Research, 187*(3), 441–453.

Cierpka, M. (2016). *Regulatory disorders in infants. Assessment, diagnosis, and treatment*. Berlin Heidelberg: Springer.

Cohen, S. (2004). Social relationships and health. *American Psychologist, 59,* 676–684.

Colclough, G., & Sitaraman, B. (2005). Community and social capital: What is the difference? *Sociological Inquiry, 75*(4), 474–496.

Cornish, F. (2004). Making 'context' concrete: A dialogical approach to the society-health relation. *Journal of Health Psychology, 9*(2), 281–294.

Curran, T. & Hill, A. P. (2017). Perfectionism is increasing over time: A meta-analysis of birth cohort differences from 1989 to 2016. Psychological bulletin. Advance online publication. https://www.apa.org/pubs/journals/releases/bul-bul0000138.pdf. Accessed January 19, 2019.

Dagnino, P., Pérez, C., Gómez, A., Gloger, S., & Krause, M. (2017). Depression and attachment: how do personality styles and social support influence this relation? *Research in Psychotherapy: Psychopathology, Process and Outcome, 20,* 53–62.

Davidson, R. J., & Begley, S. (2012). *The emotional life of your brain: How its unique patterns affect the way you think, feel, and live—and how you can change them*. London: Penguin Books.

Findlay, A. M., Hoy, C., & Stockdale, A. (2004). In what sense English? An exploration of English migrant identities and identification. *Journal of Ethnic and Migration Studies, 30,* 59–79.

Gómez, E., & Jaén, P. (2011). Transmisión intergeneracional del maltrato y aislamiento social. *Boletín de Psicología, 102,* 43–54.

González, G., Bargsted, M., Miranda, D., Carvacho, H., Tropp, L., van Laar, C., … Cheyre, M. (2017). Resultados Primera Ola Estudio Longitudinal Social de Chile (ELSOC). Módulo 1: Cohesión Social y Migración. Santiago: Notas COES de política pública. www.elsoc.cl/wp-content/uploads/2017/07/Modulo_I_cohesion_y_migracion.pdf. Accessed January 19, 2019.
Gotlib, I. H., & Hammen, C. L. (2002). Introduction. In I. H. Gotlib & C. L. Hammen (Eds.), *Handbook of depression* (pp. 1–20). New York: Guilford Press.
Güell, P., Peters, T., & Morales, R. (2012). Individuación y consumo cultural: las afinidades electivas. In P. Güell & T. Peters (Eds.), *La trama social de las prácticas culturales* (pp. 21–49). Santiago de Chile: Universidad Alberto Hurtado.
Heim, C., & Nemeroff, C. B. (2001). The role of childhood in the neurobiology of mood and anxiety disorders: Preclinical and clinical studies. *Biological Psychiatry, 49,* 1023–1039.
Hodgetts, D., Bolam, B., & Stephens, C. (2005). Mediation and the construction of contemporary understandings of health and lifestyle. *Journal of Health Psychology, 10,* 123–136.
Hildebrandt, L. K., McCall, C., & Singer, T. (2017). Differential effects of attention-, compassion-, and socio-cognitively based mental practices on self-reports of mindfulness and compassion. *Mindfulness, 8,* 1488–1512.
Keng, S. L., Smoski, M. J., & Robins, C. J. (2011). Effects of mindfulness on psychological health: A review of empirical studies. *Clinical Psychology Review, 31*(6), 1041–1056.
Kessler, R. C., & Bromet, E. J. (2013). The epidemiology of depression across cultures. *Annual Review of Public Health, 34,* 119–138.
Kim, H. S., Sherman, D. K., Mojaverian, T., Sasaki, J. Y., Park, J., Suh, E. M., et al. (2011). Gene–culture interaction: Oxytocin receptor polymorphism (OXTR) and emotion regulation. *Social Psychological and Personality Science, 2*(6), 665–672.
Kirmayer, L. (2015). Mindfulness in cultural context. *Transcultural Psychiatry, 52*(4) 447–469.
Krause, M., Güell, P., Jaramillo, A., Zilveti, M., Jiménez, J. P., & Luyten, P. (2015). Changing communities and increases in the prevalence of depression: Is there a relationship? *Universitas Psychologica, 14*(4), 1259–1268.
Krause, M., & Montenegro, C. (2016). Community as a multifaceted concept. In M. A. Bond, C. B. Keys, & I. Serrano-García (Eds.), *Handbook of community psychology* (pp. 275–294). Washington, D.C: American Psychological Association.
Kulkarni, M. (2012). Social determinants of health: The role of neighborhoods, psychological factors and health behaviors in predicting health outcomes for the urban poor in India. *Journal of Health Psychology, 18,* 96–109.
Langer, A. I., Ulloa-Jiménez, V. G., Cangas, A. J., Rojas, G., & Krause, M. (2015). Intervenciones basadas en mindfulness en educación secundaria ¿Una intervención bio-psico-social?: Una revisión sistemática cualitativa. *Estudios de Psicología/ Studies in Psychology, 36*(3), 533–570.
Luyten, P., & Blatt, S. (2013). Interpersonal relatedness and self-definition in normal and disrupted personality development. *American Psychologist, 68,* 172–183.
Mannarini, T., & Fedi, A. (2009). Multiple senses of community: The experience and meaning of community. *Journal of Community Psychology, 37*(2), 211–227.
McMillan, D. W., & Chavis, D. M. (1986). Sense of community: A definition and theory. *American Journal of Community Psychology, 14*(1), 6–23.
McLeod, J. D., & Shanahan, M. J. (1996). Trajectories of poverty and children's mental health. *Journal of Health and Social Behavior, 37*(3), 207–220.
McLeod, J. D., & Shanahan, M. J. (1993). Poverty, parenting, and children's mental health. *American Sociological Review, 58,* 351–366.
McLeod, J. D. (1991). Childhood parental loss and adult depression. *Journal of Health and Social Behavior, 32,* 205–220.
Mikulincer, M., & Shaver, P. R. (2007). *Attachment in adulthood: structure, dynamics, and change.* New York, NY: The Guilford Press.
Nisbet, R. A. (1953/1967). *Community and power (formerly "The quest for community").* New York, NY: Oxford University Press.

Olhaberry, M., Zapata, J., Escobar, M., Mena, C., Farkas, C., Santelices, M. P., et al. (2014). Antenatal depression and its relationship with problem-solving strategies, childhood abuse, social support, and attachment styles in a low-income Chilean sample. *Mental Health and Prevention, 2*, 86–97.

Pettigrew, T. F. (2018). The emergence of contextual social psychology. *Personality and Social Psychology Bulletin, 44*(7), 963–971.

Rappaport, J. (1984). Studies in empowerment: Introduction to the issue. In J. Rappaport, C. Swift, & R. E. Hess (Eds.), *Studies in empowerment* (pp. 1–7). Binghamton, NY: Haworth.

Sarason, S. B. (1974). *The psychological sense of community: Perspectives for community psychology*. San Francisco: Jossey-Bass.

Sennett, R. (2006). *The culture of the new capitalism*. Boston: Yale University Press.

Tolosa, M. (2013). *Comunidades y redes sociales. El desplome de las pirámides*. Santiago: Papyrbit.

Turró, C., & Krause, M. (2008). Beyond survival: Tracing individual empowerment processes in a poor Chilean settlement. *Journal of Community Psychology, 39*, 381–403.

UNDP. (2004). *Informe de Desarrollo Humano. El poder: ¿para qué y para quién?* Santiago de Chile: United Nations Development Program.

Veinot, T. C., & Williams, K. (2012). Following the "community" thread from sociology to information behavior and informatics: Uncovering theoretical continuities and research opportunities. *Journal of the American Society for Information Science and Technology, 63*(5), 847–864.

Way, B. M., & Lieberman, M. D. (2010). Is there a genetic contribution to cultural differences? Collectivism, individualism and genetic markers of social sensitivity. *Social Cognitive and Affective Neuroscience, 5*, 203–211.

Chapter 17
The Economics of Love: How a Meaningful and Mindful Life Can Promote Allocative Efficiency and Happiness

Felix Fuders and Vanessa Nowak

Each of you should use whatever gift
you have received to serve others
1. Peter 4:10

Abstract This chapter introduces the transcendental law of love for one's neighbor as a paradigm for economics before describing how this new economic model could be applied to enhance well-being. If there was an understanding that the purpose of life was not purely to make money, but to contribute to the common good, we would no longer need competition to force us to offer good products at good prices. We would simply do that by ourselves without any market pressure being necessary. That is to say, if people led a more meaningful and mindful life, a life in which they felt they were making a special contribution to the good of all through the use of their specific talents, we would achieve economic efficiency and, in addition, increase the 'gross national happiness'. This way, we could construct a veritable economy of neighborly love. An economy in which the wish to best serve one another, not market competition, is the principal driver behind the production of good products at good prices. Without stress and fear for economic survival, production would be efficient. People would be happy because they would feel that they made a special contribution to the well-being of all, and in so doing, provided their lives with greater meaning. We outline how such a paradigm shift could be promoted through a monetary reform and through an unconditional basic income.

F. Fuders (✉)
Faculty of Economics and Administration, Economics Institute, Universidad Austral de Chile, Valdivia, Chile
e-mail: felix.fuders@uach.cl

V. Nowak
German Chilean Competency Center for Development, Valdivia, Chile

Faculty of Engineering and Technology, Universidad San Sebastián, Valdivia, Chile

C. Steinebach and Á. I. Langer (eds.), *Enhancing Resilience in Youth*,
https://doi.org/10.1007/978-3-030-25513-8_17

Keywords Paradigm for economics · Market failure · Meaning of life · Basic income · Allocative efficiency

17.1 Introduction

This chapter introduces the transcendental law of love for one's neighbor as a paradigm for economics before describing how this new economic model could be applied to enhance well-being. If there was an understanding that the purpose of life was not purely to make money, but to contribute to the common good, we would no longer need competition to force us to offer good products at good prices. We would simply do that by ourselves without any market pressure being necessary. That is to say, if people led a more meaningful and mindful life, a life in which they felt they were making a special contribution to the good of all through the use of their specific talents—their 'comparative advantages' in the literal sense of David Ricardo—we would achieve economic efficiency and, in addition, increase the 'gross national happiness'.

While we still assume that our financial system is the main reason for market failure (e.g. Fuders, 2016, 2017) and while we still plead for a reform of our monetary system so that money only operates as a medium of exchange aimed at establishing a market economy that serves people and not vice versa, here we go even a step further: if we combined such a monetary reform with a change of consciousness, we could even shift from a market economy serving people to what might be called 'economics of love' in which people achieve true happiness and self-actualization by serving each other through the use of their individual talents. Such a sea change in thinking would require a great deal of educational work. This educational reform is outlined in Chap. 12 of this book.

17.2 Competition Compels Us to Behave as if We Loved One Another

Markets and the concept 'perfect competition' are being increasingly challenged. One plausible driver of this dissatisfaction might be the disparity in wealth observed in many countries (e.g. Bárcena, Cimoli, García-Buchaca, & Pérez, 2018). Also, the destruction of the environment, excessive egoism, individualism, and the so-called 'elbow-society' in which everyone seems to think only of themselves first are associated with competition. A frequent criticism of the competitive economy is that instead of competition, one should rely on cooperation (e.g. Latouche, 2003, 2009; Felber, 2009; Traverso, 2015). Yet, the destruction of the environment and the growing inequality are not caused by the competitive economy, but by our monetary system. In particular, it is the money rate of interest that demands constant economic growth and fuels inequality (Soddy, 1934; Creutz, 1993; Kennedy, 1990,

2011; Lietaer, Arnsperger, Goerner, & Brunnhuber, 2013; Fuders, 2009a, 2009b, 2010, 2016, 2017; Fuders & Max-Neef, 2014a). Individualism, too, is not caused by competition directly, but by a lack of love for one's neighbor, combined with the ability to conveniently store work in the form of monetary units, which our unnatural[1] monetary system makes possible (Fuders, 2017).

17.2.1 Competition Does Not Impede Cooperation

Free market competition does not impede cooperation. On the contrary, any company can be seen as a cooperation between different stakeholders to produce a certain product or service. Also, beneficial companies can cooperate among each other, to a certain extent. However, competition law prohibits cooperation in pricing or other competition parameters. There are good reasons for such restrictions. Not only does price-fixing between competitors limit the freedom of third parties (legal-philosophical justification of competition law—see e.g. Emmerich, 2001; Mestmäcker & Schweitzer, 2004; Fuders, 2011) and decrease efficiency (economic justification of competition law—see e.g. Fuders 2009b, 2011); such agreements (called collusion or cartels) also contradict neighborly love because they serve to bundle market power with the principal aim of selling a product at a higher price, but without any improvement. Price agreements between competitors thus serve to enrich the company owners unjustifiably at the expense of the consumer.

It is not only price agreements between competing companies that contradict the principle of loving one's neighbor, but any type of concerted action with the aim of restricting competition. For the same reason, competition law in many countries also prohibits agreements on advertising or research budgets as well as the division of markets (Fuders, 2009b). Companies that hold a dominant position on their own (monopolies) do not even have to compromise with competitors in order to impose prices on customers that the latter would not pay in a state of perfect competition. This is why, in addition to concerted practices, competition law usually prohibits the abuse of a dominant market position and, in many countries, even allows an *ex ante* control of corporate mergers (Fuders, 2009b). To sum up: 'workable' competition (which is the state as close as we can realistically get to the theoretical concept of 'perfect' competition; Clark, 1940; Kantzenbach, 1966) forces producers to offer the best possible products at the best possible prices, to avoid being pushed out of the market (Fig. 17.1). This should be regarded favorably, as offering good products at good prices is a behavior comparable to charity. In this way, competition causes us to behave as if we loved one another.

To further clarify this, let us examine the following example: The Ibis hotel group promises all customers that if a problem is not resolved within 15 min, the customer will be given a night's stay for free. One might think that such an offer is a realization

[1]That our money and, in particular, the money rate of interest contradict the laws of nature was already pointed out by Aristotle (1995a, p. 1258b).

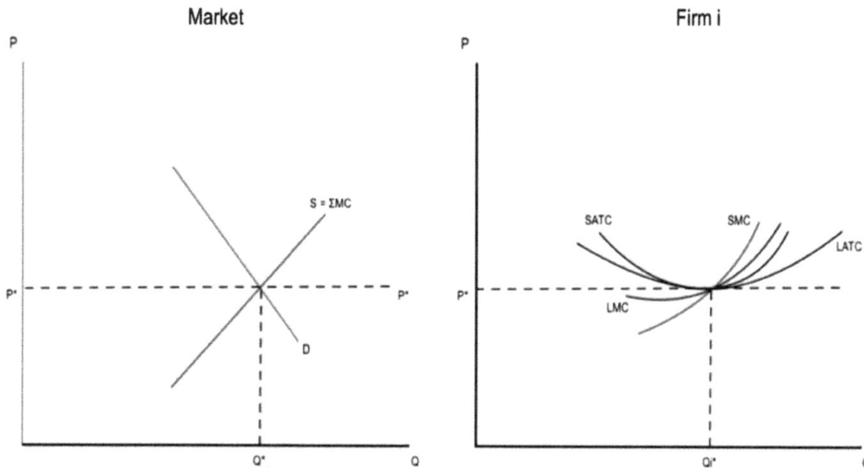

Fig. 17.1 Long-term equilibrium in perfect competition. *Source* own work. Explanation: The market price P* is at the lowest possible level (minimum Short-term Average Total Costs curve [SATC] and Long-term Average Total Cost curve [LATC])

of neighborly love. But, most probably, Ibis is compelled to make this offer by the pressure of heavy competition in the hotel market. Here, for the consumer at least, competition is wonderful. It forces us to behave in a way that, for all intents and purposes, represents neighborly love. Of course, it would be better if companies actually behaved like this out of love for their neighbor, i.e. out of eagerness to contribute to the common good and not because competition obliges them to do so. Interestingly, company owners who have realized that earning money is not an end in itself may do so (we come back to this later). For everyone else, there is competition.

17.2.2 Competition Limits Our Selfishness

That selfishness, individualism, and the so-called 'elbow society' are associated with the competitive economy may also have been reinforced by a questionable, but frequently heard interpretation of a much-cited Adam Smith quote:

> (…) and by directing that industry in such a manner as its produce may be of the greatest value, he intends only his own gain; and he is in this, as in many other cases, led by an invisible hand to promote an end which was no part of his intention. Nor is it always the worse for the society that it was no part of it. By pursuing his own interest, he frequently promotes that of the society more effectually than when he really intends to promote it. (Smith, 1952, p. 194)

Often, this statement is misinterpreted as expressing the egoistic, self-interested behavior of market participants, which, being controlled by an 'invisible hand', causes the efficient allocation of resources (e.g. Frank, 2008; Common & Stagl,

2008). In fact, the opposite is true: it is despite our selfishness that competition compels us to behave as if we loved one another: to offer the best products at the best prices, in what economists term *allocative efficiency* (in the long-term competitive equilibrium, the price is equal to the minimum point of long-term total average cost curve (LATC in Fig. 17.1), which means there is no less expensive, i.e. more efficient way to produce). It is not selfishness that drives competition. Rather, competition limits our selfishness.

17.2.3 Neighborly Love Would Render Competition Unnecessary

Selfishness is no virtue, but the opposite of neighborly love and, possibly, the transcendental cause of all evil in the world. As outlined above, competition promotes allocative efficiency even though we are egoists. Whenever the mechanism that compels us to produce the best possible products at the best prices (*allocative efficiency*) does not work, we speak of *market failures*. A monopoly, for example, is a structural market failure and the opposite of so-called perfect competition (e.g. Frank, 2008). While in perfect competition each market player earns exactly the amount that equals the opportunity cost of the production factors invested (i.e. the amount he could have earned elsewhere with his investment in capital, time, diligence, and knowledge), the monopolist can demand prices that are out of all proportion to the cost of production—obtaining a so-called 'monopoly rent'. Achieving monopoly rents is a selfish behavior. Someone who loves their neighbor will not exploit their market power even if they hold a dominant market position. Instead, they might only set a moderate price relative to production costs. Unfortunately, selfishness is hardly regarded as something reprehensible in economics today, which might, in part, be due to a questionable interpretation of Adam Smith's 'invisible hand'. Indeed, the achievement of monopoly rents is even considered desirable for entrepreneurs and makes up essential parts of business strategies (e.g. Stalk, 2004).

In fact, all market failures can be seen as a failure of the mechanism to compel us to behave in a manner consistent with the love-thy-neighbor principle. For example, those who love their neighbor will not collude with competitors to artificially create market power with the objective of imposing prices that the customer would not pay in a state of 'workable competition'—to use Clark's famous expression once again. Also, there would be no unfair competition, such as misleading advertising. The three pillars of competition law (the prohibition of the abuse of a dominant position; the ban on concerted actions regarding competition parameters; and unfair competition) would not be necessary if everyone respected and practiced the commandment to love one another. Also, our monetary system, identified as the main (but possibly least recognized) reason for market failure (see Fuders, 2016, 2017) is, in fact, the result of this lack of love for one's neighbor. This is principally seen in the urge to accumulate monetary units and thus interrupt the economic cycle or 'blackmail' an interest for putting it in circulation (Gesell, 1949, p. 344), "to exploit the scarcity-value of capital" as Keynes (1936, p. 376) put it. If we were not selfish and everyone fully practiced neighborly love, we would not need any competition law and maybe not even a monetary reform to incentivize us to produce the best products at the best prices (on this see Fuders, 2017). This leads us to venture a little utopia: to outline a model of an economy based on the love-your-neighbor principle.[2]

17.3 Neighborly Love as New Paradigm for Economics

We have outlined above how genuinely workable competition is to be desired as it forces the market to offer the best possible products at the best possible prices. But we have also acknowledged that it would be of further advantage if we were to offer the best possible products at the best possible prices without the pressure of competition being necessary.

17.3.1 Finding Our Vocation as True Meaning of Life

Those who have reflected on the meaning of life might conclude that their true purpose is to promote the common good by practicing neighborly love. For Christians, both the Old Testament and the New Testament state, as the two highest commandments and God's will, to love God and to love one another (Bible, Leviticus 19:18; Deuteronomy 6:5; Matthew 22:37–22:39; Galatians 5:14). According to Christ, both commandments are equally important (Mathew 22:40). In this chapter, we use the Christian principle of love for one's neighbor as the basis for building an economy of love. However, the commandment to love one another seems to be the cornerstone of many other religions too (for Islam see Quran, Surah 42:23; for Judaism see Tora, Lev 19,18). There is evidence in psychology showing that prosocial and altruistic behaviors can be cultivated in a secular way (e.g. Condon, 2017).

Love for one's neighbor translates into treating others as we would like to be treated; not to do onto our neighbor what we would not want to be done on us (Matthew 7:12). One could say that loving our neighbor is the perfect realization of Immanuel Kant's categorical imperative (Kant, 1868b), which in its best-known version asks us to act only according to that maxim whereby you can, at the same time, will that it should become a universal law. However, neighborly love is not just reserved for helping people in distress, proselytizing, warning people of occult practices, or observing the Ten Commandments, which, in fact, can be seen as a concretization of the wider commandment to love one another. Neighborly love also compels us to make use of our talents for the benefit of the common good. Part of

[2]The idea of an economy based on neighborly love instead of competition has already been laid down in Fuders (2017).

the realization of neighborly love is therefore also to find our vocation and make it our profession or a life's work, so that we may earn our daily bread with our skills.

Interestingly, the German word for profession is 'Beruf', which derives from 'Berufung', which means vocation. The word 'Berufung' itself contains the word 'Ruf', which means 'call'. The 'Berufung' is God's call for a special service (Kluge, 1989). In the same way, the English expression 'vocation' derives from 'vocatio', which is Latin and means invitation. 'Vocatio' itself contains the expression 'voca' most probably from 'bucca' (latin = mouth); in other words, we are called to serve.

17.3.2 Using Our Vocation Fosters Allocative Efficiency

A person's vocation is dependent on the individual, as people have different talents. That we should use these talents derives from the commandment to love our neighbor. As part of neighborly love can be regarded the promotion of the common good by bringing in our divine gifts to the community, a point already explained by both Paul (Romans 12: 1–8) and Peter (1 Peter 4:10). Consider, as an example, a conventional factory line: as much as the worker is convinced that he should be thanked for any added value produced, usually the head of a company perceives that he is responsible for such value creation. The inventor, in turn, believes that the company that has bought his patent is profitable thanks to his invention. In fact, all three are wrong. The company owner, the inventor, and the worker are *jointly* involved in the creation of value. Everyone has their place in the world. No one can do without the other. The inventor as a scientist or engineer often is not a good entrepreneur. The entrepreneur cannot produce products without someone putting them together on the production line. The worker on the assembly line might not have the talent to run a business.

In this regard, every human being can be seen as part of the great puzzle of 'love' that may not be fully explored or understood by each individual, but through which everyone can still contribute to by consistently practicing neighborly love through his or her talents. This can be deemed a principal part of the realization of neighborly love, because we help others the most by utilizing the talents we have been endowed with. In economics, this would be described as *allocative efficiency*, the form of the best allocation of resources, or, in the words of Ricardo (1911), the exploitation of 'comparative advantages', which here are our individual talents.

So, when we utilize our talents and gifts to perform the tasks we are best suited to, we will promote the common good in the best way possible. Furthermore, one might argue that we harm our neighbor if we occupy a job position for which we were not actually suited and thus prevent other people from doing this work. Here, to use an expression made famous by Abraham Maslow (Maslow, 2005, p. 173 ff.), another person could reach 'self-actualization' in this role. This could be likened to trying to force a piece of a puzzle into a place it does not belong. This way, we do not only destroy the slice, but also the puzzle will never be whole again since the slice will be missing on the location where it was planned to go by the creator of the puzzle.

In this sense the so-called *Pareto efficiency* will never be reached as long as persons occupy a job in which they do not use their special talents. Pareto efficiency (according to Italian engineer and economist Vilfredo Pareto) is another frequently used definition of efficiency in economics. A society is Pareto efficient if it is impossible to reallocate resources so as to make any individual better off without making at least one individual worse off (Frank, 2008). However, as long as there is just one person in an economy occupying a job in which they do not use their talents effectively, the society cannot be Pareto efficient. The person who holds a job they are not made for improves the well-being of all (including their own) by looking for a job in which they can actually make their special contribution to society. At the same time, the new vacancy gives another person the opportunity to self-actualize and contribute to the common good with their talents.

We can now answer the old and famous question of whether we work to live or live to work. The answer is that we live to work, at least if we agree that we live to contribute to the common good with our talents. Then, work is no punishment but a blessing (Escrivá de Balaguer, 1986). From a Christian perspective, and if we make use of our vocation, this offers us the possibility to help God in his creation, to become co-creators and participate in the divine creativity (Fernández Carvajal, 1987; Escrivá de Balaguer, 2010). Insofar, we can conclude that it is our very duty to use our gifts and talents for the benefit of all and not only as an exercise through which to earn money. We explore this idea more fully below.

17.3.3 Earning Money Is Not an End in Itself

Does it make a difference which parts of our body we make use of? Is it therefore not true that anyone who does an activity not out of love, but only for the sake of making money, is basically prostituting himself or herself? Of course, we have to earn money, but not as an end in itself. Indeed, even Aristotle (1995a) refused what he called '*chrematistics*' (the earning of money as an end in itself). Chrematistics can be seen as the opposite of what Aristotle used to call '*oikonomia*' (the efficient use of the household's resources: Aristotle, 1995a). Even though the term 'economics' finds its origin in the Greek 'oikonomia', today when we speak of economics we usually refer to what Aristotle describes as 'chrematistics'.

That earning money should not become an end in itself can actually also be deduced from the teachings of Christ, who encouraged us to do good without expecting something in return (Luke 6:35). This verse has to be read in conjunction with the request to be faithful and not worry about the future. Just as God gave the birds food, He would not allow people to starve (Luke 12:24, Matthew 6:26). This parable is not a call to idleness or to stop working, since the Holy Scripture also teaches us that those who are unwilling to work shall not eat either (2 Thessalonians, 3:10). Rather, it means that when we do our daily work, we do not need to worry about our livelihoods. Hence, this parable could be interpreted as a call to accept a job because it enables us to make a special contribution to society rather than simply because it pays well.

17.3.4 How to Find Out, What Our Talents Are?

We should, as explained above, earn our daily bread with an activity that corresponds to our vocation. This is an activity that gives us personal fulfillment and satisfaction—something we love to do. An activity we love is an activity we would undertake without expected financial reward. This is why we can find out what our vocation is by selecting an activity that we would dedicate ourselves to even if we did not get paid in monetary units for it.

Although money is the most common form of remuneration, it is not the only one. For example, a person might be conducting an activity voluntarily, yet joylessly, moved only by the recognition associated with that role. This can be seen as being as superficial as the pursuit of money. This is probably why the best way to answer the question of whether or not we are employing our talents in a certain job is to ask if we would do this work even on the last day of our life, assuming we knew what day this is. The motivation behind any activity that we perform on our last day would certainly not be the pursuit of money or recognition. On the last day of our lives, we will do only activities we love to do, and these are just activities for which we have a special talent. This is because when we feel that what we are doing something very special for the benefit of others, we feel happy. It is precisely serving others with our talents what gives us true pleasure. Indeed, serving others through an activity that someone else might do better is certainly less satisfactory as we do not feel we have given a special contribution to the well-being of others. On our last day of life, we would most probably not be pursuing such an activity.

In this very sense, the founder of Apple Computers Steve Jobs once remarked at a keynote speech at Standford University that everything in life is about love: *"You've got to find what you love, and this is true for your work as it is true for your lovers (…) the only way to be truly satisfied is to do what you believe is great work. And the only way to do great work is to love what you do. If you haven't found it yet, keep looking"*. In his address, Steve Jobs confessed that since he was 17 years old, he had asked himself every morning that if this day were his last day in his life would he do what he was going to do this day? And when the answer had been 'no' in too many days in a row, he said that he then knew he needed to change something (Jobs, 2005).

17.3.5 Neighborly Love Makes Us Truly Happy

There is no clear correlation between happiness and income. Those countries that achieve the highest marks in the so-called Happy Planet Index (Nef, 2018) are not those considered to be the most developed (Fuders, 2015). Indeed, in economics, a new discipline has sprung up in recent years: the *Economics of Happiness*. But even if we measured development alternatively from GDP (e.g. by measuring the satisfaction of fundamental human needs; Fuders et al., 2016), it is doubtful that development and happiness would be clearly correlated. At a United Nations conference in 2012 (Wikipedia, 2018b), which debated the 'Gross National Happiness', there was a sign with a wise inscription:

If you want happiness…

- for an hour - take a nap
- for a day - go fishing
- for a month - get married
- for a year - inherit a fortune
- for a lifetime - help someone else

This means that, if we truly want long-lasting happiness, we should aim to constantly help and serve others. Here, we do not refer to happiness as the superficial, materialistic joy we feel after having bought new possessions (e.g. a car), but to a deep sense of inner fulfillment that might come from the intuitive knowledge that you are contributing to the divine puzzle—to once again use this metaphor. If we appreciate that the purpose of life is not to make as much money as possible, but to earn money with an activity that we would undertake even without the promise of any monetary gain (and even on the last day of our life), then this will make us truly happy. It will make us happy because we feel that we are making a contribution to the common good. Unlike Aristotle (1995b) in his Nicomachean Ethics, we do not consider felicitousness (*eudaimonia*) to be the highest aspirational good. The pursuit of happiness as an end in itself might even be considered as superficial as the pursuit of money or recognition. Rather, true happiness can be considered as compensation for achieving the highest goal: the realization of neighborly love. This can also be derived from the German word for felicitousness (Glückseligkeit), in which the words 'happiness' (Glück) and 'soul' (Seele) are combined. Felicitousness is the state in which the soul is happy.

Among high-level business managers, it is becoming fashionable to use vacation time to work. Such a person might, for example, work as a farm hand in a traditional small family farm in the Swiss mountains. These 'working holidays' involve starting early and a day of hard work. They do this without getting paid; instead, they pay for the experience as a sort of occupational therapy. One might ask, why do not these people do this job all their life? Why are they doing this freely (and even pay for it) as a recreational occupation? One probable reason is that this work gives them the sensation, maybe more than their job as CEO, that they are contributing something truly useful. In fact, the so-called 'occupational therapy' is based on just this idea: to develop, recover, or maintain meaningful activities (*occupations*) for people with disabilities or mental health problems, especially depression (Wikipedia, 2018a). Where does their depression come from? Is it really only caused by a disorder of serotonin or other neurotransmitters in the brain of depressive people? And if so, where does this disorder come from? One aspect of this condition, notwithstanding other drivers, could be that people with depression are lacking a sense of purpose in life. Here, a meaningful occupation might provide the chance to feel they are contributing to society. In the same way, the increasing number of people with *burnout syndrome* (Maslach et al., 2001; Dorsch, 2017) could be due to precisely this. These people do not like their jobs, they intuitively recognize that they are wasting their life, and this makes them less stress-resistant.

17.3.6 Employing Our Talents Fosters Economic Success

For many, the only reason to work is to earn money and, in so doing, be 'successful'. Such a rationale fits the concept of the so-called '*homo oeconomicus*'. On the other hand, the Economics of Love, as we promote it here, is about serving each other as a way of reaching true and lasting happiness. Although a monetary reward in our model is not an end in itself, we may also be more economically successful if we make use of our talents: a person who uses their talents for a certain task will most likely perform it better than someone who does the same activity reluctantly and only for the sake of gaining money. For example, in the long run, it is foreseeable that someone with a talent for cooking will be more successful as a cook than if he tried to construct machines as a mediocre engineer.

Some readers might now criticize that there are also activities that no one enjoys doing, such as simple, boring activities. We are convinced that—as St. Paul stated (Romans 12: 1–8)—*every* person has gifts, and there are also people who are made to perform simple activities and even prefer to do those because they would be overstrained with other, more sophisticated jobs. Conversely, someone who has a talent for engineering or science will be bored with simple activities that require little concentration. This person will feel that they are wasting their life and will not undertake such an activity with joy and dedication. Instead, they would need to be incentivized with the prospect of earning money. Maybe this person would be so bored by their simple task that they would perform to a lower standard than a person who is less blessed with abilities, but who would do this job with joy, feeling that they are doing something useful and, in that, contributing to a positive development of society. That is to say, even with tasks that many would be reluctant to perform, others might realize 'self-actualization' and be economically successful. With simple tasks, one too can make a valuable contribution to the well-being of all. This is why there are no low-category jobs, all are of great importance (Escrivá de Balaguer, 1986, 2004, 2010, 2012). However, we stress here that this is only the case if one was created for this simple activity.

17.3.7 Serving Others with Our Talents to Reach Freedom and Dignity

Using our talents for the benefit of all, as the fulfillment of neighborly love—and the transcendental meaning of life—might even contribute to the realization of freedom. Freedom, as we learn from Kant, is the state of being unconstrained by other people's arbitrary choices (Kant, 1868a, 1868b). This also means that the freedom of others should not be limited by our own compelling arbitrariness. That, in turn, means we should not occupy a job other people are better suited for. We can understand that the realization of freedom is connected herewith when we recognize that freedom does not necessarily depend on external circumstances. For example, someone sitting in their office all day may be less exposed to the open air than someone in prison (who might be allowed to do sports in the prison's yard). However, this person does not necessarily feel imprisoned, at least not if they enjoy and love their job. Instead, they feel that their work is making a valuable contribution to the well-being of all. On the other hand, someone who works the whole day outside, e.g. on a construction site, may feel less free than someone sitting in the office all day if they feel compelled to work in order to survive. The difference between a slave and a free man is that the free man is doing his job out of *free will*, i.e. voluntarily and not only to survive. However, this does not mean that activities in which one uses one's talents cannot be tedious and exhausting. Certainly, an activity for which one is talented, and for which one also feels they are making a special contribution to society (and that they therefore love to do), is going to be easier than any activity that one does only for the sake of gaining money (Traverso, 2015). Nevertheless, it can still be exhausting. Indeed, this may be the reason why some argue that work dignifies man (Fernández Carvajal, 1987; Escrivá de Balaguer, 2010, 2012).

17.3.8 Serving Others with Our Talents Reduces Individualism

Recognizing that a meaningful life consists of helping one another by making use of our talents might remedy some of the deplorable characteristics of our current lifestyle. Steadily growing individualism and the 'elbow society' create communities in which many only think of themselves and in which they push fellow human beings aside in order to improve their own situation. Yet, this is not a side effect of competition, as some think (Traverso, 2015). Rather, the 'elbow society' comes about because people do not realize that their purpose in life should be to promote the common good, instead of accumulating as much, mostly 'virtual' (Soddy 1933), wealth as possible. After all, the Bible is true in that we one cannot serve God (who is love: 1 John 4: 8) and money (Matthew 6: 24). When we understand this, selfish behavior becomes contradictory. There would be no people working full-time as speculators or living on interest, as these activities do not contribute to the well-being of others, but rather exist at the expense of others (Fuders, 2017). It is precisely because most people have not yet come to this deeper understanding of the meaning of life that we need a workable competition that limits our egoism and its related vices.

We can now understand the greed for accumulating monetary units by people who have already earned so much money that they cannot spend their income in a meaningful manner: they do not like their job. It is possible they would not work at all if not for the sake of money. However, their intuition tells them that they are wasting their life. Indeed, because they only work for the money they get, any merit becomes unsatisfactory. No merit in the world can make up for lost time. Making money for those people thus becomes a kind of addiction, where the dosage has to be increased on a regular basis to achieve a short-term feeling of superficial happiness—a small compensation for the feeling of wasting their life.

17.3.9 Serving Others with Our Talents for More Justice

Using one's talents also helps to make society more just. Plato philosophized on this topic and incorporated it into his theory of justice. He found justice to be righteous when each person performs the service for which his nature is best adapted (Plato, 2011). According to Plato, "to do one's own business and not to be a busybody is justice" (Plato 2011, p. 332 ff.). In fact, one can deduce the obligation to use one's talents (and also the aspect of justice derived thereof) also from the Bible. Here we learn that God is just (Psalm 116: 5) and also that God is love (1 John 4:8). Thus, infringing against the commandment to love one another is a violation of justice. Furthermore, the Holy Scripture teaches us that there is righteousness when one lives in love and keeps God's commandments (Ezekiel 18: 9). As the use of one's talents for the benefit of all can be seen as part of the realization of neighborly love, exercising any activity solely for the sake of monetary gain and not making use of our special abilities and talents becomes a violation of the commandment to love one another and, thus, of justice. In this understanding of justice, and in accordance with Plato (2011), the government of a state should ensure that everyone carries out their tasks according to their abilities and without interfering with the responsibilities of others. In consequence, in addition to a monetary reform, we could consider it a task of the state to introduce an unconditional basic income and teach schoolchildren that earning money is not an end in itself. We will come back to this recommendation later.

17.3.10 Trust Will Rule Over Control

Mediocrity and, above all, laziness are well-known vices (Fernández Carvajal, 1987). These may come from the fact that many people would only do a job in order to earn their daily bread and not without financial gain. When they do not love their job and only work for money, they do not undertake it with real dedication and mindfulness. Without supervision, these people do little work or none at all. Such behavior occurs unrelated to pay scale. A good salary alone is hardly likely to motivate an employee to carry out their task more conscientiously if they do not feel joy in the performance of their work. Mediocrity is not found in people who do their work with joy, or is at least much less frequent. For example, we know a particular craftsman who has done all his work to a higher standard than expected. One can depend on him and trust him to the extent that it is not necessary to negotiate prices in advance. With this craftsman one can trust that he will charge a fair amount for any work undertaken. Where does this difference to other workers come from? It is possible to quickly recognize that this craftsman loves his work and the satisfaction that it brings him. He does not only work for the sake of making money. Indeed, he once remarked that positive feedback from his clients is more important to him than any monetary reward.

If all people were to do their work that conscientiously—and above all with love—control would no longer be necessary. The well-used adage "trust is good, but control is better" would be turned upside down. An economy of neighborly love would therefore also be an economy of trust. Incidentally, the aforementioned craftsman is also doing well economically, despite having no higher education. He receives big orders and builds entire houses, because word has spread that he does good work for a fair price. He also makes a happy impression, which confirms what we have already outlined above: the person who carries out their work with love and dedication ultimately also serves themselves through happiness and economic success.

17.3.11 A Completely New Entrepreneurship Would Be Possible

Business owners who have understood that making money is not an end in itself, and that their job is to contribute to society through their products and services, will behave differently to most other companies. A notable example in Chile is a company that sells "*Late*" mineral water. On the label of the bottle, the buyer is assured that 100% of the profit will be donated to charity. Indeed, the brand name comes from the phrase "late tu corazón" (your heart beats). As explained on the label, this relates to the feeling that the purchaser can expect knowing that their purchase has had a positive impact. The company's website announces that nearly 1,000,000 euros have been donated to date (Late, 2018). There is real potential for this corporate concept to pioneer a new generation of businesses. The fact that all surpluses are donated does not necessarily mean that the owners work completely free of charge. If the owners pay a fair salary to themselves, i.e. a salary the owner could gain as employee somewhere else with the same talent, time and knowledge invested, they do not contradict their charitable ambitions (as long as all other surpluses are donated or reinvested).

Could all companies operate in such a fashion? The answer is yes, they could—at least if they acknowledged that the purpose of their existence is to contribute to the well-being of society with their products. Such an entrepreneur would be happy to see people using their products because that is why they made them. If there was a surplus at the end of the year, such an entrepreneur would donate their surpluses and/or raise the salaries of their employees or reduce the prices of their products the following year. This process would truly *create shared value* (Porter & Kramer, 2011).

Of course, such an entrepreneur would not exploit a dominant position were they able to do so, or agree with competitors on prices (i.e. form cartels). Such behavior makes little sense if one sees the purpose of their existence in living and practicing neighborly love. On the contrary, the entrepreneur would endeavor voluntarily—and without competition having to force them to do so—to offer their products at lower rather than higher prices since they desire to contribute to customer well-being. Competition law prohibiting the abuse of a dominant market position, price fixing, and unfair behaviors (the three pillars of perfect competition) would no longer be necessary if all entrepreneurs thought that way. Such a market economy would serve people by allowing them the freedom to serve one another. This would truly be an economy of neighborly love.

17.4 Economic Incentives to Promote the Paradigm Shift

17.4.1 Reform of Our Monetary System

The change in personal and societal consciousness could be promoted by an educational reform as proposed in Chap. 12 of this book. Yet many of the benefits of such a new consciousness could also be fostered indirectly through a reform of the monetary system. In a monetary system as that proposed by German-Argentine businessman Silvio Gesell 100 years ago, it would be impossible to hoard large sums of money for long periods. Gesell's idea was that money should serve only as a medium of exchange and not as a means to hoard (virtual) wealth (Gesell, 1949). Surpluses would have to be consumed or invested productively. In such a monetary system, it would make less sense to accept a job only on the promise of a high salary. Furthermore, money that loses value if hoarded too long (like many tangible goods) would limit our 'preference for liquidity' (Keynes, 1936). This preference is the urge to preserve material wealth in the form of monetary units. If one cannot hoard huge amounts of money anyway, this will reduce the appeal of a particularly well-paid, but otherwise unattractive, position. Therefore, it encourages people to select a job in which they might earn less money but feel that they are making a special contribution to the well-being of all. That is to say, such a reform of our monetary system is not only necessary to avoid the many negative side effects inherent in our monetary system (our money system is, in many ways, completely unnatural, forces us to grow and with this to destroy our natural environment and can be seen as a main driver behind the steadily growing income inequality and the regular occurrence of financial and economic crises; see Soddy, 1934; Gesell, 1949; Kennedy 1990, 2011; Creutz, 1993; Fuders, 2009a, 2009b, 2010, 2016, 2017; Fuders et al., 2013; Fuders & Belloy, 2013; Fuders & Max-Neef, 2014a, 2014b) but would also significantly contribute to the establishment of an economy based on neighborly love even if we have not yet realized that this is the purpose of life. Such a monetary reform thus promotes a market economy in which not the accumulation of money, but the desire to contribute to the common good, is the driving force of our actions.

17.4.2 Basic Income Guarantee

In addition to the monetary reform, a Basic Income Guarantee could serve to promote the shift from an economy that requires competitive pressure to achieve allocative efficiency to an economy of love. The introduction of a basic income guarantee has been discussed since the 1960s (Theobald, 1967; Pechman & Timpane, 1975). Unfortunately, the concept is often misunderstood. For example, in a referendum in Switzerland (2016), the majority voted against the implementation of such a guaranteed income. This rejection may have been partly due to associations with well-known socialistic policies. However, it has little to do with socialism. On the contrary, while excessive socialism has proven to foster idleness and a severely inefficient allocation of resources, the concept of a guaranteed basic income could encourage people to choose a job in which they made use of their talents and, in so doing, improve allocative efficiency.

At this point we do not want to debate about whether or not a governmental basic income guarantee would be fundable. Rather, we would like to point out that, were it to be financially viable, it certainly would have advantages. This is not only because of the benefits of the redistribution of income some might see, but also because it encourages people to pursue an activity commensurate with their talents—even when such an employment shift would incur an initial financial cost. Such a basic income would be paid regardless of assets and other income. The idea is to reduce the jobseeker's fear that the pursuit of their desired profession (that assumedly matches their talents) is financially unviable. If there is a basic income guarantee, a jobseeker might be more willing to pursue an activity where they feel they can make a special contribution to society regardless of initial financial costs. Similar functions also characterize classic unemployment benefit programs, e.g. the German Arbeitslosengeld II (ALG II). Nevertheless, basic income has advantages over the ALG II. For example, if an ALG II beneficiary finds a job, the amount they earn will be deducted from their stipend. Consequently, if they have not yet realized the importance of employing their talents to contribute to the common good, they have little incentive to look for a position that offers less than their ALG II payment.

We suggest this would decrease their probability of discovering the enjoyment of love-based work in a position where they could contribute to the well-being of all.

17.5 Summary: Allocative Efficiency Without Competitive Pressure

In this chapter, we stressed that loving one another does not (only) mean occasionally donating money to charity or complying with the Ten Commandments. Rather, neighborly love can be lived through our daily work. The best way for us to contribute to the common good is to use our talents. On the other hand, if we perform an activity that does not correspond to our talents, we diminish our service to the well-being of society. We might even harm others by preventing someone better suited to the position from having the opportunity to self-actualize and contribute to the common good. By understanding that (i) it is important to use our talents and that (ii) the purpose of doing business is not just to make money, we may achieve allocative efficiency without the need for market pressure. Voluntarily, all people would offer the best possible products at the best possible prices. This, in turn, would nullify many of the reasons for market failure.

This way, we could construct a veritable economy of neighborly love. An economy in which the wish to best serve one another, not market competition, is the principal driver behind the production of good products at good prices. Without stress and fear for economic survival, production would be efficient. People would be happy because they would feel that they made a special contribution to the well-being of all, and in so doing, provided their lives with greater meaning. Therefore, if we only engage in the activity in which we make the best use of our talents, we serve our neighbor, the common good, and eventually also ourselves. We have outlined how such a paradigm shift could be promoted through a monetary reform and through an unconditional basic income.

References

Aristotle. (1995a). Politik 1st Book. In F. Meiner (Ed.), *Aristoteles Philosophische Schriften in sechs Bänden* (Vol. 4). Hamburg: Felix Meiner Verlag.

Aristotle, (1995b). Nikomachische Ethik. In F. Meiner (Ed.), *Aristoteles Philosophische Schriften in sechs Bänden* (Vol. 3). Hamburg: Felix Meiner Verlag.

Bárcena, A., Cimoli, M., García-Buchaca, R., & Pérez, R. (2018). *La ineficiencia de la desigualdad.* Santiago de Chile: Cepal.

Clark, J. (1940, 30). Toward a concept of workable competition. *The American Economic Review*, 241–256.

Common, M., & Stagl, S. (2008). *Introducción a la Economía Ecológica.* Barcelona: Reverté.

Condon, P. (2017). Mindfulness, compassion, and prosocial behaviour. In J. C. Karremans & E. K. Papies (Eds.), *Mindfulness in social psychology* (pp. 124–138). New York, NY, US: Routledge/Taylor & Francis Group.
Creutz, H. (1993). *Das Geldsyndrom. Wege zu einer krisenfreien Marktwirtschaft*. München: Müller/Herbig.
Dorsch, F. (2017). *Lexikon der Psychologie*. Göttingen: Hogrefe.
Emmerich, V. (2001). *Kartellrecht*. München: Beck.
Escrivá de Balaguer, J. (1986). *Surco*. Madrid: RIALP.
Escrivá de Balaguer, J. (2004). *Camino*. Madrid: RIALP.
Escrivá de Balaguer, J. (2010). *Es Cristo que pasa—Homilias*. Madrid: Rialp.
Escrivá de Balaguer, J. (2012). *Conversaciones*. Madrid: RIALP.
Felber, C. (2009). *Kooperation statt Konkurrenz—10 Schritte aus der Krise*. Wien: Deuticke/Zsolnay.
Fernández Carvajal, F. (1987). Hablar con Dios—Meditaciones para cada día del año. *Tomo 3: Tiempo Ordinario (1)—Semanas I-XII*. Madrid: Ediciones Palabra.
Frank, R. (2008). *Microeconomics and behaviour*. New York: McGraw-Hill/Irwin.
Fuders, F. (2009a). Die natürliche Wirtschaftsordnung als Option nach dem Zusammenbruch. *Aufklärung & Kritik, 16*(2), 128–145.
Fuders, F. (2009b). *EG-Wettbewerbsrecht*. Saarbrücken: SVH.
Fuders, F. (2010). Alternative concepts for a global financial system—an answer to the present world financial crisis. *Estudios Internacionales, 166*, 45–56.
Fuders, F. (2011). Zum so genannten freien Wettbewerb und dem vermeintlichen Verbot vertikaler Kartelle im EU-Wettbewerbsrecht. *Zeitschrift für Wirtschaftspolitik*, 271–284.
Fuders, F. (2015). Do Calidad Humana and happiness depend on development? In R. Mayorga (Ed.), *Calidad Humana—sharing the Filipino Spirit* (pp. 94–110). Manila: Energy Development Cooperation.
Fuders, F. (2016). Smarter money for smarter cities: How regional currencies can help to promote a decentralised and sustainable regional development. In E. Dick, K. Gaesing, D. Inkoom, & T. Kausel (Eds.), *Decentralisation and regional development—experiences and lessons from four continents over three decades* (pp. 155–185). Cham, Suiza: Springer.
Fuders, F. (2017). Neues Geld für eine neue Ökonomie—Die Reform des Geldwesens als Voraussetzung für eine Marktwirtschaft, die den Menschen dient. In G. Krämer (Ed.), *Finanzwirtschaft in ethischer Verantwortung—Erfolgskonzepte für Social Banking und Social Finance* (pp. 121–183). Wiesbaden, Alemania: Springer-Gabler.
Fuders, F., & Belloy, P. (2013). Terremoto del 27.02.2010 en Chile - Cómo el sector financiero se beneficia de la destrucción de capital real. *Realidad Económica*, 61–75.
Fuders, F., & Max-Neef, M. (2014a). Local money as solution to a capitalistic global financial crisis. In M. Pirson, U. Steinvorth, C. Largacha-Martinez, & C. Dierksmeier (Eds.), *From Capitalistic to Humanistc Business* (pp. 157–189). Hampshire, New York, Inglaterra/ USA: Palgrave Macmillan.
Fuders, F., & Max-Neef, M. (2014b). Dinero, deuda y crisis financieras. Propuestas teórico-prácticas en pos de la sostenibilidad del sistema financiero internacional. In J. Fernández (Ed.), *Economía Internacional. Claves teórica-prácticas sobre la inserción de Latinoamérica en el mundo.* (pp. 245–274). Guayaquil, Ecuador: LATIn.
Fuders, F., Mengel, N., & Maria del Valle, B. (2016). Índice de desarrollo a escala humana: propuesta para un indicador de desarrollo endógeno basado en la satisfacción de las necesidades humanas fundamentales. In R. Pérez Garcés, E. Espinosa Ayala, & O. Terán Varela (Eds.), *Seguridad Alimentaria, actores Terretoriales y Desarrollo Endógeno* (pp. 63–106). Iztapalapa: Laberinto.
Fuders, F., Mondaca, C., & Azungah Haruna, M. (2013). The central bank's dilemma, the inflation-deflation paradox and a new interpretation of the Kondratieff waves. *Economía (U. de los Andes),* 36, 33–66.
Gesell, S. (1949). *Die natürliche Wirtschaftsordnung durch Freiland und Freigeld*. Lauf: Rudolf Zitzmann.

Jobs, S. (2005). *Standford University*. https://www.youtube.com/watch?v=UF8uR6Z6KLc. Accessed January 10, 2018.

Kant, I. (1868a). Metaphysik der Sitten—Erster Theil. Metaphysische Anfangsgründe der Rechtslehre. In G. Hartenstein (Ed.), *Immanuel Kant's sämmtliche Werke—In chronologischer Reihenfolge, Bd. VII* (pp. 1–173). Leipzig: Leopold Voss.

Kant, I. (1868b). Metaphysik der Sitten—Zweiter Theil. Metaphysische Anfangsgründe der Tugendlehre. In G. Hartenstein (Ed.), *Immanuel Kant's sämmtliche Werke—In chronologischer Reihenfolge, Bd. VII* (pp. 175–304). Leipzig: Leopold Voss.

Kantzenbach, E. (1966). *Die Funktionsfähigkeit des Wettbewerbs*. Göttingen: Vandenhoeck u. Ruprecht.

Kennedy, M. (1990). *Geld ohne Zinsen und Inflation—Ein Tauschmittel, das jedem dient*. Steyerberg: Permakultur.

Kennedy, M. (2011). *Occupy Money—Damit wir zukünftig alle die Gewinner sind*. Bielefeld: J. Kamphausen.

Keynes, J. (1936). *The general theory of employment, interest and money*. New York: Hartcourt.

Kluge, F. (1989). *Etymologisches Wörterbuch der deutschen Sprache* (22nd ed.). Berlin, New York: De Gruyter.

Late. (2018). Late. https://late.cl. Accessed January 12, 2019.

Latouche, S. (2003). *Would the West actually be happier with less?* (p. 1). Le Monde Diplomatique: The world downscaled.

Latouche, S. (2009). *Farewell to growth*. Cambridge: Polity Press.

Lietaer, B., Arnsperger, C., Goerner, S., & Brunnhuber, S. (2013). *Geld und Nachhaltigkeit*. Berlin: EuropaVerlag.

Maslach, C., Schaufeli, W., & Leiter, M. (2001). Job Burnout. *Annual Review of Psychology*, 397–422.

Maslow, A. (2005). *El hombre autorealizado*. Barcelona: 16. ed. Kairós.

Mestmäcker, E., & Schweitzer, H. (2004). *Europäisches Wettbewerbsrecht*. Munich: Beck.

Nef (2018). *Happy Planet Index*. Retrieved from http://www.happyplanetindex.org.

Pechman, J. A., & Timpane, P. M. (1975). *Work incentives and income guarantees: The New Jersey negative income tax experiment*. Washington D.C.: The Brookings Institution.

Plato. (2011). Politeia. In W. Ursula (Ed.), *Platon—Sämtliche Werke Band 2* (pp. 211–537). Reinbek: Rowohlt.

Porter, M. E., & Kramer, M. R. (2011). Creating shared value how to reinvent capitalism and unleash a wave of innovation and growth. *Harvard Businees Review*, 1–17.

Ricardo, D. (1911). *Principles of political economy and taxation. (Reprinted 1996 by Prometheus Books. New York)*. New York: J. M. Dent & Sons.

Smith, A. (1952). An inquiry into the nature and causes oft he wealth of nations. *Great Books of the Western World, No. 39*. Chicago: W. Benton.

Soddy, F. (1933). *Wealth, virtual wealth and debt—the solution of the economic paradox*. New York, USA: Dutton.

Soddy, F. (1934). *The role of money*. London: Routledge.

Stalk, G. (2004). *Harvard business review: Estrategias de crecimiento*. Buenos Aires: Deusto.

Theobald, R. (1967). *The Guaranteed income—next step in socioeconomic evolution?*. New York: Doubleday.

Traverso, M. (2015). *Economía Consciente—La transformación espritual de la economía que comienza por uno mimso*. Buenos Aires: Kier.

Wikipedia. (2018a). *Occupational therapy*. https://en.wikipedia.org/wiki/Occupational_therapy. Accessed January 12, 2019.

Wikipedia. (2018b). *World happiness report*. https://en.wikipedia.org/wiki/World_Happiness_Report. Accessed January 12, 2019.

Kolibri 360 GmbH
Ferdinand-Jühlke-Straße 7
99095 Erfurt, Deutschland
produktsicherheit@kolibri360.de